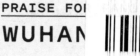

T0115697

"This is an important and dignified book. . . . [*Wuhan Diary*] is most scorching in Fang Fang's calls to hold to account the leaders who downgraded and minimized the virus."

—*New York Times*

"Fang Fang's account makes clear that as the geopolitical differences between the Chinese regime and the United States grow by the day, the lives of middle-class Chinese meanwhile seem ever less exotic and ever more similar to those of Americans."

—*The Washington Post*

"The go-to unofficial account of events unfolding in Wuhan."

—*Financial Times*

"Imagine this: the author Fang Fang did not exist in today's Wuhan. She did not keep records or pen down her personal memories and feelings. . . . What would we have heard? What would we have seen?"

—Yan Lianke, author of *Three Brothers: Memories of My Family* and *The Explosion Chronicles*

"Voices like Fang Fang's . . . remain increasingly rare in China. But in the context of larger conversations being had about China and its place in the world, American readers would do well to remember they exist."

—*NPR*

"As the rest of the world went into lockdown, what her diary documented saw grim repetitions elsewhere. . . . [*Wuhan Diary*] remains a glimpse into a distressing future."

—*The New Yorker*

"Essential reportage with hard-won lessons for residents of every place on the planet on how to survive the pandemic."

—*Kirkus Reviews* (starred review)

"This is a book that will be referred to in the future when people want to know how many Chinese felt about the pandemic."

—Ian Johnson, author of *The Souls of China* and *Wild Grass*

"A literary work of distinction: pithy, acerbic, and sometimes funny; compassionate thoughtful and nuanced. It's the kind of book that rewards a second reading; it will outlast the virus and its aftermath."

—Hong Kong Review of Books

"[*Wuhan Diary*] is the personal account of a layperson reacting to confusing, conflicting, and distressing circumstances in real time. It is an emotional work that finds its charm in its spontaneity and wit."

—*South China Morning Post*

"There will be plenty written about this strange time but right now this has a message that deserves to resonate around the world."

—*Evening Standard*

WUHAN
DIARY

WUHAN DIARY

DISPATCHES *from a* QUARANTINED CITY

FANG FANG

Translated by Michael Berry

HarperVia

An Imprint of HarperCollins*Publishers*

This diary contains discussions of various treatments of COVID-19 that took place early on during the outbreak in Wuhan. They are not to be taken as medical advice. For treatment advice concerning COVID-19, please consult your medical provider.

HarperCollins books may be purchased for educational, business, or sales promotional use. For information, please email the Special Markets Department at SPsales@harpercollins.com.

FIRST HARPERCOLLINS PAPERBACK EDITION PUBLISHED IN 2022

Designed by Yvonne Chan
Concentric circles image by Artsem Vysotski / Shutterstock

Library of Congress Cataloging-in-Publication Data is available upon request.

ISBN 978-0-06-327354-2

22 23 24 25 26 LSC 10 9 8 7 6 5 4 3 2 1

CONTENTS

Introduction

THE VIRUS IS THE COMMON ENEMY OF HUMANKIND

I

When I first logged on to my Sina Weibo account to write my initial diary entry, I certainly never imagined that there would be 59 more entries to follow; nor could I ever have imagined that tens of millions of readers would be staying up late each night just waiting to read my next installment. So many people have told me that they could only finally get to sleep after reading my entry for the day. I also never imagined that this collection of diary entries would be collected in book form and published overseas so quickly.

Just as I completed my final installment of the diary, the government coincidentally announced that on April 8, 2020, the city of Wuhan would reopen.

Wuhan was under lockdown for a total of 76 days. April 8 also happened to be the date that websites in the United States uploaded presale information for the English edition of *Wuhan Diary*.

The whole thing seemed something like a dream; it was as if the hand of God had been silently arranging everything from behind the scenes.

II

Starting on January 20 when the Chinese infectious disease special-ist Dr. Zhong Nanshan revealed that the novel coronavirus was being spread by human-to-human transmission and news broke that 14 med-ical workers had already been infected, my first reaction was shock, but that later turned into anger. This new information was completely at odds with what we had seen and heard earlier. Official media sources had been consistently telling us that this virus was "Not Contagious Be-tween People; It's Controllable and Preventable." Meanwhile, even more rumors were circulating that this was in fact another SARS coronavirus.

Once I learned that the approximate incubation period for this virus was around 14 days, I started to calmly make a list of whom I had been in contact with over those previous two weeks to see if there was any risk that I might have been infected. The scary thing I discovered was that during this period I had been to the hospital three different times to visit sick colleagues. I didn't wear a face mask during two of those visits. On January 7th I attended a friend's party and later went out to dinner with my family. On January 16th I had a serviceman come to my apartment to install a new heater. On the 19th my niece visited Wu-han from Singapore, so my big brother and his wife took us all out to dinner, including my second brother and his wife. It was a good thing that there were already all those SARS rumors floating around by then, so I made sure to wear a face mask every time I went out.

Given my occupation and what my normal schedule looks like, it is actually quite out of the ordinary for me to have gone out so many times during such a short period. I suppose I was going out more be-cause this was the time just before the Lunar New Year when people hold a lot of parties and host get-togethers to celebrate. Once I put ev-erything together, it was really hard for me to say definitively whether or not I might have been infected during that period. The only thing I could do was work backward to try to rule out an infection by counting down, day by day, until I had passed that two-week period. During that time, I was feeling quite depressed.

My daughter returned from Japan on January 22, the night before the quarantine was announced. I went to pick her up at the airport that night at 10:00 p.m. By that time, there were hardly any cars or pedestrians on the streets. When I got to the airport, almost everyone standing outside waiting to be picked up was wearing a face mask; there was a heavy feeling in the air and everyone seemed extremely stressed out. There were no signs of the hubbub, chatter, and laughter that you normally see there. Those few days were when panic and fright were at their very height in Wuhan. Just before going out I left an online message for a friend of mine, telling her I was reminded of a line from that old poem, "the wind whistles by as a chill descends on Yishui." Since her plane was delayed, my daughter didn't come out of the terminal until after 11:00 p.m.

My ex-husband had dinner with my daughter the previous week. Then, just a few days before I picked her up, he called to tell me that something was wrong with his lungs. My guard immediately went up; if he was infected with the novel coronavirus, then there was a possibility that my daughter might also be infected. I told my daughter and we decided that she had better self-quarantine at her apartment for at least one week before going out. That meant that we wouldn't spend the Lunar New Year together. I told her I would bring her some things to eat (since she had been on vacation abroad, she didn't have any fresh groceries in her apartment). We both wore face masks in the car and although she is usually always excited to tell me all about her trips, she barely said a word about Japan during our drive. We were both silent the whole way there. The anxiety and stress that were permeating the entire city were also there in the car with us.

I dropped my daughter off at her place and then had to stop for gas on the way back to my apartment. I didn't get home until 1:00 a.m. As soon as I returned home I turned on the computer and immediately saw the news: The quarantine would be going into effect the following day. Although a few people had suggested shutting down the city, I remember thinking "how are you supposed to lock down a city as big as Wuhan?" So when the order came down, I really didn't expect it. The quarantine order also made me realize that this infectious disease that had been spreading must have already gotten to an extremely serious point.

The next day, I went out to buy some face masks and groceries. The streets were very quiet. I don't think I'd ever seen the streets of Wuhan so wide open and deserted. Seeing those desolate streets made me very sad; my heart felt as empty as those abandoned avenues. That was a feeling I had never before experienced in my life—that feeling of uncertainty about the fate of my city, that uncertainty about whether my family members and I had been infected, and all the uncertainties about the future. All that left me with a strange feeling of confusion and anxiety.

I went out again for the next two days in search of face masks, but the only people I encountered out on those empty streets were a few solitary street sweepers. Since there were so few pedestrians out, the streets were not even very dirty, but they kept frantically sweeping. For some reason, that scene gave me a strange sense of consolation and really set my heart at ease.

On my way home, I kept wondering, since I had first heard about this virus back on December 31, how come everyone had such a lax attitude about it for the following 20 days? We should have already learned our lesson from the SARS outbreak back in 2003. This "why" is also a question that a lot of people had been asking themselves. *Why?*

To be perfectly frank, part of the reason is that we had been too careless, and there are also objective life situations that contributed to that. But more important is the fact that we have placed too much faith in our government. We had faith that there was no way that the governmental leaders in Hubei Province would adopt such a lax and irresponsible attitude when it came to such a critical event where lives were in the balance. We also had faith that they would never hold fast to their "political correctness" and old ways of doing business in the face of a new threat that could affect the lives of millions of people. And we had faith that they would have better common sense and exercise better decision-making skills when a real threat was afoot. It was owing to that faith that I even sent a message to one of my WeChat groups saying: "The government would never dare to try to conceal something so huge." But in reality, as we now see how things have evolved, we know that a portion of the blame for this catastrophe lies with human error.

Deeply ingrained habitual behaviors, like reporting the good news while hiding the bad, preventing people from speaking the truth, forbidding the public from understanding the true nature of events, and expressing a disdain for individual lives, have led to massive reprisals against our society, untold injuries against our people, and even terrible reprisals against those officials themselves (a group of high-ranking Hubei officials have already been dismissed from office, while others who should bear additional responsibility still remain in office). All this, in turn, led to the city of Wuhan's falling under a 76-day quarantine, with its reverberations affecting untold numbers of people and places. It is absolutely essential that we continue to fight until those responsible are held accountable.

III

Beginning on January 20, Wuhan would be gripped by a cloud of fear and anxiety for the next three days as we quickly approached the quarantine order. Locking down an entire city with a population of millions in order to stop the spread of an epidemic was a historically unprecedented action. It was certainly also a very difficult decision to make on such short notice, because a quarantine order would certainly affect the lives of every citizen in Wuhan.

However, to impede the spread of this virus, the city government of Wuhan gritted its teeth and made the hard choice that needed to be made. This was also a decision that was unique in Wuhan's thousands of years of history. But, looking at it from the perspective of how we changed the course of the virus's spread, this was clearly the correct decision, even if it came a few days late.

During the five-day period lasting from three days before the quarantine order went into effect through the first two days after the restrictions were imposed, most people in Wuhan were in a state of utter panic. Those were five terrifying days that seemed to last forever; meanwhile, the virus was quickly spreading throughout the city, and even the government appeared as if it was at a loss as to what to do.

On January 25, Day One of the Lunar New Year, people finally started to settle down a bit. The media reported that China's top-level leaders were closely following the outbreak in Wuhan and that the first team of medical experts from Shanghai had arrived in Wuhan. Those reports gave the people of Wuhan some solace and helped calm their spirits. That's because everybody knows that once something in China is taken up at the national level, everyone will step up and do what needs to be done. From that day forward, the frantic and confused people of Wuhan could dispel all their fears. And that was the day that I began my diary.

But that was also when the period of true suffering arrived here in Wuhan—the number of people infected with the coronavirus exploded during the Lunar New Year. Because the local hospitals couldn't cope with the surge of new patients, the entire system was brought to the brink of collapse. As it happens, that was precisely the period of the Chinese New Year when families normally come together for the holiday; it is a time of year that is usually filled with joy. But instead the world froze over; countless people became infected with the coronavirus, and they ended up traipsing all over the city in the wind and rain searching in vain for treatment. After the quarantine was imposed, all public transit in the city shut down, and since most residents in Wuhan don't have their own automobiles, they had to walk from one hospital to another in search of a place that might admit them. It is hard to describe how difficult that must have been for those poor patients. That is also about the time that short videos of patients appealing for help began to appear online; there were also videos of people lining up all night long outside hospitals, hoping to get admitted, and clips of doctors on the brink of exhaustion. We all felt completely helpless in the face of these patients crying out, desperate for help. Those were also the most difficult days for me to get through. All I could do was write, and so I just kept writing and writing; it became my only form of psychological release.

Once we got through that most difficult period, several top officials in Hubei and Wuhan were removed from office, 19 provinces from all over China sent medical relief teams to provide aid to Hubei, and we constructed a series of temporary hospitals to handle the influx of patients. Eventually, the new quarantine procedures that were put in place helped to completely turn the tide away from the tragic and chaotic state that things had been in. All patients were divided up into four groups: patients with severe symptoms, confirmed coronavirus patients, suspected coronavirus patients, and those who had close contact with confirmed patients. Those with severe symptoms were admitted to the main hospitals designated to treat coronavirus patients; those confirmed patients with mild symptoms were sent to the temporary hospitals; all suspected cases were admitted to local hotels where they would be kept under quarantine; and close contacts were also quarantined in hotels or other facilities, such as school dormitory rooms. All these methods were immediately put into place and quickly began to yield results. Once they got into the hospital system, a good majority of the mild cases were able to see a quick recovery. Day after day, we were able to personally witness the situation improving here in Wuhan. You can see that gradually taking place in my diary.

During the early stage of the quarantine, the challenge of taking care of the daily needs of nine million people was taken care of by neighborhood groups that self-organized and used online services to make group purchases in order to provide daily necessities. Later the government mobilized all its civil servants to each and every community to help serve the needs of local residents. Wuhan's nine million residents worked together to cooperate with all the government's requests; their restraint and patience helped to ensure that Wuhan would be able to contain this virus; they are deserving of whatever recognition we can muster to acknowledge their collective sacrifice. Spending a full 76 days in quarantine was not an easy thing for people to do. But the amount of energy the government later put into the quarantine and various other measures was indeed extremely effective.

By the time I got to my 60th diary entry, the situation in Wuhan had already completely turned around. And then on April 8, the 76th day of the lockdown, Wuhan officially reopened. That was an unforgettable day. The moment the quarantine order was lifted, there was barely a dry eye in the entire city.

IV

What I never imagined was that just as the coronavirus outbreak in Wuhan was starting to ease up, the virus began to spread throughout

Europe and the United States. These tiny virus droplets that are invisible to the naked eye quickly brought the world to its knees. The entire world, both East and West, were all tortured in horrific ways by this coronavirus.

Meanwhile, politicians from both sides pointed fingers at each other, while never facing up to the fact that everyone had taken missteps along the way. China's lax attitude early on and the West's arrogance shown in its distrust of China's experience fighting the coronavirus have both contributed to countless lives being lost, countless families being ripped apart, and all humanity having been dealt a heavy blow.

A Western reporter asked me: "What kind of lesson should China learn from this outbreak?" My response was: "The spread of the coronavirus is not limited to China; it is something affecting everyone all over the world. The novel coronavirus has not just taught China a lesson, it has taught the entire world a lesson; it has educated all of humanity. This lesson is: Humankind cannot be allowed to continue on lost in its own arrogance, we can no longer think of ourselves as the center of the world, we can no longer believe that we are invincible, and we can no longer underestimate the destructive power of even the smallest things—like a virus."

The virus is the common enemy of humankind; that is a lesson for all humanity. The only way we can conquer this virus and free ourselves from its grip is for all members of humankind to work together.

V

I would like to extend special thanks to my four doctor friends; throughout the course of my diary, they provided information and medical knowledge about the coronavirus.

Thanks to my three brothers for their assistance and love, along with all my family for always lending me their full support. When people started attacking me online, one of my cousins said: "Don't worry, your family always will have your back." Another one of my cousins kept constantly sending me information. My extended family's support warmed my heart along the course of this journey.

I also thank my old college and high school classmates. They too provided so much strong support to prop me up throughout this process. They sent me all kinds of information about what was going on in our society during the outbreak, and during those moments when I wavered, they were the ones who cheered me on. And then there are my colleagues and neighbors; I thank them all for providing help with my everyday life affairs throughout the process of writing this diary.

Finally, I would like to thank my translator, Michael Berry. If it hadn't been for his suggestion, I never would have thought of trying to publish this book overseas; and it certainly never would have been brought out at such a rapid speed.

This is a book dedicated to the people of Wuhan. It is also a book for those people who came to Wuhan's aid during my city's darkest hour. All my proceeds from this book will be used to aid those people who put their lives on the line for this city.

Fang Fang
April 13, 2020

JANUARY

*Technology can sometimes be every bit
as evil as a contagious virus.*

I'm not sure if I'll be able to send anything out through my Weibo account. It wasn't too long ago that I had my account shut down after I criticized a group of young nationalists who were harassing people on the streets with foul language. (I still stand by my position: There is nothing wrong with being a patriot, but that shouldn't be an excuse to act like a hooligan—it comes down to basic civility!) I tried to complain to Sina, the company that runs Weibo, yet there is really no way to get through to them. After that, I was so disappointed in Sina that I decided to completely give up on using Weibo.

But at that time I never imagined that something so serious would befall the city of Wuhan. What happened led Wuhan to become the focal point of the entire nation, it led to the city being locked down, the people of Wuhan being subjected to prejudice, and me being quarantined here in this city. Today the government issued another order: Starting at midnight tonight all motor vehicles are prohibited from operating in the downtown district of Wuhan. That is precisely where I happen to live. A lot of people have been sending me text messages to ask how I'm doing; everyone is quite concerned, and they are sending in their warm wishes. For those of us quarantined here in the city, those heartwarming messages mean a lot. I just received a message from Cheng Yongxin, an editor for the literary journal *Harvest*, suggesting that I start writing a series that we could call "Wuhan Diary," or "Notes from a Quarantined City." My first instinct is that, if my Weibo account is still active and I'm able to post, perhaps I really *should* start writing about what is happening. It would be a way for people to understand what is really going on here on the ground in Wuhan.

But I'm not sure if this will even be able to be posted. If any of my friends are able to view it online, please leave a comment so I know it went through. Weibo has a special feature that makes the user believe their post was successfully uploaded when it actually remains invisible to other users. Once I learned about this programming trick, I realized that technology can sometimes be every bit as evil as a contagious virus.

Let's see if this post is able to be uploaded.

JANUARY 26, 2020

> *What you are seeing from government officials*
> *in Hubei is actually what you can expect*
> *from most cadres throughout China.*

Thank you, everyone, for your attention and support. The people of Wuhan are still in a critical phase of this outbreak, even though a lot of folks have already emerged from that initial state of fear, helplessness, and anxiety. We may be much more settled and at peace than we were a few days ago, but we still need everyone's comfort and encouragement. For a while now, everyone in Wuhan seemed to be in a state of paralysis, frightened and not knowing what to do, but as of today it seems that people are starting to emerge from that. I originally wanted to run through the cycle of emotions that I have gone through since December 31, ranging from a state of heightened alert to the more relaxed psychological space I am in now, but as soon as I began to write it down I realized it would be too long. So, instead, I will focus on what I'm going through emotionally right now, based on what is happening, and then gradually get to this "Wuhan Diary."

Yesterday was Day Two of the Lunar New Year and it is still cold, windy, and rainy outside. There is some good news but also a lot of bad news. The good news is that the state is lending more and more support to the effort to fight this virus; there are more medical personnel rushing to Wuhan to join the efforts here, etc., etc. All this gives the people of Wuhan some peace of mind. But I'm sure you all already know about this.

As for myself, one bit of good news is that up until now, not a single one of my relatives has been infected. My middle brother lives very close to the epicenter of the outbreak—his apartment is right next to the Huanan Seafood Market and Hankou Hospital of Wuhan. My brother is not in the best of health; even before the outbreak, he was often in and out of the hospital, so I am quite thankful that he and my sister-in-law are both okay. My brother already prepared enough fresh food and vegetables to last them for a week, and he doesn't plan on leaving the apartment. My oldest brother and his family, along with my daughter and me, are all across the river in Wuchang. Over here the risk seems a bit lower and we are all doing all right. Although we are stuck at home all day, we don't feel particularly bored. I suppose we are all homebodies, anyway! The only ones in our family who seem to be a bit worried are my niece and her son, who returned from out of town to visit my brother. They were originally supposed to leave Wuhan on high-speed rail on the 23rd to meet up with the rest of their family in Guangzhou. (Even if they had been able to get there, I'm not sure that things would have been much better for them in Guangzhou.) But on the day they were supposed to leave, the city was locked down and they didn't make it out. It is unclear how long this quarantine will last; right now we are still in the middle of the Chinese New Year holiday, but it could get complicated when things start to affect work and school. Since my niece and her son are both Singapore passport holders, yesterday they received a notice from the Singapore government that arrangements were being made for a plane to take them back there. (I suspect that there must be a considerable number of ethnic Chinese Singaporeans living in Wuhan.) Once they return to Singapore, they will need to be quarantined for 14 days. The fact that they are implementing a quarantine is a good sign and allows us all to breathe a bit easier. I also received some pretty good news about my ex-husband; he had been hospitalized in Shanghai and had a chest X-ray that showed some spots on his lungs, but yesterday they ruled out anything serious and it seems to be nothing more than a common cold. He has not been infected by the novel coronavirus and will be discharged from the hospital today. That also means that our daughter, whom he had just gone out to dinner with, doesn't need to be strictly segregated to her own room anymore. (A few days ago I even drove out in the pouring rain to bring her some food!) I really hope that tomorrow will bring more good news like this! Although the city is shut down and we are stuck inside our homes, those bits of good news go a long way toward brightening our mood.

Yet the bad news continues. Yesterday my daughter told me that the father of one of her friends seemingly contracted the virus (he was also suffering from liver cancer); they took him to the hospital but there was no one available to treat him and he died three hours later. This must have happened sometime within the past two days, and my daughter's friend was still really emotional when they spoke on the phone. Last night my colleague Xiao Li called to tell me that two people from the Provincial Literary and Arts Federation housing complex where I live have been infected. They are from the same family and are both in their thirties. Xiao Li told me to be careful. The infected couple's apartment is probably only around 300 meters away from where I live. However, my building has a separate entrance and a separate courtyard from them, so I'm not overly concerned. But I'm sure those neighbors in the same building are getting a bit nervous. Today my colleague called again and told me that they both have mild cases of the coronavirus, so they are just self-quarantining and treating themselves at home. In general, young people have better constitutions and tend to only suffer from mild infections, so that couple should be able to rebound quickly. I pray for their speedy recovery.

Yesterday's press conference in Hubei about the coronavirus has become a trending topic on the internet. There are a lot of people roasting those officials online. The three representatives from the government all looked utterly exhausted and depressed, and they kept making mistakes during their presentations; but this shows just how chaotic things are for them. Actually, I kind of feel bad for them. I'm sure they have family members here in Wuhan, and when they attempted to take the blame for what was happening I really felt like they were speaking from the heart. But how did things get to this point? Looking back and going through everything in my head, it is pretty clear: During the early stage of the outbreak, officials from Wuhan didn't take the virus seriously enough. Both before and after the quarantine went into effect, those officials were at a loss trying to deal with what was unfolding, which led to a great wave of public fear and really hurt a lot of people here in Wuhan. These are all aspects of the situation that I plan to write about in detail. But right now what I want to say is that what you saw from those government officials in Hubei is actually what you would expect from most government cadres in China: They are all basically on the same level. It's not that they are somehow worse than other Chinese officials; they simply got dealt a worse hand. Officials in China have always let written directives guide their work, so once you take away the script they are at a complete loss as to how to steer the ship. If this outbreak had happened in another Chinese province, I'm sure the performance of those officials wouldn't be much different than what we are seeing here. When the world of officialdom skips over the natural process of competition, it leads to disaster; empty talk about political correctness without seeking truth from facts also leads to disaster; prohibiting people from speaking the truth and the media from reporting the truth leads to disaster; and now we are tasting the fruits of these disasters, one by one. Wuhan is always vying to be first at everything, but now it is first in line to taste this suffering.

(This was a make-up entry written on January 27, 2020)

JANUARY 27, 2020

We don't have enough face masks.

I would like to again express my thanks to everyone out there who has been lending their attention and support to what is happening in Wuhan, and also to the residents of Wuhan.

For the time being, most people are not too concerned with the big issues. What's the use of worrying about those problems, anyway? Most people who are not infected are trying to remain optimistic.

One thing that citizens are more concerned about right now is the shortage of face masks. I saw an online video report today about a man in Shanghai who went to the pharmacy to buy a mask, only to find the price inflated to 30 yuan[1] each. This guy was so infuriated by the markup that he lost his temper and started yelling at the employees; he recorded the whole thing with his cellphone. At the end of the day, he still bought some, but he insisted that the pharmacy give him a receipt so he would be able to prove how badly they were overcharging customers. I would never have thought of doing that; I really admire his bravery.

These disposable masks are quite wasteful and people go through them quickly. According to the medical professionals, only N95 masks are effective when it comes to stopping the spread of the virus. But in reality there is absolutely no way to get your hands on those types of masks. The ones for sale online are all out of stock. One of my brothers had better luck; his neighbors have some relatives who sent them more than 1,000 N95 masks! (How wonderful their relatives are!) They gave 10 masks to my brother's family. "You see, there are still kindhearted people in the world," my brother told me. But my eldest brother was not so lucky—they couldn't get their hands on a single N95 mask. All they have are some disposable masks that my niece brought them. But even those are in limited supply. The only option is to wash them and disinfect them with a hot iron before reusing. It is actually a bit pathetic. (By the way, my niece wanted me to announce on Weibo that she still has not received any confirmation as to when Singapore citizens will be evacuated from Wuhan.)

I'm holding up about the same as before. I was supposed to visit a patient in the hospital on January 18th, but I could only go if I wore a face mask. But I didn't have a single one on hand. Then I remembered that my old classmate Xu Min had given me one when I visited Chengdu back in mid-December, to protect me from the air pollution there. The air in Wuhan probably isn't much better than in Chengdu, and I've long grown accustomed to breathing bad air, so I never wore that mask. Thanks to him, I found a way out of this bind. And it turns out it was actually an N95 mask! I wore that mask to the hospital, to the airport, and even when I went out to buy face masks! I wore that same mask for days on end, since I didn't have any other choice.

Besides me, I also have a 16-year-old dog at home. On the afternoon of the 22nd I suddenly discovered that I was out of dog food. I quickly called the pet store to put in an order, I figured that I could also pick up some extra face masks while I was out. I went to the local pharmacy on Dongting Road (I won't post the name of the store) and they had some N95 masks in stock, but they were selling them for 35 yuan each (five yuan more than that store in Shanghai!). A box of 25 masks was selling for 875 yuan. I asked them how they could be so cold-hearted as to price gouge their customers during a time like this. The storekeeper explained that their suppliers raised their prices, so they had no choice but to raise theirs. But since masks are a necessity, I was prepared to cave in and just buy a few, even at that inflated price. I was about to buy four masks from them when I discovered that the face masks all came in a big box with no individual packaging; when I saw the saleswoman reaching in with her bare hands to fish them out, I decided I had better not buy them after all. It's better not to wear a mask at all than to wear one that has not been hygienically handled.

On the eve of the Lunar New Year, I went out again to try to buy some face masks, but all the pharmacies were closed. The only stores still open were a handful of small mom-and-pop markets. I found some N95 masks for sale at one store; they were gray Yimeng Mountain brand masks, each individually packaged. 10 yuan each. I bought four. Only then could I finally heave a small sigh of relief. Since I had heard that my big brother didn't have any masks for his family, I also decided to save two for him. I was going to take them over to him the following day, but then he called and told me not to risk going out. It's a good thing that we are all basically relegated to our apartments and don't go outside, so we don't really have a pressing need for that many masks.

I was just texting with a friend on WeChat; everyone is now talking about the shortage of face masks as the single most pressing issue. After all, all of us still need to occasionally leave our homes to buy food and supplies. One colleague had a friend send him some, but the package never arrived. Others have no choice but to purchase masks by fishy manufacturers. Online they are also talking about people selling used face masks that are "refurbished," but no one dares to use those. Most people I know are down to their last mask or two, so we keep encouraging each other to use them sparingly. One joke I saw online was right on point: Face masks have indeed replaced pork as the most precious commodity for the Chinese New Year!

I'm sure that it is not just my eldest brother, my colleague, and me who are short of face masks. There must be many people here in Wuhan without any face masks. But I am confident there isn't a real shortage of supplies; it's more a problem of the logistics of how to get them into people's hands. Right now I just hope those express delivery companies can resume work soon and speed up the delivery of supplies into Wuhan; we need some help to get through these tough times.

JANUARY 28, 2020

The virus doesn't discriminate between
ordinary people and high-ranking leaders.

It finally stopped raining and the weather has been improving since yesterday. The sun even came out for a little while today. The sky is clear, which usually brightens one's mood, but after being stuck at home for so long it just makes you even more frustrated. It has already been close to six days since the lockdown went into effect. Over the course of the past five days, people have had a lot more opportunities for real conversations with each other, but they have probably also had more opportunities to get into real arguments with each other, too. Most families have never spent so much time all clustered up together like they are now, especially those living in tiny apartments. Most adults can handle being forced to stay inside for so long, but small kids are bouncing off the walls—it is torture for them. I'm not sure if there are any psychologists out there who have any special advice on how to console the people of Wuhan. But no matter what happens, we need to hang on and get through these 14 days of isolation. They keep saying that the virus should reach full outbreak level within the next two days. I heard one doctor repeatedly urging people, "As long as you have something to eat at home, just stay in! Do not go outside!" Okay, then; I suppose I had better follow the doctor's orders.

Today there is again a mix of good and bad news. Yesterday my old schoolmate Xia Chunping, who is now deputy chief editor of the China News Agency, did an interview with me over WeChat, and today he came over with a photographer to take a few photos for the story. The big surprise was that he brought me 20 N95 masks! It was like receiving a bag of coal on a cold winter's day; I was ecstatic. As we were standing outside the main entrance to the Literary and Arts Federation building, talking, we ran into Old Geng, another former classmate, who was just returning from a trip to the store to buy rice. Old Geng looked us over with a suspicious gaze. I almost thought he might yell at us in that stern Henan accent of his: "Hey! Who are you people? Why are you standing in the entrance like that?" So when I saw that expression on his face I immediately called out to him and the look in his eyes instantly softened up. Old Geng became quite warm and cordial. He acted like we hadn't seen each other in forever, even though we often interact with each other online in one of our mutual group chats. Xia Chunping was a history major in college; back then, all the Chinese majors and history majors lived in the same dorm. So as soon as I introduced the two of them, they immediately hit it off. Old Geng lived in the same courtyard compound as me in both Wuhan and Hainan. But this year, we are both stuck in the same boat—neither of us made it down to Hainan, and instead we are both locked-down here in these dormitory-style apartments amid the quarantine. Old Geng told me that the two infected people from Building 8 had both been admitted to the hospital. All the neighbors seem to be breathing a bit easier since they left. I'm sure that couple will be better off getting professional medical treatment than just self-isolating at home. But I continue to pray for their swift recovery.

I saw Xia Chunping off and, just as I entered my apartment, my old friend Xiao Yuan came by. Xiao Yuan had edited some of my early books, like *The Villas of Lushan* and *The Foreign Concessions of Hankou*; he read my post about the scarcity of face masks and delivered three packages of masks right to my doorstep! I was so moved. It is good to have old friends you can count on. All of a sudden I have found myself with an overabundance of face masks. I've made sure to share them with my colleague who only yesterday was complaining about the shortage of masks. Just now she came to pick them up and brought along some fresh vegetables for me. It really does feel like we are a little community working together to get through these difficult times. My colleague has three generations under one roof, so she has to take care of ailing in-laws and little kids. Because she has so many people to feed, she has to go out every other day to buy vegetables. She was born in the 1980s, and I'm sure it's not easy for her and people of her generation. And on top of everything, she still has to deal with work. I saw a thread online where she was discussing whether or not they should still send out manuscripts for the next issue of their journal. When you have hardworking people like her in Wuhan, I'm sure we can get through anything that life throws at us.

But of course the bad news is circling everywhere. A few days ago when I first saw the news of a public banquet gathering at Baibuting attended by 40,000 families, I immediately sent out a text to my friends group criticizing it. I was quite harsh with my words. I even said that hosting a large-scale community gathering like that during a time like this "should effectively be considered a form of criminal action." That is what I said back on the 20th but I never imagined that on the 21st the provincial government would then go ahead and host a massive song-and-dance concert. Where has people's common sense gone to? Even the virus must be thinking, *Wow, you people have really underestimated me!* I don't want to say too much more about this issue. The bad news today is coming from where else but Baibuting, which now has several confirmed cases of the novel coronavirus. Although I haven't authenticated this new information yet, based on my own intuition I don't see any reason for my source to be lying. Just think about it; if you put 40,000 people together in a closed space, how can you expect people *not* to get infected? Some specialists have pointed out that the death toll from this type of new virus is not too high; everyone wants to believe that, myself included. However, some of the other news coming through is quite alarming. For those officials attending all those government meetings between the 10th and the 20th, please take care, because the virus doesn't discriminate between ordinary people and high-ranking leaders.

While I'm writing, I'd like to say a little bit about Mayor Zhou Xianwang's hat. For the past two days everyone online has been roasting him alive over his hat.[2] During ordinary times I may have also gotten a good laugh out of this, but right now Mayor Zhou has been running all over the city, trying to lead an army of Wuhan city officials in the fight against this outbreak; you can see the exhaustion and anxiety written all over his face. I suspect that he may have even realized what will probably befall him once this thing has settled down. In times like this, people usually face a mixture of guilt, self-blame, uneasiness, and a sense that they should have done more, even though now it is all too late—I'm sure that Mayor Zhou is experiencing all these complex feelings. But he is, after all, still the man running our municipal government; he needs to pull himself together and focus on the pressing tasks ahead that we are going to have to face. He is, after all, just an ordinary person. I have heard people say that Mayor Zhou is a disciplined and pragmatic man; people usually have a very good impression of him. He started out in western Hubei and worked his way up the bureaucratic ladder, one step at a time. He has probably never encountered anything on this scale in his entire life. All this makes me think that we should perhaps look at this "hat incident" from a more sympathetic perspective. Perhaps it is something as simple as his wanting to wear a hat because it was so cold outside, but when he saw that the premier wasn't wearing a hat he got nervous. After all, he is younger than Premier Li Keqiang and maybe he thought that if he wore a hat but the premier wasn't wearing one, it might be interpreted as impolite? Perhaps that is why he suddenly took off his hat and handed it to his assistant. Perhaps it is better if we just look at it from this perspective?

Anyway, that's all I have to record for today.

JANUARY 29, 2020

Taking care of oneself is one way to contribute to the effort.

I decided to let everything go today and just sleep until noon. (It is actually not uncommon for me to sleep in like that, but in normal times

I would blame myself for being so lazy. These days, however, everyone in Wuhan is saying: "On those sunny days when we till the crops, It's hard to get a good night's rest! We sleep all morning; we sleep all afternoon."[3] When people are all sleeping in like that, it is hard not to just let things go!)

I was still lying in bed flicking through messages on my phone when I saw a text one of my doctor friends sent me: "Take care of yourself and, no matter what, don't go out! Don't go out! Don't go out!" I felt a bit jittery as soon as I saw the way he repeatedly emphasized the phrase "Don't go out!" I figured this must mean that the outbreak is hitting its peak. I quickly called my daughter, who was about to go out to the local neighborhood supermarket to pick up a few boxed lunches. I told her not to go. Even if the only thing you have left to eat at home is plain white rice, don't go out. Back on the first day of the Lunar New Year, when I first heard that the downtown district was shutting down the traffic, I immediately went over and brought her enough supplies to get her through at least 10 days. I suspect she was just too lazy to cook and that is why she wanted to go out. A good thing my daughter has a good fear of death ingrained in her! The second she heard what I had to say, she agreed to stay at home. She called me back a bit later to ask how to cook cabbage (can you believe that she actually put a head of cabbage in the freezer?). I don't think my daughter has ever cooked a proper meal in her apartment. Usually she just comes to my apartment for dinner, or simply orders takeout. Perhaps this was a good way to get her to finally start using her kitchen. But I'm not sure if my daughter's finally forcing herself to learn how to cook should be considered the silver lining in this situation. Compared to her, I've got it much easier. One of my neighbors just brought over a plate of steaming hot buns for me. We were both wearing face masks when she dropped the buns off; although it's risky, I decided to just brave up and dig in.

The sun is glorious today. The most comfortable weather during the Wuhan winter is when the sun beams down like this, so soft and warm. If not for the coronavirus, I'm sure that the streets around my apartment would be jammed with traffic right now. That's because East Lake Garden Lane, one of the Wuhan locals' favorite destinations, is right around the corner. But these days East Lake Garden Lane is completely deserted. Two days ago my old classmate Old Dao went there for a jog. He said that he was the only person out there. If you want to figure out where the safest place in the city is, I suspect that East Lake Garden Lane might be it.

For those of us here in Wuhan who are quarantined at home, most of us are fairly at ease—that is, as long as no one in our family is sick. But those patients and their families are really having a rough time. Right now it is extremely difficult to get a bed at any hospital, and many people are still suffering. The construction site for Huoshenshan Hospital[4] is really kicking into high gear, but, as the old saying goes, distant water can't put out a nearby fire. Those patients without a place to go are the greatest victims of this tragedy. So many families have been torn apart by this. But a lot of media outlets have been reporting on these stories. Freelance journalists have been even more active in covering this topic, many of them quietly documenting what has been happening from the very beginning. All we can do is record what is happening. This morning I read an essay about a family whose mother just died from the coronavirus on the first day of the Lunar New Year and both the father and the elder brother were infected. Reading that essay really tore me up, and this was basically a middle-class family. But what are all those lower-income people supposed to do? What will their lives be like? A few days ago, I actually saw some video clips of exhausted medical workers and patients collapsing, and I can tell you that I don't think I have ever seen that kind of helpless sadness in my entire life. Professor Liu Chuan'e from Hubei University said that he feels like crying every day. Don't we all?! I've been telling my friends that what we are seeing today allows one to clearly appreciate the true gravity of this human calamity. After pondering things, I really feel that there is no way to forgive those irresponsible workers; they should all pay a price for their incompetence. But for now all we can do is put all our efforts into this fight to get us through these hard times.

I should say a bit about what has been happening with me. Besides the fact that I'm in a very different state of mind than normal, my everyday life is actually not that different from before. During previous years, I spent the Lunar New Year in basically the same way as I'm spending it now. The only thing different is that I normally visit my great-uncle Yang Shuzi to pay my respects and join him for a New Year's lunch, but this year the luncheon was canceled. My great-uncle is getting on in years and isn't in the best of health, so we need to take special care not to expose him to the virus. So in the end, I basically didn't go anywhere during the holiday this year. I actually have acute bronchitis and it usually acts up during the winter months. There was one period of time when I ended up being hospitalized for my bronchitis three years in a row during the Lunar New Year. So these past few days I have been repeatedly reminding myself to do everything possible to ensure that I don't get sick. I did have a little headache a few days ago, and yesterday I had a slight cough; but today I'm feeling much better. A long time ago, Jiang Zidan[5] (she is something of a specialist in traditional Chinese medicine) told me that, based on my illness, I have a condition referred to as "cold encapsulating fire." From that point on, every winter I would prepare a traditional medicinal potion of milk vetch root, honeysuckle essence, chrysanthemum, Chinese wolfberry, red dates, and American ginseng, boiled in a pot of mulberry leaf tea. I

gave my little potion the nickname "hodgepodge brew" and made sure
to drink several large glasses each day. Once the coronavirus outbreak
started to get serious, I added a morning vitamin C supplement, a glass
of fizzy vitamin C drink, and a few glasses of hot water to my daily regimen. For my evening shower I made sure to let my back soak under
the hot water, which was on the verge of scalding. I also went through
an entire package of Lotus Flu Capsules. One of my classmates even
taught me the "mantra of the closed door" to chant silently to myself:
"Close up all of your body's openings! If you stave off the cold wind, the
hundred evils will not befall you! Store up the proper *qi* inside yourself, so the evil will be unable to assail!" He told me in a manner of all
seriousness that this was a chant that had been secretly passed down
for generations and was not at all "superstitious." We had a good laugh
about that one! I wonder if anyone really does chant it. In any case, I
have already picked up whatever tricks I can from all sorts of people
on how to protect myself from this virus, and I am employing them
all, except, that is, for chanting the "mantra of the closed door"! But I
think all those other tactics seem to be working. I'm in a pretty good
state for the time being. Taking care of oneself is one way to contribute
to the effort.

By the way, two days ago one of my posts on Weibo was taken
down. It actually had a longer lifespan online than I originally thought
it would. I didn't expect it to be forwarded by so many people. I've
grown accustomed to writing in that small status window afforded one
on the Weibo platform, so when I publish things online they tend to be
quite informal (I always had a preference for a more informal style!). I
just post whatever pops into my mind. I don't spend much time editing
my posts before uploading them, so there are often grammar and spell-
ing mistakes (which is embarrassing, considering that I'm a graduate
of the Wuhan University Chinese Department!). I hope readers will

excuse me for my carelessness. I actually had absolutely no intention of criticizing anyone during this outbreak. (Isn't there an old Chinese saying about "Best to wait until autumn to settle your scores"?) After all, right now our main adversary is the virus itself. I am dedicated to standing side by side with the government and all the people of Wuhan, fully committed to battle this outbreak together. I am also 100 percent committed to accommodating any and all requests made of me by the government. However, as I write about this I also feel that reflection is required. And so, I reflect.

JANUARY 30, 2020

There is no way for them to shirk responsibility on this issue.

The sky is clear and it feels like one of those perfect winter days. This is the kind of weather that really allows you to appreciate the winter season. But the virus has completely destroyed all of that. It may as well be the most gorgeous day in a thousand years, yet there is no one outdoors to admire it.

The cruelty of reality continues to dangle before me. After I got up, I saw a news story about a peasant traveling in the middle of the night who was prohibited from going to his destination. People had built a dirt wall to block the road and no matter how he pleaded, the people guarding the road would not let him pass. Where else could that peasant go in the middle of a cold winter night? It was really difficult to watch. The regulations that they have put in place to prevent the spread of the disease are pretty good, but you can't enforce them with an iron will that overlooks the basic principles of what is humane.

Why is it that all these different levels of government officials are able to take an official document and turn it into something so dogmatic and inflexible? Why couldn't someone just put on a face mask and take that poor man to an empty room where he could spend a night in isolation? What would be so wrong with that? I also saw a report of a child with special needs whose father was ordered into isolation; the child was forced to live on his own for five days and ended up dying of starvation. This outbreak has exposed so many different things: It has exposed the rudimentary level of so many Chinese officials, and it has exposed the diseases running rampant through the very fabric of our society. These are diseases that are much more evil and tenacious than the novel coronavirus. Moreover, there is no cure in sight. That is because there are no doctors willing to treat this disease. Just thinking about this leaves me with an indescribable sadness. A few minutes ago a friend told me that a young man from our work unit got sick about two days ago and has been having difficulty breathing. He thinks he has the coronavirus but hasn't been properly diagnosed and there are no hospital beds for him. He is really a good, honest, hardworking young man and I'm quite close to his whole family. I really hope it is just a common cold, and praying that he hasn't been struck down by this evil virus.

I've been getting a lot of messages from people who saw my interview with China News Agency and really appreciated the things I was saying. Of course, a lot of the original content was censored, which is understandable. However, there are a few things that I think should be worth preserving. When I was discussing the topic of "self-treatment," I also said: "The most important group we should be paying attention to are those who are infected and the families of those people who have died from the coronavirus. They are the ones who are worst off and suffering the deepest pain. Many of them will never truly recover from what they have experienced here. They are the ones most in need of the government's support. . . ." When I think back and reflect on that peasant who was turned away in the middle of the night, when I think about that boy who starved to death at home, those countless everyday people calling out in vain for help, those people from Wuhan (including children) who have been discriminated against and driven out onto the streets like a pack of stray dogs, I have a hard time imagining how much time will have to pass before they can heal their pain. And that is not even to mention how much we have lost on a national scale.

For the past two days, the internet has been abuzz with news about how that group of specialists behaved when they visited Wuhan. That's right, these are the same well-respected "specialists" who lowered their guard and nonchalantly told us that it was "Not Contagious Between People" and "It's Controllable and Preventable"; they have truly committed heinous crimes with their irresponsible words. If they had even an ounce of decency left, I wonder what sense of guilt they might feel when they see all those people suffering. Of course, the political leaders of Hubei have the basic responsibility to ensure the safety and security of the people who live here. Now that we have arrived at a time when the people are no longer safe or secure, how could they not share some of the responsibility? The coronavirus getting to this point is the result of multiple forces coming together. There is no way for them to shirk responsibility on this issue. But right now what we really want is for them to stand up and lead the people of Hubei out of this dark place, with a sense of repentance and responsibility. That is how they can win back the people's understanding and forgiveness. If Wuhan can make it through this, the rest of the country can, too.

All my relatives live here in Wuhan. I am quite thankful that up until now everyone has remained healthy. Actually, most of my family members are getting old. My eldest brother and his wife are already in their mid-seventies, and my middle brother is also about to hit 70. Staying infection-free is the best thing we can do to help our country. I'm happy that my niece and her son were finally able to make it safely back to Singapore, where they are now being quarantined in a resort area. For that, I need to express my deepest thanks to the Hongshan Department of Transportation. When my niece received the notification yesterday, it read: "The flight to Singapore will depart at 3:00 a.m.; please arrive early to the airport." But my brother doesn't drive, and with public transportation shut down, they had absolutely no way to get to the airport. That's where I came in. Since Huazhong University of Science and Technology where my brother works is located in the Hongshan District, I checked with the Hongshan District Traffic Office to see if I would be allowed to drive there. There are quite a few officers who work at the station there that are actually my readers. They insisted that I just stay home and focus on my writing; they told me that they would take care of the rest. Officer Xiao was assigned to help get my niece to the airport. My entire family is grateful for his help. When you are in a bind, you can always go to the police for help! That's something you can always count on. But the fact that my niece and her son were able to get out safely is the only thing I have to be happy about today.

It is already Day Six of the Lunar New Year, eight days since the quarantine began. What needs to be said is that although the people of Wuhan tend to be naturally optimistic, and things around the city are becoming increasingly orderly, the reality here inside the city is growing grimmer by the day.

For dinner I had a small bowl of millet congee. In a little bit I'll go on the treadmill to get some exercise. Little by little, bit by bit, I'm recording everything here in my little file.

JANUARY 31, 2020

If you are just going to fawn all over the officials,
please restrain yourselves.

It is the seventh day of the Lunar New Year and the weather is bright and sunny. Might this be a good omen? This week will be the most critical stage in our fight against the virus. The specialists are all saying that by the fifteenth day of the Lunar New Year, all infected individuals should start showing symptoms. That should be the turning point. So we just need to hang in there for one more week. After this week, all the infected patients should be segregated, and those not showing symptoms should be free to leave their homes; then we'll be free—at least, that is how they are imagining it. It has now been nine days since the city went into quarantine, and we have already gotten through the bulk of it.

I grabbed my phone before even getting out of bed and immediately saw some really good news: That young man that I work with sent a group text saying that he has "not been infected after all. I'm now completely back to normal. I had an upset stomach yesterday and must have taken too much medicine, which caused those symptoms! I know I'm a stupid kid! Anyway, once this whole virus business is over, I'm treating everyone to dinner to make up for giving everyone such a scare!" I was still giggling from that message when I saw another bit of news. There is a guy from the provincial song-and-dance troupe that a lot of my friends know; after he fell ill, he got on the wait-list to be admitted to the hospital, but by the time notice arrived that they had a bed for him he had just passed away. I also heard that quite a few government officials from Hubei have been infected and a few have already died. My god, how many families here in Wuhan are being destroyed by this disaster? And up until now I still haven't heard a single person stand up to take responsibility or apologize. Instead, I just see an endless number of people writing essays or giving speeches that shirk the responsibility onto others.

Who can the families of the deceased cry out to? Who can they curse? I saw an interview that a reporter did with a Chinese writer, and in the interview he talked about "winning a resounding victory against the virus." I was speechless. Take a look at Wuhan! Take a look at the entire country! Millions of people are living in fear, thousands of people are hospitalized with their lives hanging by a thread, countless families have been destroyed. Where is this "win"? Where is this "victory"? Where is the end to all this? This writer is a colleague of mine in the same profession, so I feel bad cutting into him like this. But don't these people think before they speak? But that's not it. They are just trying to say something to please the higher-ups; he definitely thought it through. I was happy that right after that, I discovered another essay by another writer also criticizing those comments. The essay was extremely critical and really took that other writer to task. This tells me that there must be a lot of writers out there with a conscience. I may no longer be the chair of the Hubei Writers Association, but I am still a writer. I wanted to remind my fellow Hubei writers that while many of you may be asked to write essays and poems celebrating all the great achievements of the government, I hope that before you pick up your pen you are able to reflect for a few moments about who it is that you should really be celebrating. If you are just going to fawn all over the officials, please restrain yourselves. I might be old, but I will never tire when it comes to speaking out.

I have been rushing around the kitchen all morning cooking for my daughter; I plan to take some food over to her tonight. She returned from a trip to Japan on the 22nd and didn't get back to her apartment until after midnight. As soon as she returned, the quarantine was imposed so she never had time to go shopping or make any proper preparations. I delivered some food to her just before the Lunar New Year and again on the first day of the New Year. That lasted her a few days, but now she is running out and was talking about ordering some takeout. Her father and I are both vehemently opposed to her ordering takeout, so I decided to take her some food myself. I don't live that far from my daughter; it is usually just a 10- or 15-minute drive. I checked with the police and they said it is no problem to go out on the roads. So I decided to cook some things for her and take them over myself. I feel a bit like "I'm bringing rations to the Red Army!" They don't allow people to enter her neighborhood, so I had to meet her at the entrance to her neighborhood and hand the food off to her there. She is the only one from her generation in my family who decided to remain in Wuhan, so no matter what, I have to protect her.

The gate to our building is on the second ring of the city, and it is usually bustling with traffic and crowded with pedestrians. These days there are very few cars and even fewer people. The main roads are all decorated with lights and lanterns for the Chinese New Year, yet all the stores along the side streets are closed, making everything appear dark and desolate. All the buildings along the main roads are decorated with lights for the Military World Games, which flicker from every direction.[6] Back when the games were being held, I found those flashing lights incredibly irritating; they were really quite the eyesore. But now as I drive down these empty streets, those festive, sparkling lights somehow give me a sense of comfort. Things have indeed changed.

Some of the smaller supermarkets are still open. There are also a few vegetable peddlers set up on the sidewalk. I bought some vegetables from one of those peddlers and went to the supermarket to pick up some milk and eggs (I actually had to go to three markets before I found one with eggs in stock). I asked the storekeeper whether or not she was afraid of getting infected by staying open during the outbreak. She answered frankly: "We've got to go on living; so do you!" That's right, they have to carry on, we all have to carry on; that's simply all we can do! I always admire those working-class people and often strike up a chat with them; somehow that always gives me a strange sense of security. Even during that two- or three-day cold spell when it was windy and rainy and the outbreak was really out of control, the streets were almost completely empty. Yet even then there would always be at least one sanitation worker out there, meticulously sweeping the streets. Whenever I caught a glimpse of one of them, I would immediately start to feel guilty for feeling so scared and anxious; one sight of them is always enough to immediately set me at ease.

FEBRUARY

And as he is saving them, I hope he saves himself, too.

The weather is still clear today. It is now Day Eight of the Lunar New Year and I'm feeling a bit nostalgic for all the excitement that normally fills our courtyard area this time of year. Once again, I started looking at my phone before getting out of bed and saw some statistics that were just published yesterday. The result of those figures were: There continues to be an increase in both the number of confirmed cases as well as the suspected cases of coronavirus infection; however, the rate of infection has clearly begun to slow down. Moreover, it has continued to slow over the course of the past three days. The number of patients with critical symptoms has also begun to decline. The mortality rate is holding steady at around 2 percent, as before. And the number of patients who have recovered and suspected cases that have been ruled out has also increased. This is all great news! All of this demonstrates that the quarantine measures taken of late have been very effective. My eldest brother sent this news out to our family group chat this morning; I can't confirm that all these statistics are accurate, but I certainly hope so! And so I keep coming back to say, if Wuhan can make it through this, the rest of the country can, too.

Now that I think back, it was actually my eldest brother who first told me that this virus was contagious. There are actually just us four siblings in that family group chat. Not even my sister-in-law and niece are in the group. Since two of my older brothers are university professors, they often have access to really good information from their colleagues and friends. That is especially the case for my eldest brother; he is a graduate of Qinghua University and teaches at Huazhong University of Science and Technology, so he often gets a lot of valuable information. At 10:00 a.m. on December 31st, that brother forwarded me an essay entitled "Suspected Case of Virus of Unknown Origin in Wuhan" and then in parentheses was the word "SARS."

My brother said that he wasn't sure if this news was authentic. But my other brother immediately chimed in and suggested that none of us go outside. My youngest brother works in Shenyang and offered for us to come visit him for a while so we could huddle down and wait things out there. He said: "It is 20 below in Shenyang, and no viruses can survive here for long." But my eldest brother reminded him: "It was actually hot climates that hindered the spread of SARS. Don't you remember what happened in 2003?" A bit later my eldest brother sent another text confirming that the news of this new disease was true and that a group of specialists from the National Health Commission had already arrived in Wuhan.

My middle brother was quite shaken by this news, since he lives very close to the Huanan Seafood Market,[1] which is the epicenter of the outbreak. I didn't see those texts until around noon and when I did, I immediately told them both to avoid hospitals for the time being. My brother isn't in the best of health, and he often goes to Wuhan Central Hospital for his appointments, which is where there is a concentration of patients with flu-like symptoms. He quickly sent another text saying he just looked outside and Central Hospital looks quiet as always. There were no reporters outside, as he had originally suspected there would be. It wasn't long after that that I started to receive videos from friends reporting on the situation at the Huanan Seafood Market and Wuhan Central Hospital. I immediately forwarded the news to my family group chat. I even reminded my brother to be sure to wear a face mask if he goes out. I even suggested that he just come to my apartment after the New Year to get away from that area for the time being. After all, I live in the Jiangxia District, which is a bit further away from Hankou. But he just said he would sit tight for the time being and see what happens. He didn't think it would turn out to be anything to be too concerned about. He also didn't think that the government would block information about what was happening; that would be a true blow to the people. My thoughts on the matter were pretty close to my brother's. I figured that there was no way the government would censor news about something so important. How could they possibly stop the public from learning the truth about what was happening?

On the morning of January 1, my elder brother reposted a story from the *Wuhan Evening News* about the Huanan Seaford Market closure. My middle brother said that things around his neighborhood were still about the same and everyone was going about their normal business as usual. As concerned citizens, we were all really tuned into the news that was happening that day. The protective measures they recommended that day were actually about the same as right now: Wear a face mask, stay home, and don't go outside. I'm sure that most Wuhan residents who had lived through the terror of SARS are just like me and took this news quite seriously. However, it wasn't long before the official government line came down. Based on the findings of specialists, they boiled everything down to a little eight-word maxim: "Not Contagious Between People; It's Controllable and Preventable." As soon as we heard that, everyone breathed a collective sigh of relief. After all, we never consume exotic wildlife and had no plans to go to the Huanan Seafood Market, so it appeared that there was nothing to be concerned about.

The reason that I am recounting all these details is that this morning I read an interview with Mr. Wang Guangfa.[2] Mr. Wang was part of the second team of specialists sent to Wuhan to investigate the outbreak. Shortly after he declared "it's controllable and preventable," he himself became infected with the coronavirus. Of course, that early statement might not have been directly coming from him; after all, it was a collective decision of the team. But I expected him to at least show some sense of remorse, self-reproach, or—dare I say?—reflection. As members of the team of specialists, they, at the very least, were responsible for giving the people of Wuhan information that severely underestimated the nature of this virus. Not matter how useless and bureaucratic those officials from Hubei and Wuhan might be, and no matter how many people attempt to cover up the truth in order to show how prosperous and powerful our country is, as a doctor, couldn't Mr. Wang have been a bit more prudent when he made that initial statement? Instead, he made that proclamation with such resolution and decisiveness. By the time that Mr. Wang was infected on January 16, it was already quite clear that this virus "*Was* Contagious Between People." Yet for some reason we did not hear Mr. Wang's timely revision of that earlier statement; nor did we hear him sound the alarm for people to start taking precautions. It was only three days later when Zhong Nanshan[3] from the Chinese Academy of Engineering arrived in Wuhan that the truth was finally revealed.

Mr. Wang's interview was from yesterday. The people of Wuhan have just gotten through their incredibly pathetic Lunar New Year (we might be optimistic, but it really *was* a pathetic New Year), patients are in a terrible state, the dead are leaving behind shattered families in their wake, the quarantine has led to massive losses nationwide, and the entire country has seen the bravery and hard work of Mr. Wang's fellow doctors. And yet in his interview Mr. Wang, who bears a certain degree of responsibility for how things were conducted, didn't express even one ounce of regret over how things were handled. There wasn't a hint of an apology. Not only that, but he behaved as if he had done the people a great service. He said: "If I had only come to Wuhan to take a cursory look at what was happening there, I would have never gone into those patients' rooms and visited those sick wards, and I wouldn't have been infected myself! But now that I'm sick, everyone now knows just how serious this coronavirus truly is!" I was truly dumbfounded after I heard those words. I suppose Mr. Wang isn't afraid of the Wuhan people cursing him to hell.

The Chinese people have never been fond of admitting their own mistakes; nor do they have a very strong sense of repentance, and they are even less likely to stand up and truly accept blame for something. Perhaps this is connected to our customs and culture? But as a doctor, his job is to cure the sick and help the injured; how could he see so many people struggling with illness and dying in desperate circumstances because of some irresponsible statements he made and not have any sense of the role he played in this? Even if the people haven't placed the blame on him, what about he himself? Is he able to just psychologically walk away from this free and clear? Isn't there even an ounce of guilt in this man's heart? Didn't he talk about charity? And now here he is going on and on about his own great sacrifice. In ancient times when the state faced great calamities, even the emperor knew enough to issue an imperial decree blaming himself for the suffering of the people. But what about Mr. Wang and the other members of that team of specialists? Don't they plan on issuing an apology to the people of Wuhan? Don't they feel that this is an important lesson for them in their careers as medical professionals?

Forget it, I don't want to go on anymore about this right now. I'll just pray that from today onward Mr. Wang does a better job of curing the sick and helping the injured. And as he is saving them, I hope he saves himself, too.

FEBRUARY 2, 2020

*When an era sheds a speck of dust it might not
seem like much, but when it falls upon the shoulders
of an individual it feels like a mountain.*

It is Day Nine of the Lunar New Year. How many days has it been that we have been hanging on? I'm not in the mood to even count. Someone wanted to come up with a trick question and asked if you can identify what day it is without looking at your cellphone—and you have to respond immediately without thinking about it. Now that is a mind zinger right there! How can anyone be expected to remember what day of the week it is? The fact that I know it is Day Nine of the Lunar New Year is already something of a miracle.

The weather is starting to turn a bit gloomy, and it even rained this afternoon. Those patients running around town to different hospitals trying to get treatment are going to be in even more desperate straits. When you go outside to take a look around Wuhan, everything seems to be orderly and normal just like always, except for the fact that there are hardly any people outside and all the lights in all the buildings are turned on. Most people don't seem to be lacking food or supplies, so as long as nobody is sick in your family, things are fairly stable. The city isn't the purgatory that a lot of people seem to be imagining it to be. It is instead a rather quiet and beautiful, almost majestic, city. But all that changes the second someone in your family falls ill. Immediately everything is thrown into chaos. It is, after all, an infectious disease. But hospital resources are limited. Everyone knows that even when doctors' family members get sick, they usually don't get admitted to the hospital unless it is a particularly serious case. These past few days we are in what the specialists predicted to be a period of "viral outbreak." I expect I will be seeing or hearing even more grim news in the days to come. The video I found most difficult to watch today was a news clip of a daughter trailing behind her mother's funeral car, screaming through her tears. Her mommy was gone and now her remains were being driven away. The daughter will never be able to give her mother a proper burial; she probably won't even know what they did with her mother's ashes. In Chinese culture, the rites of death are so central to who we are, perhaps even more important than how we live, which makes this all the more heartbreaking for a daughter to face.

But there is nothing we can do. Actually, there is nothing anyone can do. Our only choice is to grin and bear it. Even though it is getting to the point that most of the patients can't bear it anymore, nor can their families. But if you don't bear it, what else is there you can do? I once wrote somewhere that when an era sheds a speck of dust it might not seem like much, but when it falls upon the shoulders of an individual it feels like a mountain. The first time I wrote those words, I don't think I fully grasped the depth of what it represented. But now those words are etched in my heart. Earlier in the afternoon I was in touch with a young reporter. He told me he felt utterly helpless. He felt like all anyone was paying attention to was the numbers, how many were infected, how many were dead—but what about what was behind those numbers? It is really a shame what these young people have to go through. They are just starting out in life and now they have to face the cruel reality of what it means to truly struggle and face death, not to mention all those restrictions that have been placed on them. I too feel helpless. But then again, when I think about it from another angle, besides standing up and putting on a brave face, what else can we do? We are not trained to help the sick. All we can do is face what lies before us and shoulder what is coming. And when we have the wherewithal to help others, we help them shoulder it, too. But no matter what, I need to bear another week.

One bit of good news comes to me via a statistic that I just saw. Official accounts are reporting that there is a reduction in the number of people infected outside of Hubei Province. Moreover, for those patients outside Hubei the recovery rate is quite high and the mortality rate is very low. The reason the statistics for Hubei are inaccurate and the death rate is so high clearly has to do with the fact that we are desperately lacking in terms of treatment resources. To put it more bluntly, the problem isn't that this illness cannot be treated. If you get good medical care during the early stages, it can be quickly controlled. I also saw a report that suggested the healthcare facilities in neighboring provinces have been gearing up in preparation for what is coming but in the end, there haven't been that many patients coming in. There are some cases of patient A transferring the illness to patient B, but there seem to be very few cases of patient B infecting patient C. There have been a few suspected cases of this type of third-level transmission, but no one is completely sure yet. So some have suggested that trained healthcare professionals should transfer some of the patients via ambulance from Wuhan to neighboring provinces so they can get better treatment. Wuhan is, after all, a city that is centrally located and a major traffic hub; there are several provincial capitals that are just three or four hours away by car. If these patients get treatment, many of them will be able to escape the hand of death. I'm not sure if this suggestion will end up being a practical one, but I think it seems to make sense. But just now I heard from an old classmate of mine who said that the new Huoshenshan Hospital will start accepting patients tomorrow (I'm not sure if that is accurate). If these patients can get out of Hubei, there are a lot of hospital beds available elsewhere; the treatment conditions elsewhere would be better too, and there are also a large number of doctors and healthcare workers ready to provide support. But if Huoshenshan opens tomorrow, then the whole idea of sending patients to other provinces will be abandoned. Anyway, it feels like my wish list has grown quite modest: I only wish that these patients can have a hospital to go to. I pray for them.

I would also like to say something in support of the young people in Wuhan. There are tens of thousands of young volunteers working on the front lines to battle this outbreak. They are all doing this completely of their own volition. They use social media platforms like WeChat to organize, and they do virtually everything under the sun. They are truly amazing! People of my generation used to always worry about this younger generation's becoming increasingly self-centered, but now that I see them springing into action, I realize that old farts like me were worried about nothing! People of each generation are actually all the same in some way, and the older generation shouldn't worry too much about the younger generation's not finding their way. Last night the writer Chen Cun[4] sent me a link to some videos by a young Wuhan native who was recording scenes from daily life after the quarantine. The videos documented several days of life here in Wuhan, and I watched them all in one sitting. Those videos were really something to behold. If I ever meet this young director, I hope I can give him copies of a few of my books as a way of expressing my admiration for what he has done. I'd also like to tell him that once upon a time, on a cold and wretched night, his videos helped brighten my spirit.

FEBRUARY 3, 2020

Lamenting our difficult lives,
I heave a deep sigh and wipe away my tears.

Day Ten of the Lunar New Year. Another bright and sunny day. Yesterday I thought it might continue to rain, but today it suddenly cleared up. Perhaps those people hoping to get medical attention will have just a little more warmth thanks to the sun making its appearance. But many of them are infected, and they are dragging their sick bodies all over the city in search of treatment. Everyone knows that none of them wanted to be in this position, but they have no choice; this is what they must do in order to survive. There is no other path for them. I suppose that the sense of cold abandonment they are feeling must be much worse than the actual cold this winter season. But as they toil around the city in search of help, I hope that they don't suffer too much along the way. There may not be a sickbed for them, but at least the sun is still shining down on them.

Flipping through my cellphone in bed again. The first thing I see is the news about an earthquake in Chengdu. The quake took a lot of people off guard, but it didn't seem to put anyone in real danger. Some of the online jokes about it were quite funny, though. One of them was: "Thanks to the earthquake, all 20,000 people from Wuhan currently in Chengdu have finally been located. Since all the Chengdu locals just stay inside soaking their feet in hot water, it was easy to identify the Wuhanese; they were the ones who rushed outside in a state of panic when the quake hit!" I couldn't help but burst out laughing when I read that. I'm sure that these Chengdu comedians gave the people of Wuhan a "moment of laughter" this morning. Sichuanese have an even better sense of humor than people from Wuhan. Thanks to the comedian who came up with that one!

There are a few videos online that I can no longer bear to watch; they are just too heartbreaking. But we need to be calm and collected and understand that we can't let the sadness of the situation consume us. The departed are gone, but the living must go on as before. I just hope we can remember: Remember those everyday people who have passed, remember those who suffered a wrongful death, remember these grief-stricken days and sorrowful nights, remember just what it was that interrupted our lives during what should have been the joyous Lunar New Year holiday. As long as we are able to scrape by and stay alive, we need to fight for justice for those who have suffered and died. We need to hold those people in charge who were negligent, irresponsible, or simply failed to act accountable for the harm they caused. These cases need to be rigorously pursued, and none of those parties responsible should be allowed to weasel their way out of this. If we do not take action, how are we supposed to give justice to those people—those fellow Wuhan residents with whom we once worked side-by-side and enjoyed life together—whose bodies ended up being carted away in body bags?

Today I watched an educational documentary about Wuhan that was pretty good. When describing Wuhan's current state of wide-open streets and utter quiet, the narrator said it was as if someone had "hit the pause button" on the entire city. That's right, the entire city is on pause, but for those people whose bodies have already been carted away in bags, it is already over. My heavens! Those undertakers at the crematoriums have never before had to deal with anything like this. But they say it is the doctors who really need our attention, as they are the ones taking care of the living.

This afternoon I got in touch with a doctor friend of mine to try to get a better understanding of what is happening in the city. He has been working right there on the front lines of this epidemic. He took a few minutes to answer some of my questions when he had a short break from his work. We talked about all kinds of things, but I can sum up our conversation in a few points. Number one: It is difficult to be optimistic about the state Wuhan is in right now, as the situation is still quite critical. Medical supplies are in a state of "tight balance"—that was the first time I heard that term, but I figure it must mean "tight supply" and that they are close to running out of many supplies, but for the time being they are just getting by. The doctor said that they should have enough supplies to get through another two or three days. Number two: Smaller local hospitals are facing some really challenging times right now. The basic conditions at many of those hospitals is not great to begin with; they aren't getting much attention, and their treatment facilities are quite limited. My friend asked me to send out an appeal to my readers to start paying attention to those local hospitals and do what you can to provide them with support. At the same time, he said that many of these smaller local governments in villages and more suburban areas have taken strong steps to enforce segregation and quarantines, and in many cases they have done a better job than here in Wuhan. Number three: Sending patients with fevers who are suspected of having the virus back into the community is not an appropriate action. Those local communities lack the professional knowledge and protective gear to properly handle patients. How are they expected to cope with what is happening? Moreover, people in those small local communities are also quite afraid for their own safety. There is nothing they can do to solve any of these problems. I agree that it was a series of bad decisions that led to the widespread increase in the number of infections in Wuhan; and once one person became infected their entire family also became sick. Number four: Doctors at every hospital are all overworked, and specialists from various departments have all been transferred to the front lines. Right now doctors are still busy treating that first wave of patients, all the while the number of new patients and suspected cases coming in for diagnosis continues to rapidly increase. (I didn't have the courage to ask him if they would be able to provide proper treatment for all these newly diagnosed patients just coming in.) Number five: My doctor friend suspects that the final tally of infected patients will end up being a terrifying number. He spoke with authority when he said: "The only way we are going to get a handle on this outbreak is if we get everyone who needs treatment admitted to a hospital and everyone who needs to be quarantined confined at home." No matter how you look at it, this is the only way forward. Based on some of the new procedures the government started to put in place today, it seems that they have also finally started to realize this.

The coronavirus is here, and from its early phase to its period of expansion and all the way up to the point where it began to get out of control, our response has gone from being completely wrong to being delayed and ultimately to its current flawed state. We were unable to get ahead of this virus and stop it; instead, we have been frantically chasing after it, and paying a heavy price in the process. This is not the time to slowly cross the river by gradually feeling for the stones; there have been so many previous outbreaks that we could have referred to, so how come we haven't learned from them? Couldn't we just copy what people have previously done to successfully control outbreaks like this in the past? Or perhaps I'm just oversimplifying things?

There was another video I saw today of a family driving over a bridge from Chongqing to Guizhou. In the car was a married couple with what looked like two children (I couldn't quite see it clearly in the video). The man was from Chongqing and the woman was from Guizhou. Their car set out from the Chongqing side and was headed to the border of Guizhou. In the end, the guards said they would let the wife through since she was from Guizhou, but no matter what, they refused to let her husband through; in the end, he had no choice but to turn the car around and go back to Chongqing. Once they got back to the other side of the bridge the guards on that side told them that since they had already left the city limits of Chongqing, only the husband could go back in, but the wife was not permitted through. The husband who was driving said: "They won't let us through on that side and now you won't let us through here; what do you want us to do? Live on this bridge?" Watching that video, I really didn't know whether to laugh or cry. I once wrote a novel entitled *The City of Wuchang*,[5] which was set nearly a hundred years ago when warlords had surrounded the city. (What a coincidence that I now find myself also quarantined here in Wuchang!) During the siege, countless numbers of people inside the city of Wuchang starved to death. People from Hankou and Hanyang worked together to try to save the people in Wuchang, and eventually the warlords worked out an agreement allowing residents three days to leave the city to search for food. During that time, the forces surrounding the city vowed not to attack, and the army guarding the city agreed to let the residents out. All this happened back in 1926. During that time there were two armies at war, and yet these two opposing forces were able to work out an agreement; and here we are today, a hundred years later, and we can't even stretch the rules a little bit for the sake of a family?! It is not as if the sky were falling! There are many ways to resolve a problem. In the end, I don't know if that family ever made it to Guizhou or ended up going back to Chongqing.

"Lamenting our difficult lives, I heave a deep sigh and wipe away my tears."[6] These days there are a lot of people expressing this sentiment.

FEBRUARY 4, 2020

Fate must have again smiled down on me.

Today the weather continues to be good. The Wuhan people continue to hold steady. We are feeling a bit stifled from being stuck indoors, but as long we can stay alive we can handle the rest.

This afternoon I heard about another person going into panic mode while at the supermarket picking up a few things; this man said he was afraid that the store would shut down and there would be no new supplies of food coming in. I felt like that was an unrealistic fear. The municipal government already issued a proclamation assuring citizens that supermarkets would stay open. Just to think through this logically: Right now, the entire country is standing behind Wuhan, and China isn't the kind of nation facing any true shortages of material goods, so I'm sure it won't be too difficult for the country to ensure that the people of Wuhan have enough food and supplies. Of course, there will certainly be some elderly people living alone who might be going through some hard times (even without the coronavirus, they don't have it easy), but I'm confident that there will be many community volunteers who will be there to help them out. Even if the government made some mistakes early on, no matter what, we now have no choice but to put our faith in our leaders; we need to believe in them. Otherwise, what is the alternative? Who else can we believe in? Who else can you rely on? Those people who are easily frightened are the kind of people who are always on edge anyway; there is really nothing you can do to help them. Just now I went out to throw away the garbage and noticed a sign posted on my front door that read "Disinfection Complete." There was also a flyer that said if you discover you have a fever, please call the following phone number for Wuchang District. From that you can tell how meticulous is the work being done on the community level. The coronavirus is a great enemy that everyone is united against; no one dares to slack off, so let's just hope the policymakers don't have any more missteps.

The question of how many people will end up being infected by this virus remains an extremely sensitive topic. I'm also anxious about how big this number will eventually be. Yesterday I posted something on Weibo that mentioned the number 100,000, which is a number most doctors have long been bracing for, even though none of them will say that publicly. Then there was actually one doctor who, while appealing to the public for help, actually said the number out loud. Today another doctor friend told me that he thought that estimate was right on. "There will indeed be that many people infected. But one thing to keep in mind is that not everyone infected shows symptoms. Perhaps only 30 to 50 percent of the people infected will actually develop symptoms." I then asked him a follow-up question: "And if you are infected but remain asymptomatic, does that mean that you gradually just recover on your own?" My doctor friend affirmed that: "That is correct." If this is true, I suppose that counts as good news?

But the fact should be reemphasized that, according to what doctors are saying, the novel coronavirus may be extremely contagious, but as long as patients receive standard treatment, the death rate is not too high. Patients who have received treatment outside of Hubei Province have already proven this to be true. The reason the death rate has been so high here in Wuhan is that there are a large number of patients who cannot get access to hospital care; without proper treatment, mild cases turn serious and serious cases lead to death. Another contributing factor is tied to the fact that the quarantine procedures were flawed early on, which led to many cases of a single person infecting their entire family. This, in turn, led to a dramatic increase in infections and sparked a whole series of other tragedies. My doctor friend told me that if they had been better prepared early on, based on the number of beds available, Wuhan should have been able to treat all the serious cases that came in. But things were just too chaotic during the early stages of the outbreak, people were consumed with fear, and a lot of people who weren't even sick flooded into the hospitals, making things even more frenzied. Now the government is consistently tweaking its response procedures. The next step will be to see if we can reach a turning point; I hope that moment comes sooner rather than later.

Besides this, yesterday some people online started to raise some questions about those "temporary hospital stations"[7] that have just been set up; they were worried that isolating large numbers of patients together would actually lead to a huge spike in cases of cross-infection. But my take on it is that those temporary hospitals are based on a model typically seen in battlefield situations during wartime. The first thing that must be done is to segregate suspected carriers together as quickly as possible, and then send doctors to provide treatment. As that is taking place, they can then gradually work to improve the conditions for those quarantined patients. If these steps are not taken, those infected individuals will continue moving around the city and every day they are out there means that more people will become infected. If that continues, there is no way this virus will ever be able to be contained. Although the conditions in those mobile hospitals are far from ideal, I imagine that the next step will be to divide those large open spaces up into smaller rooms. But that is just my guess; I'm not sure if that is the actual plan. But no matter what, quickly separating those infected individuals from the general population is the most pressing issue at the moment.

I saw a "selfie" video today that was shot by one of the patients at Huoshenshan Hospital. From the video I could tell that the treatment facilities there are quite good and the patients there seem to have a positive outlook. That is exactly the kind of video I was hoping I might be able to see. I hope they all recover soon, and I hope that everything will move forward from here in a more rational and organized manner.

This outbreak is the result of several forces coming together. The enemy is not just the virus itself. We ourselves are also our own worst enemies in this fight, or, at the very least, we are accomplices to the crime. I'm told that there are a lot of people who are now suddenly waking up to just how meaningless it is to go around every day shouting empty slogans about how awesome our country is; they know that those cadres who go around giving speeches on political education but who never take concrete action are utterly useless (we used to refer to them as people who "live off the labor of their mouths"); and they certainly know that a society that lacks common sense and fails to pursue the facts as they present themselves not only ends up harming people through words but can actually result in the loss of human lives—many, many human lives. This is a lesson that resonates deeply and also comes with a heavy weight. Even though we have all lived through the SARS epidemic of 2003, it seems we have all quickly forgotten the lessons we supposedly learned then; now fast-forward to 2020—will we forget again? The devil is always on our heels and if we aren't careful, he will catch up to us again and torture us until we finally wake up. The real question is: *Do we even want to wake up?*

Thinking back to the year of SARS, that disease began to spread in March but the government initially tried to cover it up. At the time, I had an old classmate in Guangzhou who was about to undergo a big operation. I went with a few dozen old friends from all over China down to Guangzhou to support her during her surgery; we all descended on the very hospital where the SARS outbreak was fiercely raging, but none of us knew that at the time (and none of us were wearing face masks). We all traveled there roundtrip by train. Once what was happening was finally exposed, everyone all over the country was in a state of panic. We in particular were sweating bullets; amid the chaos, I told myself that fate must have smiled down on me to allow me to have escaped infection. This time I made three trips to the hospital between January 1st and the 18th, each time to visit colleagues who had been hospitalized for surgery. During two of those visits I didn't even wear a face mask. Now that it has passed, I cringe when I think about it and, once again, I think that fate must have again smiled down on me.

FEBRUARY 5, 2020

All us ordinary people have paid a price
for this human catastrophe.

Yesterday marked the first day of spring and today the weather indeed feels like spring. Across from our house is a row of old camphor trees, two osmanthus trees, and one *yulan* magnolia; the rich blanket of leaves makes one feel as if winter was never even here.

Today we are still in the middle of what the experts had predicted to be the peak period of the coronavirus outbreak. It is said that the number of confirmed cases is continuing to climb. A famous painter who I know is right now in critical condition due to the virus. My friend YL told me that she knows three cinematographers who got infected while on a shoot and all of them have since died from the coronavirus. My circle of friends is quite small and I'm so thankful that they are doing well so far. The situation in Wuhan is still grim, but not as chaotic as before. At the same time, things have not really eased up. Those depressing online videos and desperate cries for help that were circulating all over the internet seem to have died down quite a bit, and they have been replaced by positive messages online that are encouraging everyone to move forward. I'm not sure if those earlier issues have really been resolved or if they've just been censored from the internet. After experiencing so much censorship, I have come to grow numb about the whole thing. Yesterday I said that we are our own worst enemies; this process of becoming enemies of ourselves probably begins with that feeling of numbness. For the time being we need to be on guard, we need to be particularly aware of what's going on with our own bodies. I'm still continually nagging my friends: Be sure not to go outside! Be sure not to go out! I know we have been locked up inside for a long time and we might end up quarantined for much longer, but we can't worry about any of that. We might not have a lot of great food to eat at home but once this outbreak has passed, we can go out to a restaurant and order all those things we have been craving. We'll be happy and those restaurants will finally be able to start making some money again.

I saw a report this afternoon that I thought was interesting. Although the title, "The First Shots in the Battle Against the Coronavirus in Wuhan Have Already Been Fired," sounded like an official government media report, the content was actually very much worth reading. I'll provide a quick summary of the major points: (1) patients have been divided into three quarantine categories; (2) Huoshenshan Hospital, Leishenshan Hospital, and other designated hospitals are Level One facilities responsible for isolating and treating critical patients; (3) the 11 newly constructed mobile hospitals are designated Level Two facilities responsible for the isolation and treatment of patients with mild infections; (4) hotels and Chinese Communist Party Schools will be designated as Level Three facilities in charge of isolating suspected cases of infection and members of the population who have been in close contact with infected individuals; (5) once these three groups of individuals have been isolated, a comprehensive, city-wide sterilization process will be put into play; (6) all hospitals will resume their normal operations (and all departments previously closed will reopen); (7) other businesses will be able to reopen and resume commerce; (8) patients will be continually monitored and their treatment will be updated based on their condition. For instance, once patients with critical symptoms turn mild, they will be transferred to mobile hospital units and if mild cases turn critical they will be moved to Level One facilities. We will follow this protocol until this catastrophic illness is completely eradicated! I'm not able to confirm whether all the details in this article were factual, but based on what I know, it seemed accurate. Ever since the military entered Wuhan, there seems to have been a clear improvement in terms of the overall efficiency with which they are facing this outbreak. The way they are fighting this virus really does feel a bit like a military campaign—clean and direct. I have a lot of high hopes for what this stage of the situation will bring. But what I really hope is that, no matter what level patients have been designated as, they are all given high-quality, effective, and reliable care.

Virtually all aspects of people's lives have been turned upside down by this outbreak; the effect on hospitals has been even worse. Doctors from all different departments have all been busy fighting this virus. Actually, even without this coronavirus outbreak there are already a huge number of patients who need to be cared for. But now all those patients have patiently stepped aside so that their doctors can fight the coronavirus; meanwhile, they continue to silently suffer from their illnesses. Many of those patients are quite anxious about what the ultimate consequences will be of their deferring their own care for so long, but they all put their needs aside so their doctors could join the fight against the coronavirus. I have great admiration for all those amazing patients. I have a colleague who was facing some major health issues and unfortunately had to undergo two major surgeries back-to-back this past January. The coronavirus outbreak erupted just before the Chinese New Year and she had just returned home from the hospital. After being discharged she still had to keep going back to the hospital for her medicine and shots, so she had no choice but to grit her teeth and drive over to the hospital to take care of these things. Her incision wasn't healing that well and was starting to show signs of purulence. Since the hospital was so overcrowded with people suffering from all kinds of illnesses, her doctors told her she'd better not come every day as she was originally supposed to. Instead they gave her some supplies to take home so she could change her own bandages. When she ran out of bandages, she had to go to the pharmacy to buy more. But once her incision started to get inflamed, she had no choice but to go to the local community hospital near her apartment for her shots. You can get anxious, upset, or even cry out through your tears, but what's the point? She herself said, "I just need to deal with it, at least until the threat of this virus has passed." I have another colleague whose father is suffering from cancer. This year she made special arrangements to bring her parents out to spend the Chinese New Year together in Wuhan. Now this entire family—all three generations—are locked down together in her apartment. They can't go anywhere and her parents are bored out of their minds; all she can do to entertain them is play cards with them every day to help them pass the time. Just now she called and complained to me that she is going crazy playing cards with them all the time. It is actually a big stress on her family. Those women in the city who are pregnant are also in a terribly stressful situation. Even if they are willing to be patient, that doesn't mean their babies will be. It is not a good time to be giving birth. These babies' arrivals, which should be filled with joy and celebration, have instead become occasions of extreme anxiety and uncertainty. This may not be a perfect world, but since these babies are brave enough to enter it, well, come on in then! Although this is the epicenter of an outbreak, I need to have faith that you will be received into a place that is warm and clean.

I am recording all the fragmented stories so that those criminals know: Besides the infected patients and the dead, there are a lot of other victims of this calamity. All us ordinary people have paid a price for this human catastrophe.

FEBRUARY 6, 2020

Right now everyone in this city is crying for him.

It started to rain again today in Wuhan. The sky is gray and overcast, the kind of windy and rainy day that leaves people feeling cold and depressed. When I went outside, the cold wind assaulted me, sending a shiver through my body.

There has been a lot of good news today, some of which is probably the most exciting news I have heard in many days. On the radio today someone who is supposedly a specialist in infectious diseases said that the outbreak would start to ease up very soon. What he was saying sounded believable to me. The other bit of news that has been circulating like crazy all over the internet is that the American pharmaceutical company Gilead Sciences has developed a new drug called remdesivir (Chinese specialists are calling it "the people's hope") and they have already begun clinical trials at Wuhan Jinyintan Hospital. Word has it that so far it has been extremely effective. Everyone in Wuhan is excited about this development; I'm sure that if we weren't all following the rules of the lockdown we would all be out dancing in the streets to celebrate. We have been stuck at home for so long, hoping for so long; now we finally have gotten a glimpse of something positive. That hope arrived so suddenly, and just in time, because we were all starting to grow increasingly depressed. Even if this news later gets refuted as a rumor or the drug turns out to be ineffective against the virus, I'll still take this bit of good news for the time being. Perhaps in another couple of days our hopes will be confirmed.

Those mobile hospitals that everyone has been so closely following have officially opened. There are already some patients who have been admitted there who have begun uploading videos, photos, and posts about their experience there. Some of them think that the conditions are really inferior and are complaining about how bad it is. There are quite a few posts like that. But I figure that you have to expect the conditions to be a bit messy at first; after all, these temporary hospitals were hastily constructed in just a single day's time. However, I'm confident that those other details will fall in place soon and things will improve. Whenever you put a large number of people together, it can be difficult to please everyone, especially when they are all suffering from an illness. It is only natural for people to feel anxious or annoyed; after all, being quarantined there is not nearly as comfortable as being in their own homes. This afternoon I received a text from cultural history professor Feng Tianyu from Wuhan University; he said that according to Yan Zhi,[8] they will be responsible for the two temporary hospitals being set up at the Wuhan International Conference & Exhibition Center and the Wuhan Keting Expo area. Mr. Yan said that he would do everything in his power to ensure that everything would go smoothly. "We are going to install a lot of television sets, set up a small library area, a charging station, a fast-food area, and make sure that each patient gets at least an apple, a banana, or some other fresh fruit every day; we want the patients to feel like we care." So you can see that they are really taking these little details into consideration. I'm sure that all the other temporary hospitals also have a system set up to properly delegate responsibility. If Yan Zhi is able to do it, I'm sure the other administrators in charge can do it, too. Wuhan has made it this far; we have already gotten through the most difficult stage of this, so this is not the time to start getting anxious about things. Let's just let those patients who have been running all over the city trying to get help finally just lie down and get some good rest; they may be quarantined, but they are also finally getting professional medical treatment, which is a good thing for them and everyone else in Wuhan. Otherwise, on a cold day like today, I'm sure a lot of them would have gotten worse or even just collapsed on the street. We have no choice but to steady ourselves and bear with the situation for now; only after things are under control will everyone be able to get back a true sense of peace and stability.

This morning I also saw a video interview with a pulmonologist from Zhongnan Hospital of Wuhan University. He himself was infected but somehow managed to recover. He made a lot of jokes as he recounted his experience; he became infected through direct contact with a patient. As his condition worsened and he grew dangerously close to dying, his wife continued to care for him. She also ended up getting infected, but it was a rather mild case. He tried to assure viewers not to panic. He said that the truly serious cases that result in death are almost all elderly people with underlying medical conditions. But if you are relatively young and get hit by this virus, as long as you are healthy, you just need to take some medication, drink a lot of water, and get a lot of rest. You should be fine if you do these things. He also discussed some of the unique properties of the novel coronavirus, such as the way in which the virus infects both lungs, starting from the outer areas of the lungs, without necessarily causing obvious symptoms like a runny nose. As someone who actually had the coronavirus, he is the most trustworthy source of information you could hope for. And so we need to stay inside and do our best to remain calm. We shouldn't go crazy; even if we get a light fever or a little cough, we need to deal with those symptoms rationally and calmly. Today the government issued a statement recommending that everyone should regularly check their temperature. Even that announcement caused a flurry of panic; some people were worried that they might get infected by an unsterilized thermometer. But as I understand it, only people suspected to be infected with coronavirus need to have their temperature checked in person at a clinic; everyone else can just check their temperature at home and report the results in by phone to their local community office. There is really no need for anyone to break out into a state of panic. Just like normal times, during this outbreak there are still a lot of foolish people doing foolish things; but these days it is not just the foolish committing those foolish acts.

I should report what has been happening with me. When I woke up I saw a text from my neighbor; she said that her daughter went out to buy some groceries and brought a few things back for me. They left a bag of items on my doorstep and told me not to forget to bring them inside after I wake up. As soon as I brought the groceries in, I got a call from my niece who wanted to come by to drop off some sausage and fermented bean curd; she said she could just hand it off to me at the front gate. When she came she actually brought a whole pile of things. I took one look and realized that even if I have to spend a whole other month in quarantine, I probably still wouldn't be able to finish all this food. We are all in the same boat amid this calamity, and people have really come together to help each other. For this I express my thanks and from this I feel the warmth of the human spirit.

As soon as I wrapped up today's blog entry [blog entry for February 6 was completed in the early hours of February 7], I heard the news that Dr. Li Wenliang[9] has passed away. He was one of the eight doctors who were penalized for speaking out about the virus early on, and later he himself was infected with the novel coronavirus. Right now everyone in this city is crying for him. And I am heartbroken.

FEBRUARY 7, 2020

During this dark, heavy night, Li Wenliang will be our light.

It has now been 16 days since the quarantine was imposed. Dr. Li Wenliang died overnight and I am broken. As soon as I heard the news I sent out a text to my friends group chat that said: "Tonight the entire city of Wuhan is crying for Li Wenliang. I never imagined that the entire country would also be crying for him. The tears people shed for him are like an unstoppable wave inundating the internet. Tonight Li Wenliang will sail away to another world on a wave of tears."

Today the weather is overcast and gloomy; I wonder if that's heaven's somber way of paying its respects to Dr. Li. Actually, we have already run out of things to say to heaven or any kind of higher power; after all, heaven, too, is helpless. During the afternoon someone here in Wuhan was heard screaming: "The people of Wuhan will take care of Li Wenliang's family!" There are many people who share that sentiment. To commemorate Dr. Li, tonight everyone in Wuhan plans to turn off their lights, then at exactly the time he passed away overnight, we will shine flashlights or cellphone lights into the sky while whistling for him. During this dark, heavy night, Li Wenliang will be our light. This quarantine has been going on so long now, what else can the people of Wuhan do to release the depression, sadness, and anger in their hearts? Perhaps this is all we can do.

At first the disease control specialists said that we might reach a turning point by the Lantern Festival on Day 15 of the Lunar New Year, but now that doesn't seem likely. In the middle of the night came the news of Li Wenliang's death; today came the news that the quarantine has been extended an additional 14 days. Anyone not here in Wuhan has no way of understanding what those of us here in the city are going through. The pain we suffer far exceeds just being trapped at home and being unable to go outside. The people of Wuhan are in desperate need of comfort and an outlet to release our feelings. Perhaps this is why Li Wenliang's death broke the entire city's heart? Perhaps all they needed was an opportunity to let it all go and just cry out? Perhaps it also has to do with the fact that Li Wenliang was just like the rest of us—he was one of us.

The outbreak is currently much worse than what had initially been predicted. The rate with which it is spreading is also much more rapid than what people had expected. And the strange and mysterious way in which the virus is behaving is leaving a lot of experienced doctors at a loss. They have been seeing patients who were clearly improving and then, in the blink of an eye, their condition rapidly deteriorates to the point that their lives are in danger. Then there are patients who have tested positive yet seem 100 percent symptom free. Meanwhile, this virus continues to roam the city like an evil spirit, appearing whenever and wherever it pleases, terrorizing the people of this city.

Those who have been suffering the most are our medical personnel. They were the first to come into contact with infected patients. At Wuhan Central Hospital where Li Wenliang worked, he was not the only casualty. I heard that besides Dr. Li, at least three other doctors also succumbed to the virus. One of my doctor friends told me that an internist from Wuhan Tongji Hospital whom he knew also died. Virtually every hospital has several medical professionals who have fallen ill. They have all sacrificed their own health and, in some cases, their lives to save these patients.

One tiny detail to be thankful for is that most of those medical workers infected were struck down during the early stages of the outbreak. My goodness, didn't they originally say that "it couldn't be transmitted between people"? Well, working under that assumption, how could you expect those doctors early on to wear those biosuits? When they finally figured out that person-to-person transmission was indeed happening, there happened to be a series of high-level government meetings taking place in Wuhan; because of those meetings, there was a strict government order not to publish any negative news. This led to a delay in this news of person-to-person transmission getting out, and many medical workers and their families ended up becoming infected. My doctor friend told me that most of the serious cases are all from that period. However, now that the hospitals all have the proper supplies and preventive measures in place, the rate of infection among doctors and nurses is much lower. Recent infections among medical personal also seem to be mild cases. My friend then went on to another topic; he said: "Later when all those doctors started to get sick, they all knew that this was a 'contagious disease,' but no one dared to speak out because they were being gagged. But just because someone told you not to do something, does that mean you shouldn't speak out? Isn't there a fundamental problem when everyone knows something is wrong but no one dares to speak out? How come the hospital administrators didn't allow their doctors to speak up? If they don't permit us to speak, does that mean that we should just keep silent? As doctors we have a responsibility." He was posing this question directly to himself and his fellow doctors. I really admired him for his willingness to reflect on what was going on.

I realized that this was precisely why we were all so angry about the death of Li Wenliang. After all, he was the first to speak out, even if all he did was warn his own friends, but by doing that he revealed the truth. But after he spoke out, Dr. Li Wenliang was punished, forced to sign a confession, and later he sacrificed his life—no one ever apologized to him before his death. When that is the result of speaking out, moving forward, how can we expect anyone else to speak the truth? People like to say "silence is golden" as a way of showing how deep and profound you are. But what was the cost of silence in this case? Will we again be in a place where we need someone to speak out, but all we hear is silence?

Everything in the city of Wuhan is still quite orderly. But, compared with a few days ago, the optimistic people of Wuhan seem to be a bit more stifled and depressed. Everyone has been locked up in their tiny, cramped apartments for too long. Sure, everyone has the boundless resources of the World Wide Web to explore, but you can only surf the internet for so long before you get bored of that, too. Besides that, everyone is facing their own set of problems in life. Take my two older brothers for instance: They both suffer from diabetes and their doctors want them to get in enough walking each day. My oldest brother used to keep track of his steps on his phone and would often walk more than 10,000 steps a day. My middle brother was even more strict, and he would go on two walks a day, one in the morning and one in the afternoon. But now it has been 16 days since either of them has been able to even leave their apartments. Even me, I have some medication that I'm supposed to take daily. For the last few days I have been just taking one pill every other day because I am running out. Now I only have one pill left for tomorrow. Should I make a trip to the hospital to get more? I hesitate about that.

I just saw a video of a group of Wuhan citizens driving a motorcade of eight cars as final send-off for Dr. Li Wenliang. Those eight cars represent the eight whistleblowers who were disciplined for speaking out. People's eyes are overflowing with tears and many are so choked up that they can barely speak. Not everyone is a tough guy and not everyone is able to remain completely calm and logical all the time. I'm afraid that during the days to come the people of Wuhan will be facing a lot of mental health issues that will require professional support. The witty black humor we all enjoy reading online can only go so far in distracting us, and it certainly cannot solve the devastating problems to come.

FEBRUARY 8, 2020

The war against this plague continues. We are still holding on.

Today marks the Lantern Festival, the fifteenth day of the Lunar New Year. Originally I thought that we would have reached a turning point by now, but it is now obvious that this is not the case. The war against this plague continues. We are still holding on. Even though I am locked down at home, I continue to write and record what I am seeing. Even though each one of my posts ends up getting deleted by the censors shortly after being posted, I continue to write. A lot of my friends have been calling to encourage me to keep going; they all support what I am doing. I also have some friends who are worried that things will get difficult for me, but I think everything will be fine. I even joked with my friends by telling them that even in the old days those underground Communist workers somehow managed to sneak their intelligence reports out from behind enemy lines; now that we are in the age of the internet, how hard can it be to get an essay posted online? Moreover, our enemy this time is a virus. I always stand on the same side as my government, cooperating with all official actions, helping the government in convincing people who are not quite on board with various policies, and aiding the government by consoling all those anxious citizens. The only difference is that I use an alternative method and, occasionally, over the course of writing, I also reveal some of my personal thoughts on various issues; but that is really the only difference.

It should be stated that the overall situation has greatly improved from before. Both the community leaders and people in charge at the cultural unit I work with have been very thorough. Yesterday someone from the local government office called to ask some basic questions like whether or not I had a fever and how many people were here living with me. I patiently answered all their questions. Today Xiao Li from the office at the Hubei Writers Association called to check on how I was doing and whether or not I was sick. One of my colleagues heard that I had run out of medicine and volunteered to refill my prescription for me. But today I received the sad news from my oldest brother that one of the best professors on his campus passed away because of the coronavirus; he was only 53 years old. It is such a shame. The university president, Li Peigen, sent me a text saying that the deceased was a diligent professor who often worked so late that he would just sleep in his office sometimes—a true honest and hardworking "scholar-type." I send my condolences and hope he rests in peace.

The sky is much brighter than yesterday, and in the afternoon I finally mustered up enough courage to make a trip to the hospital. If you suffer from diabetes, it is always best not to interrupt your treatment regimen. The endocrinology department was not open but a doctor there helped me get the medicine I needed from the pharmacy. There were many fewer people in the hospital than normal, and I had never seen the parking lot there so empty. There was a big delivery truck parked outside the entrance to Building 4 that was unloading supplies donated from other provinces. There were a lot of people helping unload the supplies, and I couldn't really distinguish the physicians from the workers. The nurses in the lobby were all lined up waiting for the elevator, and they were all pushing medical carts filled with fruit and snacks, which also looked like donations from other provinces. I suspect that they were bringing these items to the patients upstairs. I didn't see many patients wandering the halls of the hospital; mostly it was just medical professionals who were bustling around. I asked someone about the situation there, and the answer I got was that everyone at the hospital was busy fighting the war on this virus. I suppose that is indeed the only important thing facing us right now.

Outside in the streets everything was just as orderly as always. There were still some cars and pedestrians, but many fewer than normal. I took some time to take everything in and realized that most of the people I saw fell into three categories: The first were food delivery boys; most of them were weaving through the streets on mopeds. The second group were policemen; the majority of them were stationed at various intersections, and there were a few standing at the hospital entrance. It was freezing outside so I can't imagine how hard it must be for them to just stand there all day long. Those cops working the beat really have it tough; they have to face all kinds of different people and carry out their required tasks. I even heard about a patient so sick that she couldn't walk down the stairs at the hospital, so a policeman carried her down on his back. When they got downstairs the patient was already dead and the police officer broke down in tears. The third group of people I noticed were the sanitation workers; they are really something else. Since there aren't too many pedestrians outside, there isn't much garbage in the streets, besides some leaves on the ground, but those sanitation workers still carry out their jobs sweeping the streets with such zest in order to keep the city clean. From the moment the coronavirus outbreak began all the way up until now, I have noticed their consistently calm attitude. They are the group that always gets overlooked as they quietly carry out their jobs, but somehow they are always there to set the heart of this city at ease.

I looked at the most recent report on the spread of the coronavirus and it seems that cases outside Hubei are clearly dropping and things are easing up a bit. But here in Hubei we are still in a critical state. The number of confirmed and suspected cases continues to increase, which is primarily a result of not restricting the movements of contagious individuals early on. Those temporary hospitals are all up and running now, so we should be able to start seeing the results of that soon. By now most people are more bored than scared. And as the conditions in those temporary hospitals improve, the patients are beginning to adapt to things there. Today I saw a comedian talking about the temporary hospitals. He said: "A young guy gets admitted to one of the temporary hospitals and strikes up a friendship with the old man in the adjacent bed. When the old man learns the young guy doesn't have a girlfriend, he tries to play matchmaker. He introduces the guy to a female patient in the same hospital. And the two begin to date." And then the comedian said, "This is what you call 'a temporary love story.'" This was the most heartwarming story I heard today. It is, after all, a holiday today; we all need something to warm our hearts a bit.

Not long ago someone reached out to me to ask if CCTV's Lantern Festival Special should be canceled due to what is happening in Wuhan. But I told them they should go on with the show. Even though Hubei has become the epicenter of an outbreak, other people still have to live their lives. Other people need to try to get on with their normal lives. People still need to celebrate the Lantern Festival; and so many people look forward to the colorful displays they see each year on the CCTV special. The people of Hubei have shouldered this disaster so that the rest of the people in China can go on with their normal lives; seeing people able to go on would actually make those of us in Hubei feel better about our sacrifice, don't you agree? Moreover, those of us in Hubei are all locked down in our homes; we really need a celebration to cheer us up. Earlier today, I really brightened up when a friend of mine told me that the Hubei Network show *I Am a Singer* was about to start.

You see, that's who we the people of Hubei are. That's what the people of Wuhan are made of.

I wonder if this post will also be deleted by the censors.

FEBRUARY 9, 2020

Life is tough, but we always find a way.

According to Chinese custom, today marks the true end of the Lunar New Year. I got out of bed, opened the curtain, and the sunlight was so bright and strong that it felt like it was early summer. It really felt refreshing to just let it shine down on me for a moment, and we really need the sunlight to drive away that dark cloud that has enveloped the entire city and to release the pain that has built up inside our hearts.

I scrolled through my cellphone as I ate breakfast and the news wasn't too bad; there was actually a lot of good news for a change. What I mean by so-called good news are headlines like: "Although the coronavirus situation is still grave, there has been a turn for the better."

Summarizing some of the main points, you could list them as follows: (1) the number of suspected cases outside Hubei Province has dramatically decreased; (2) the numbers of confirmed cases and new suspected cases in Hubei have continued to decrease; (3) the number of new critical cases nationwide (including Hubei) has significantly dropped off. This last item is something that we are all really ecstatic about. As far as I know, almost everyone suffering from mild infections is able to fully recover; most people who have died from the disease had serious infections that were not immediately treated; (4) the number of patients cured has continued to increase; in fact, according to some, it has already surpassed the number of confirmed cases, although I am not sure that is accurate. But no matter what, the fact that so many people have recovered has brought a lot of hope to all those who are currently infected; (5) the American antiviral drug remdesivir has been very effective in treating patients in a clinical setting. Even cases of serious infection have seen improvement with this drug; (6) it is quite likely that we will see a turning point with the virus in about 10 days. This final point is most encouraging for us. This is all the information that I have collected from several of my friends in different fields. As far as I can tell, all of this information is reliable. At the very least, I believe it all to be true. But I regret to report that the death rate has not fallen. Most of the deceased are people who were infected early on but were unable to be hospitalized or get access to effective medical treatment; some of them died before ever even being properly diagnosed. How many people are we talking about here? I'm not quite sure. This morning I heard a recorded phone call between an investigator and a female employee at a mortuary. The woman was clear-minded and quick-witted and spoke with a certain directness; in some ways she reminded me of Li Baoli, the protagonist in my novella *A Thousand Arrows Piercing the Heart*.[10] She said that none of the employees had been able to rest and even she was on the brink of collapse. Through her anger, she called out various government officials by name, cursing them and calling them dogs. She really let out all of her pent-up anger. That's two recordings of people completely losing their tempers that I have heard today.

People from Wuhan tend to be quite straightforward; they value friendship, honor, and brotherhood and think it is important to always do the right thing. They are also always willing to step up and help out their government; after all, there are usually only two or three degrees of separation between your average person and local government officials, so how can we refuse to help them? In the face of a calamity like this, even if you feel like you can't carry on anymore, you have to just dig in and keep moving forward. This is a quality that many Wuhan people have that makes me feel very proud. But even if you keep pushing forward, there are still going to be times when you can no longer hold in that oppressive feeling inside you. During those times other people need to sometimes carry the burden for you, and you have to let others release their anger and frustration. When Wuhan people really go off on somebody, they can be extremely vicious; they won't leave the other person with any dignity, and they certainly won't think twice about pulling the other person's ancestors into the dirt along the way. I'm sure that they are going to be torn to pieces by the curses the people of Wuhan unleash on them. And if your ancestors get dirty along the way, please don't blame the people of Wuhan; just blame yourself for not taking your responsibility to the people seriously.

Over the course of the past few days, the people dying from this virus seem to be getting closer and closer to me. My neighbor's cousin just died. A good friend of mine just lost his younger brother. Another friend lost his parents and wife to coronavirus, before he himself succumbed to the disease. The people don't have enough tears left to mourn all these deaths. It is not like I've never lost a friend before; who hasn't known someone who fell ill, received treatment, but eventually passed away? We all experience that. In times like that, families come together to support their sick relatives, doctors do their best to save their patients, but, in the end, sometimes none of those efforts work. You feel helpless, but we face it and the patient gradually accepts their fate. But this coronavirus outbreak is different: Those people infected early not only die but they face hopelessness. Their cries go unanswered, their attempts for medical intervention are useless, their search for effective treatment proves fruitless. There are simply too many sick people and not enough beds; the hospitals simply cannot keep up with the demand. For those unlucky enough to be denied a bed, what can they do other than just sit by and wait for death? There are so many patients who thought their days would just continue to go on as peacefully as always; they assumed that if they got sick they would just go to the doctor; but they were completely unprepared for the fact that they would be facing death so unexpectedly, not to mention the experience of being denied medical care. The pain and helplessness they faced before death were deeper than any abyss you could ever imagine. Today I even asked my friend, "How could you possibly *not* be sad and depressed after living with these stories every day?" "Not Contagious Between People; It's Controllable and Preventable"— those eight words have transformed Wuhan into a city of blood and tears filled with endless misery.

To my dear internet censors: You had better let the people of Wuhan speak out and express what they want to say! Once they get these things off their chests, they will feel a bit better. We've already been locked down in quarantine for more than 10 days and have seen a lot of terrible things. If you won't even allow us to release some of our pain, if you can't even permit us to complain a little bit or reflect on what is happening, then you must be intent on driving us all mad!

Forget it. Going mad won't solve our problems. If we drop dead, they won't care anyway. Better to simply not talk about these things.

For the next few days, things will go on as they have. We will still fully support our government by hunkering down at home and following this through to the very end. I just hope things turn around soon; I'm waiting for the quarantine to be lifted, but praying even harder for those patients to recover.

As this drags on, the issue of feeding everyone is becoming more pressing. The amazing thing is the number of capable people in various communities who have suddenly appeared to help address this problem. My middle brother told me that his neighborhood established its own group to purchase food and vegetables. Everyone who joins gets a number and then they put in a wholesale order with a vendor. Each family gets one bag of vegetables. The bags are delivered to an open courtyard area in the neighborhood and people pick them up one by one, according to their assigned number; that way no one has to have direct contact with anyone else. If you have an issue with the quality of the food delivered, you just take it home with you anyway, but there is a number you can call to request an exchange. They even devised an entire strategy for purchasing food so that the entire process would be as streamlined and orderly as possible. That way, no one needs to go out to the supermarket and the issue of getting fresh food into people's homes is solved. Today I also learned of a colleague whose neighborhood also set up a similar system for purchasing pork, eggs, and other items. They provide all kinds of options, such as shredded pork, ground meat, lean meat, ribs, etc., with prices and quantity all clearly marked. All you need is to get 20 people on board to form a group and they will deliver; you just need to pick it up. My colleague asked me if I was interested in signing up. How could I not?! After all, we still have at least another two weeks to get through before the quarantine is lifted. I ordered Pork Option C, which was 199 yuan. Life is tough, but we always find a way.

FEBRUARY 10, 2020

We can expect the overall situation to
start improving at any moment.

Another gloomy day, although the sky is still fairly bright. I'm still talking to friends, hoping to get some good news. I saw one video that said, "What do you think the people of Wuhan will do when Zhong Nanshan gives the green light for people to leave their homes?" And then they cut to a montage that featured footage of several flocks of roosters and ducks soaring into the air, shots of several stylish people making a grand exit out of doorways, and people walking around in all kinds of crazy, exaggerated, and arrogant poses. I guess that the people of Wuhan have many talents; besides being able to push through a crisis and being experts when it comes to cursing at people, they also have quite an imagination.

Sixteen Chinese provinces have volunteered to each sponsor one of Hubei's 16 cities. Medical professionals have been lining up to volunteer; they are cutting their hair, some even shaving their heads completely,[11] and saying goodbye to their friends and family to come here to help. The videos of those volunteers are so moving. I'm told that besides the volunteers coming to Hubei, they are also bringing all kinds of medical supplies and protective gear with them. They are even bringing their own supplies of salt, cooking oil, soy sauce, vinegar, and other basic supplies like that so as not to add to the burden of these already-stressed cities. Their selflessness has really brought so many people here in Hubei to tears. More than 20,000 medical workers have volunteered to come to Hubei. You can only imagine the dedication and solidarity behind their sacrifice.

The human losses that Hubei doctors and nurses have suffered have been particularly devastating, which I had heard about some time ago and mentioned in one of my entries a few days ago. Now a massive infusion of backup troops has finally come to the rescue. Thanks to their help, the medical professionals and citizens of Hubei can finally heave a collective sigh of relief. All those local doctors who are no longer able to sustain the exhaustion of this protracted warfare can finally get some rest. Those comedians who have fallen silent these past few days are starting to post their jokes again online.

This dramatic turn of events was dependent on the country's standing up to lend its support. Thanks to the expansion of temporary hospitals, the increase of sickbeds, the arrival of backup medical workers, effective quarantine policies, well-organized administration, and the cooperation and tenacity of the citizens of Wuhan who all worked together, this virus's ability to spread has finally begun to show clear signs that it is waning. All this will probably be much clearer over the course of the next few days. My doctor friend also believes that we are close to a breakthrough. In the end, the reason this quarantine has lasted so long is primarily due to: (1) we lost precious time during the early days of the outbreak, which allowed it to spread; (2) some isolation procedures put in place early on were not effective, which led to further infections; (3) hospital resources have been exhausted and medical workers have fallen ill, which has hampered the ability to provide aid to those who need it.

But now that we are seeing a change for the better on all these fronts, we can expect the overall situation to start improving at any moment.

I saw a message online from a patient at the temporary hospital set up at Hongshan Auditorium. He said that all three members of his family are at the hospital and they should be able to be discharged within the next two days. He also said that there are a lot of other patients there with mild symptoms that will probably also be released soon. They are using a combination of treatments from both Chinese medicine and Western medicine to treat the patients there, and they are taking both traditional Chinese herbs and Western drugs. All their meals have been provided by Sunny Sky, which is a well-known restaurant here in Wuhan. The food there is excellent and this patient said that it was even better than what he usually eats at home; he even gained a lot of weight! His post gave a lot of people encouragement. I keep hearing that there are a lot of patients who are still afraid to be admitted to one of the temporary hospitals; they are all worried about the conditions there and would rather just stay home. But now that they have had time to address a lot of the details at those temporary hospitals, they don't seem so bad, after all. At the very least, people can get the professional medical care that they need there, and it is much better than just staying at home. Those temporary hospitals are large, open structures; you could even hold a dance party in one! Since there are a lot of "old aunties" who love to do community dancing admitted there, of course they are going to take advantage of that open space! The video I saw of those aunties dancing in the hospital really brightened me up to no end; those Wuhan aunties are so amazing, not only in their ability to tenaciously fight this disease, but also in their ability to tenaciously get in their ballroom dancing! Shall we call this the "temporary hospital dance"?

Fearful of being censored, it seems as if I am turning into someone who only reports the good news but ignores the bad. In actuality, these bits of good news are things that I genuinely want to share with my readers. We have been yearning for some good news for so long. Online, there are all kinds of discussions and scary controversies that people are sharing; there are also all these experts trying to analyze everything logically, and then there are all those ridiculous rumors floating around. For those of us here in Wuhan, we really don't want to hear about any of that stuff. All we worry about is ourselves; we worry about whether or not the number of infected patients has declined, whether or not people who need to be admitted can get a bed in the hospital, whether or not they have received effective treatment, whether or not the number of fatalities has decreased, when will the next food delivery come, and when we can finally leave our apartments.

The bad news continues to worry me. This afternoon Professor Lin Zhengbin, an organ transplant specialist from Tongji Hospital, passed away. He was 62 years old, full of energy, and had an incredible wealth of experience in his field; it is such a terrible shame to lose him. Tongji Hospital is connected to Huazhong University of Science and Technology. They have lost two top professors in just three days; everyone on campus is quite heartbroken. I also heard that Central Hospital—that is where Li Wenliang worked in the ophthalmology department—now has two more doctors whose conditions have deteriorated to the point that they both had to have breathing tubes inserted. Even worse, because of lingering anger over the death of Li Wenliang, I heard that some donations have come with stipulations not to give any supplies to Central Hospital because of the way they treated Dr. Li. (I'm not sure of the accuracy of this yet.) Right now Central Hospital is in desperate need of more supplies. My goodness, if Li Wenliang were able to hear this news, he would be more upset than anyone else.

FEBRUARY 11, 2020

> *The arrival of a new life is the best hope that*
> *heaven can give us for the future.*

The weather today is just like yesterday—still gloomy, but not quite as overcast.

This afternoon I saw a photograph of some of the donations coming in from Japan, and the boxes had a couplet from an old classical Chinese poem printed on them: "A mountain may separate us, yet we share the same clouds and rain; The bright moon belongs to both my village and yours."[12] I was so moved to see that. I also saw a clip of Joaquin Phoenix's Oscar acceptance speech where he seemed to be fighting back tears to say how he wanted to use "the opportunity to use our voice for the voiceless," which also really touched me. I also read a line from Victor Hugo today: "It is not so easy to keep silent when the silence is a lie." But this time I wasn't moved; instead I felt a sense of shame.

That's right; I have no choice but to go with shame.

Seeing how many videos there are online of people crying out for help just makes you want to scream; but I can't stand watching them anymore. I know that no matter how rational I may be, I too have my breaking point. And those people who might be somewhat less rational than me are even more prone to losing it. Right now, the single most pressing thing for us to do is to raise up our heads and look toward wherever we might find a glimmer of hope. I hope we can look toward those people who continue to move forward even in the face of danger, like those who built the Huoshenshan and Leishenshan Hospitals. I hope we can look toward those people who continue to do their best even when they themselves are struggling, like those people with so little to their name yet who commit to leaving their life savings to help the poor (I also approve of those appeals *not* to accept their money). I hope we can look toward those people who stand by their post even when they are on the brink of exhaustion, such as those medical professionals who continue working even with the threat that they themselves might get infected. And I look to those people out there day and night in the streets volunteering to help with all kinds of tasks that need to be done. And then there are so many more. . . . Looking at what they do helps me understand that, no matter what, we cannot be scared and we cannot fall apart. If that happens, everything we have fought for will be for nothing. So no matter how many heartbreaking videos you see and no matter how many terrifying rumors you hear, you must not be afraid and you must not break down. The only thing we can do is to protect ourselves and take care of our families. We need to follow instructions and cooperate completely with whatever is asked of us. Just shut the door, grin and bear it. No one will blame you if you want to have a good cry to just let it out or even stop following the news about the outbreak. Watch some TV or put on a movie, watch some of those lousy variety shows, do whatever you have to do to get through this. Perhaps that is our contribution.

Things are gradually starting to take a turn for the better, even though everyone knows it will still take some time, but isn't a slight improvement already a form of hope? Besides Hubei, almost all other provinces in China have begun to see a marked improvement. But now with the help of so many people, Hubei is also headed in the right direction. Just today quite a few patients were discharged from the temporary hospitals. Some of those who have recovered had smiles on their faces as they left the hospital; you could tell they weren't just hamming it up for the media, those were smiles of genuine happiness. It wasn't that long ago that you would often see people smiling like that on the street, but it has now been a long time since I have seen that. But I figure this is just the beginning; perhaps before too long we will see the streets filled with smiling faces again?

Now that I mention it, I have been living here in this city of Wuhan for more than 60 years. This city has been my home ever since my parents brought me here from Nanjing when I was two years old, and I have never left. I went to kindergarten here, elementary school, middle school, high school, university, and even stayed here to work after graduating. I have worked here in this city as a porter (I worked at Baibuting!), a reporter, an editor, and a writer. I lived in Hankou, just north of the river, for more than 30 years and south of the river in Wuchang for another 30 years. I lived in Jiang'an District, I went to school in Hongshan District, I worked in Jianghan District, eventually settled down in Wuchang District, and spent a lot of time writing in Jiangxia District. In the 30-odd years since I graduated from college, I attended countless conferences in a variety of capacities. My neighbors, classmates, colleagues, and fellow writers are spread out deep in every corner of this city. When I'm out I run into people I know all the time. There was a girl writing an online diary who was crying out for someone to save her father; I suddenly realized that I actually know her father, he is a fellow writer. I once met him back in the 1980s at a television station. For the past few days I've been having trouble getting the image of her father out of my head. If it hadn't been for his death, I probably would have never remembered him. I'm always saying that all my memories are deeply rooted in this city, each memory planted by the people I met in this city from my childhood all the way into my old age. I'm a Wuhan native, through and through. Two days ago an internet friend of mine sent me an instant message with a short essay attached. Contained in that document were words that I had completely erased from my mind. One year sometime during the last century, Chen Xiaoqing hosted a documentary series on CCTV called *One Person, One City*;[13] I wrote the script for the episode on Wuhan. I wrote: "Sometimes I ask myself, compared to other cities in the world, why is Wuhan such a difficult place to live? Perhaps it has to do with the terrible weather here? Then what is it that I like about this city? Is it the city's history and culture? Or is it the local sites and customs? Or is it the natural scenery? Actually, it is none of that. The reason I like Wuhan starts with the fact that this is the place I am most familiar with. If you line up all the cities in the world before me, Wuhan is the only place I really know. It is like a crowd of people walking toward you and amid that sea of unfamiliar faces you catch sight of a single face flashing you a smile that you recognize. To me, that face is Wuhan." I remember when that episode first aired, the painter Tang Xiaohe[14] called me to tell me how much he admired those lines I wrote for the show's narration. That's because Mr. Tang and his wife, Mrs. Cheng Li, understood exactly what I was trying to say; the two of them have lived in this city even longer than me; they are true Wuhan natives.

It is only because we have lived in this city for so long and have so many deep connections with the people here that we are so very concerned about this city's fate and feel so deeply sad by the difficulties the city is now facing. You have people here who are carefree and happy-go-lucky, always smiling for no reason; there are people who speak so loudly and quickly that when visitors from out of town hear them, they think there is an argument going on; and those worldly people who know what it means to fight for honor and seem to have a confidence that comes out of nowhere. Once you get to know them, you begin to understand just how warm and sincere they really are, and how much they love to look cool. But today so many of them are suffering, wrestling with the god of death. And here I am—here *we* are—utterly helpless to do anything. At the most, we can go online and gently ask, Is everyone okay? But sometimes I don't even dare to ask—I'm afraid at some point I won't get a response.

Unless you have lived your entire life in Wuhan, I'm afraid it might be difficult for you to understand this or the feeling of pain that we are going through right now. For more than 20 days now, I have been relying on sleeping pills to fall asleep each night. I blame myself for not having enough courage to face everything.

I can't go on about this anymore.

This afternoon I cooked four dishes for myself; it should hold me over for the next three days. For the previous few days, I've just been eating whatever I had left over around the house. I also cooked some extra rice. My 16-year-old dog is out of dog food. He was born on Christmas Eve of 2003; I suppose you could call him my Christmas present. I had just had an operation at the hospital. My daughter was home alone and she had a mix of fear and excitement when she saw our dog give birth right before her eyes. One of the puppies was a cute little white dog that looked like a stuffed animal, so we kept him. Just like that, he has been in my life for a full 16 years now. Just before the Chinese New Year I ordered him some dog food on Taobao, but it never arrived. The seller apologized but told me there was nothing they could do. The day before the quarantine began, I picked up some food at the pet store, but I never imagined it wouldn't be even close to enough. I called the vet at the animal hospital to ask what to do and he told me I could feed the dog rice. So from now on, whenever I cook rice, I need to cook an extra portion for him.

As I was cooking, my colleague called to tell me that her classmate just gave birth to a 4.5 kg fat baby boy by C-section. She told me that the arrival of a new life is such a happy occasion.

That is the best news I heard today. That's right; the arrival of a new life is the best hope that heaven can give us for the future.

FEBRUARY 12, 2020

Shouting political slogans is not going to ease the pain
that the people of Wuhan are going through.

It has been 21 days now since the city went on lockdown. It's almost as if I'm living in a daze. It is hard to believe that we have been quarantined for this long. I'm somewhat amazed that we are somehow still able to do mundane things like share jokes with friends and poke fun at one another over group-chat threads and talk about what we are eating each day. I was even more amazed when I read a thread of messages on my phone and saw a message from a colleague who jogged three kilometers just by running back and forth between her kitchen and bedroom! Now *that* is amazing! Trying to jog around your apartment like that is a completely different level! Compare that to taking a run alongside East Lake in Wuhan. No comparison. I figure I must indeed be getting old; I'm sure I would pass out if I tried to run around my apartment like that.

The sky is really glowing today; the sun even came out for a bit in the afternoon, brightening up this winter day. Yesterday the lockdown order was extended to every district. Now no one can go outside. This order was sent down so that the quarantine can be more strictly enforced. After seeing so many tragedies over the course of what has happened, we all understand why this needs to be done and calmly accept it.

Realizing that every household needs a supply of food, each neighborhood has set up a series of practical measures so that every three to five days, one person from each household is allowed to go outside to purchase groceries and supplies. So from here on out, every few days the people of Wuhan will take turns making supply runs to stock up on food. Today one of my colleagues sent her husband to play the role of the do-gooder Lei Feng[15]—he not only picked up supplies for his household, but also brought back a bag of groceries for me and another for my neighbor Chu Feng. He even delivered the groceries right to my doorstep! I fall into the category of people who are at particularly high risk of contracting the virus, and Chu Feng has a back injury that makes it difficult for him to get around; so we both have a lot of people looking out for us. In the bag was meat, eggs, chicken wings, and some fresh fruit and vegetables. I don't think my kitchen was this stacked even *before* the quarantine! I told my colleague that for someone like me who only eats a small bowl of rice and a simple dish each day, this will be enough to last me for the next three months!

My eldest brother told me that there is only one gate in his neighborhood that they have open and only one person from each household can go out once every three days to purchase supplies. My middle brother said that there is this delivery boy in his neighborhood who runs around every day delivering food to everyone. Every family writes up its own shopping list and hands it off to him, and he takes care of the rest. His family gave the kid a list that included a bunch of vegetables, eggs, some cooking sauce, disinfectant, and instant noodles. Everyone goes down to the main gate of their development for pickups. My middle brother said, "Now we get to stay home for a few more days without having to worry about going out again." He lives just across from Central Hospital, which for the past several days has been the number one most dangerous area in all of Wuhan in terms of the number of infections. He said: "We need to stand firmly together against this, and let's hope that by late February everything will be back to normal!"

That is indeed what most of us are all hoping for.

There are always a lot of kindhearted people who do incredible things during difficult times. The Yunnan writer Zhang Manling[16] sent me a video of the people from Yingjiang prefecture sending nearly a hundred tons of potatoes and rice to be donated to the people of Hubei. Zhang Manling had spent time in Yingjiang as an educated youth during the Cultural Revolution, and that is the place she wrote about in her novel *Sacrificed Youth*.[17] The film adaptation of *Sacrificed Youth* was a movie that everyone of my generation saw. In some ways, it served as a record of our collective coming-of-age story. I have been to Yunnan Province many times over the years, but never to Yingjiang, but now I will always remember that place.

I surfed the web on my phone as I ate lunch but most of the news was more of the same items from the previous few days. Much of it is those fearmongering essays that friends keep forwarding, often the same content, just with different headlines. My phone doesn't even have enough memory to download all these stories, so I find myself deleting a lot of this content, just like the internet censors.

But there isn't really that much that is new. The outbreak seems to be heading in a positive direction, and the virus that was once exploding seems to be showing signs that it is getting tired. Perhaps the turning point will come any day now, even though those infected early on continue to die at an alarming rate. But I have a kind of uneasy feeling inside. Those patients crying out for help may indeed be fewer than before, but there is also a lot of self-ridicule floating around out there among the Wuhan people. This has left me of two minds: On the one hand, things are finally more organized and the entire system is getting on track. As soon as a patient calls out for help, they are getting medical attention. But at the same time, the people of Wuhan are starting to grow more depressed about the overall situation.

Here in Wuhan it is hard to find anyone who isn't experiencing some form of psychological trauma from all this. This is something that I'm afraid none of us can avoid. Whether it be those still-healthy individuals (including children) who have been stuck at home for more than 20 days, those patients who have spent time wandering the city in the cold and rain trying to find a hospital to take them in, those relatives who have been forced to watch their loved ones tied up in a body bag and shipped off to a crematorium, or those medical workers who helplessly watch as patient after patient dies while they remain unable to save them. And there are so many more traumatic stories that will continue to be a psychological burden on people for a very long time to come. Once this plague has passed, I'm afraid that Wuhan will need an army of counselors and psychologists to help the people get through the aftermath. If possible, each district should allocate psychologists to visit each and every resident for treatment. People will need a release, they will need a good cry, they will need a place to scream out their accusations, and they will need to be consoled. Shouting political slogans is not going to ease the pain that the people of Wuhan are going through.

Today I am actually feeling quite bad, and I think I really need to get some things off my chest.

Several cities have already sent aid workers to provide support to all the local Wuhan funeral homes. All those aid workers have been showing up with Chinese flags, taking pictures in front of the funeral homes, and then posting the photos all over the internet. There are quite a large number of these volunteers, and seeing their images flood social media has left me somewhat beside myself. As soon as I see those images pop up, I can feel my hair standing on end; it is so painful to see. Of course I am thankful that they have come to help, but I really want to tell them: Not all situations call for you to get all patriotic and wave your flags. Is it really necessary to intimidate us with all of that?

I think it is a great thing that the government has asked public servants to go and help those requiring the most basic needs and services. But then a friend sent me a video link to a group of these public servants carrying a bunch of Chinese flags as they marched down to serve those disenfranchised people. Usually when we take a photo in front of the Chinese national flag it is because we are visiting some famous scenic site while on vacation; it is not the kind of thing you do when you are rolling up your sleeves to volunteer in a region rampaged by disease and suffering. Once they took their pictures, they then just threw their protective gear into a trash can on the street. My friend asked, "Just what are they doing?!" How would I know? I suppose this is just how they are accustomed to operating. Everything they do starts with a good show to prove just how important they are. If going down to the underprivileged classes and helping them out was part of their daily work routine, would they need to wave those flags around? Just as I was writing the previous sentence, another video just appeared in my friend's feed—it made me even more uncomfortable. One of the temporary hospitals received notice that a certain local political leader was about to visit the hospital, and so several dozen people lined up at the hospital entrance, including officials, medical professionals, and probably even some patients. They were all wearing face masks and went one by one singing to all the patients in their sickbeds, "There Would Be No New China Without the Communist Party!" It is a song that everyone knows, but is there really a need to bust out in full chorus like that for all these suffering patients? Have they even considered the feelings and needs of those patients? Isn't this a contagious disease we are dealing with? Doesn't it affect the lungs, making it difficult to breathe? And here you want them to sing?

Why has the outbreak turned so deadly here in Hubei? Why are those Hubei officials being castigated by everyone online? Why have the measures taken to control the outbreak in Hubei been repeatedly marred with errors? Each and every step along the way has been a series of blunders that have only added to the suffering of the Hubei people. And now, after all this time, do you mean to tell me that there is still not a single person in the government who is willing to reflect on any of this? The turning point we keep hearing about still has yet to arrive and our people are in pain, everyone is still trapped inside their homes, yet here they are so quick to raise up their red flags and sing patriotic songs about how great the nation is?

I also want to ask: When will those public officials go do their work without taking any more commemorative photos? When will our political leaders go on a survey trip to a hospital without expecting people to sing songs of gratitude or put on big performances for them? My people, only when you understand common sense will you be able to truly understand how to take care of practical matters. Otherwise, how can we expect the people's suffering to ever end?

FEBRUARY 13, 2020

> *Perhaps then they will finally understand what*
> *ordinary people are going through.*

I opened the window in the afternoon and noticed that the sun had come out again. I believe that today marks the Seventh Day[18] since the passing of Li Wenliang? The Seventh Day is when those who have embarked on their distant journey return one last time. When Li Wenliang's soul in heaven comes back to this place of old one final time, I wonder what he will see.

After two quiet days with virtually no real news online, last night things suddenly came to life again. In particular, there were three rather miraculous short essays published in the *Yangtze Daily* newspaper that really got under the skin of a lot of readers. It seems like everyone got a new injection of energy after reading those essays. This energy comes from the fact that we are all aching for the opportunity to really let someone have it. Actually unloading all our anger on someone or something would be a productive psychological outlet for most of us. My daughter once asked her 99-year-old grandfather what his secret to a long life was. His response: "Eat a lot of fatty meat, don't exercise, and be sure to curse out anyone who deserves it." And so the third secret to a long life is cursing people. The people of Wuhan are all locked up at home, bored out of their minds with nothing to do—we all need a release. We can't get together to talk because of the risk of infection; we can't open our windows and sing together because we are afraid airborne particles of saliva can still spread the virus; we can't collectively mourn the loss of Dr. Li Wenliang, due to the fear it might impact social stability; the only thing left for us to try is to start unleashing our curses on those people who caused us so much pain. What's more, the Wuhan people have always had a special talent for putting people in their place. Once you have gotten it out of your system, your entire body feels completely refreshed; kind of like the way northerners feel after they have spent time at the bathhouse on a cold winter day. But I have to say that the views portrayed in those three essays were all right on point. So I have to express my thanks to the *Yangtze Daily* for giving all of us who have been pent up for so long a chance to really just unleash our screams! What's more, after the death of Li Wenliang even newspapers as far away as Shanghai put commemorative essays about Dr. Li on the front page; and here you are, your editorial office is just steps away from Dr. Li's hospital, and how much coverage have you devoted to Dr. Li? I suspect that there are a lot of people in Wuhan who are secretly holding a grudge, and I'm sure they will remember this. Of course, at the same time, I know that there are a lot of things we can't criticize, but we can criticize you guys! When I woke up, the first thing I did was go online to see if the internet authorities had posted a notice stating that they had deleted the post. Guess what, there wasn't anything! That means that the *Yangtze Daily* had themselves deleted those essays! Now that really leaves you with something to think about.

Things are still quite tense due to the outbreak, yet online the headlines keep changing, alternating between depressing stories and uplifting ones. The commander-in-chief responsible for spearheading the fight against this outbreak in Wuhan has finally been replaced. Actually, as far as the people are concerned, it really doesn't matter who they send here. It only matters if that person has the ability to control this outbreak, if that person is able to avoid making the mistakes that keep repeatedly being made, if that person can refrain from those meaningless displays, and if that person can avoid repeating that same old empty bullshit over and over again. If they send someone who can do that, it will be enough.

As for those Hubei government officials who have been removed from office, they never lived up to fulfilling their most basic responsibility of protecting this land and keeping the people safe. They allowed this city and the people here to go through such terrible pain; I don't see any way they could have quelled the people's anger, short of firing them. But it is still unclear if they will simply be transferred to another location where they can start all over again. In traditional China, the emperor used to have a policy of "never again employing" government officials who had committed grave mistakes that led to catastrophic consequences for the people and the nation. I think that, at the very least, this approach should be adopted here—those officials would actually be getting off easy. I figure they might finally understand what everyday people are going through if they themselves get stripped of their power and get a taste of what being an average person is like.

One bit of news today left me particularly sad; that was the news of the death of the famous master of traditional Chinese painting Mr. Liu Shouxiang.[19] I had heard that the virus got him, but I still didn't expect things to come to this. I also know Mr. Liu through my next-door neighbor, who is also a painter. Even more heartbreaking was a photo that a doctor friend texted me. Seeing that image suddenly brought back all the sadness that has been surrounding me these past several days. The picture was of a pile of cellphones piled up on the floor of a funeral home; the owners of those phones had already been reduced to ash. No words.

Instead, I had better talk about the outbreak. For nine days straight now, the number of people infected in all regions outside of Hubei has been on the decline. Hubei, on the other hand, continues to go in the opposite direction, and today alone the number of confirmed cases continued to multiply. The expanding numbers are enough to make anyone following the outbreak shudder. The reason for this is clear; this is what the specialists have been referring to as "stockpiled patients." What that means is these are the people who originally could not even get into the hospital system due to overcrowding so they were all simply sent home and told to self-quarantine as "suspected cases." Now the government is doing everything possible to get everyone officially diagnosed into a hospital and trying to make sure that all suspected cases are properly quarantined. Perhaps the numbers we are seeing today will be the peak? I suspect that from here on out, we won't see another influx like this. There are, of course, all kinds of objective reasons that account for the missteps taken early on; however, as far as your average person is concerned, all those objective reasons resulted in real human lives being lost. Shirking responsibility is useless when millions of netizens are keeping a clear tally online. At least those heart-wrenching videos of people wailing out to the heavens for help have disappeared. This time I am confident that the situation is really improving and that it wasn't just another case of internet censors erasing those videos.

But one thing clear is that the government actions taken to control the outbreak are proving to be increasingly effective. Over time, they are also gradually finding methods that are more humanistic. Large numbers of public servants have been sent to help out local communities on a grassroots level. Entities like my work unit of the Hubei Writers Association have a number of people they have sent out. Even Chinese Communist Party members who are skilled professionals are being sent out to help. Each person is assigned to oversee a group of families in order to help the government understand their current health condition and what they might be lacking in their daily lives right now in terms of supplies and other items. One of my friends is the assistant editor at *Yangtze Arts Magazine* and even though she is an MA graduate of a top school, she still makes a lot less than most public servants; yet even she was assigned to oversee a block of six families. Hearing her recall the details of those families and what they have been going through leaves one speechless. These days most families only have one child and there are usually several elderly people at home to care for. One family, for instance, was composed of a middle-aged husband and wife, each of whom had a set of elderly parents they had to care for; in addition to that, the wife also took care of their kids and the husband took care of all the shopping for everyone. Wuhan is a large city; even if you have a car, driving around to deliver food to all these people is itself an exhausting job. During normal times people would all comment on how difficult they had it, but these days they seem lucky as compared to all those families suffering from sickness and death. At least they are all still alive to take care of one another. They all keep saying that they will be able to hang in there and that they believe in what the government is doing.

A never-ending supply of aid provisions continue to flood into Hubei. This evening my middle brother told me that the [US] city of Pittsburgh's donation of 180,000 face masks had just arrived in Wuhan via a China Air shipment. "They are still making arrangements for even more medical supplies to be sent over. Why don't you mention this in your blog today?" Pittsburgh and Wuhan are sister cities; of course I'll mention it, I told him. I actually visited Pittsburgh twice many years ago, and I really liked the atmosphere in that city. But as far as my brother was concerned, he really couldn't care less whether or not we were sister cities; what is important is that his son and grandchildren all live in Pittsburgh. As someone living in the center of this plague zone, he just wanted to find a way to express his appreciation to the city of Pittsburgh.

By the way, there is one item I want to clear up: Several years back, Writers Publishing House published an illustrated book that described animals like the masked palm civet as being "edible." The editor credited was someone named "Fang Fang." A few people have been putting images from that book with the editor's name crossed out online and using that as an opportunity to attack me. I just want to say that the "Fang Fang" responsible for that book is a completely different person and is in no way related to me. Today I even half-jokingly bragged to one of my colleagues, "Wow, I didn't even know I was a book editor! Yet somehow I published this book as lead editor without even knowing it!"

Let me wrap up today's entry with a quote from one of those online memes: "I long not for my trip down to Yangzhou to enjoy the spring scenery in March, I crave only to be able to finally go downstairs by March."

FEBRUARY 14, 2020

The problem is that your so-called humanistic
spirit hasn't allowed you to think about things
from someone else's perspective.

The weather today is rather strange. It was perfectly clear this afternoon and then, in an instant, it suddenly started to rain; queer weather indeed. I just went down to the Hive Box express delivery locker to pick up a package (my daughter figured out a way to order some dog food, since she knew I was all out). As I got there the wind was picking up and before long I started to hear thunder. Now the sky is filled with a mixture of thunder and lightning and this night that started out so quiet is now bursting with all kinds of sounds, which, at the same time, feel so perfectly pure. Yesterday I had heard that a cold front would be coming through; I was told the temperature would drop by at least 10 degrees and it might even snow. I am assuming that the government must have already taken the necessary steps to provide blankets and other provisions for the patients quarantined in those temporary hospitals.

When I looked at WeChat this morning, I immediately saw the news about an entrepreneur friend of mine who was busy leading a group of volunteers distributing donations. For the past few days he has been doing this kind of work nonstop; he also managed to mobilize a group of other entrepreneurs to also make donations. I have never seen him look so haggard as he did in those photos. We actually have a mutual friend, a painter who lives in America, who also donated 100,000 yuan. There was a comment he left that read: "I know that this small amount of money is far from enough; I'm a bit embarrassed by how little it is compared to the challenges we are facing. The group of volunteers that you have been leading have all been working selflessly day and night and they are truly an example for all of us to aspire to. We are all the way on the other side of the ocean, but our hearts are with you and we feel the same pain; but unfortunately, we are unable to be there to help out in person. Please accept this humble donation on behalf of Judy and me as a way to express our thoughts and sympathy for the unprecedented suffering that this ancient city that reared me is currently enduring. We are thinking of those brave warriors and angels in white on the front lines who are selflessly racing against time to save innocent souls from the clutches of this devilish disease. With support, respect and love." This painter is a native of Wuhan who actually grew up in

Hankou; he has been closely following news of the outbreak every day. He is one of us.

The outbreak is still at a crucial juncture, but things are starting to take a turn for the better. The cadres in charge no longer dare to slack off, which means the public is now in much better shape. One of my high school classmates shared a slogan that a lot of people have been saying about government officials: "If you are not going to get to work, might as well find a different line of work!" Basically it means that if you aren't going to be 100 percent committed to battling this outbreak, you'd better just resign now! Just today there were two local officials from the Wuchang District who were fired. One man who is still in quarantine told his childhood neighbor: "It is only these past few days that I finally got to hear from a government official who speaks with a reasonable tone of voice! All those previous officials did was shout back and forth!" His neighbor responded: "I can understand why they are always shouting like that. There are too few of them and they simply can't handle all the people continually seeking them out for help! They are all going crazy! But on the other hand, I am also quite moved just hearing someone speaking to us in a calm and normal tone of voice." In times of crisis, those patients don't really have a lot of requests; they really just want to get a kind answer to their questions. But during the previous couple of days, even that was considered a luxury. I basically grew up in Hankou, but these days I can barely stand to keep in touch with my old friends from there. As soon as I hear from them, the first thing out of their mouths is always a long narrative about how tragic their lives have been. After hearing those stories a few times, it starts to trigger my own anxiety!

I had better change the topic: Because the fight against the outbreak is such an important task, all other patients have been deferring their care. However, as time goes on deferring care for some patients with chronic health issues eventually becomes a death sentence. For many patients on dialysis or those in need of immediate surgery, they are often just a day or two away from being in grave danger. Owing to the overflowing numbers of infections, there are many hospitals that have cleared out their hospital beds to reserve them exclusively for the treatment of coronavirus patients. Most other medical departments have closed down, triggering a flood of patients with other disorders and illnesses to seek treatment elsewhere. Yesterday I saw footage of a cancer patient from Hubei Cancer Hospital recounting her challenges with this issue; she had to fight back tears as she spoke. Watching that, I couldn't help but think that it was as if someone had fastened a tight knot around her neck. . . . I wondered if there would be any way for her to get out of it. Some patients end up just going back home to wait for death. But how can there really be nothing else that can be done for these people?

They say that other hospitals outside of Hubei are not willing to accept novel coronavirus patients due to the high risk of spreading the disease; but what about these other patients with other chronic medical conditions here in Wuhan? If both parties agree, why don't they send ambulances to pick up these patients and provide them with treatment? Perhaps it is a bit complicated and there might be additional costs involved, but these patients are also part of the big picture of what is going on; I'm sure the government can come up with some kind of subsidy to cover the extra costs. After all, we are talking about human lives here. We are talking about saving people, and we need to do whatever is necessary. Even if we have to call on volunteers to help out or put out a call for donations; I'm sure people would step up to help—how could they not? Just yesterday I heard that two members of my kidney dialysis chat room died. Although we still have not reached that elusive turning point, the backup troops have arrived, a new commander-in-chief has assumed the reins, and our battle against this virus is clearly now on a proper path; however, aren't there some finer points to this that can be handled with a bit more finesse and care? There are people out there suffering from all sorts of illnesses and maladies, and they are all people, too.

I also want to point out that this coronavirus outbreak has allowed us to get a clear picture of our society's level in terms of how we humanely deal with a catastrophe. Once this outbreak has finally passed, I'm afraid there will be people making all kinds of appeals about how important it is for the public to improve on their humanistic moral education. But this should have been a fundamental part of our basic education from the get-go. We often see scenes in war movies where medical personnel are treating wounded soldiers on the battlefield, and they never play favorites based on someone's race or where they are from, often providing the same care to both enemy soldiers and their own troops. As long as they are human, they are deserving of salvation. This comes out of the most basic fundamentals of what the humanistic spirit is all about. But now we find ourselves amid an outbreak that is akin to a battlefield, and yet the level of humanism that we have displayed is so low, so low. I'm simply at a loss for words as to how to describe it.

People often have reasons that they use to describe their actions, such as "we were just carrying out written directives." But reality is filled with all kinds of unpredictable changes, whereas written directives are often prepared hastily with only broad guidelines. Moreover, those written directives are mostly composed with common sense in mind, so they are usually not in direct contradiction with the basic principles of humanitarianism. All we need is for the people assigned to enforce these principles to have just a little more humanistic spirit; just enough so that a driver who had been stuck out on the highways for more than 20 days wouldn't end up with his life in danger; just enough so that when someone is infected with coronavirus, a crowd of people doesn't end up sealing their front door with a steel rod so that everyone is locked inside; just enough so that when an adult is forced into mandatory quarantine, their children don't end up starving to death alone at home. That is all I am asking for.

If our humanistic spirit had been broad and embracing enough, we wouldn't have to abandon our sick and weak as we do battle with this terrible virus. If our humanistic spirit had been more fully formed, it would have told us that we must do everything within our power to ensure that these other patients who are also suffering are able to continue receiving the care they need. There has to be a way forward that no one has come up with yet. After all, that's what people do; we find new ways forward. Our social resources are strong, and this is not a weak nation by any means; there must be a way to resolve this issue. The problem is that your so-called humanistic spirit hasn't allowed you to think about things from someone else's perspective. If you did, then you would have taken all this into consideration already. Look how I find myself always complaining about these commonsense issues. Adhering to the principles of humanism is the most basic and fundamental type of common sense. We are part of the human race, after all.

Today I would like to reach out to my childhood friend who was with me from elementary school all the way up through high school and wish her a speedy recovery. I would also like to extend my thoughts to one of my middle school classmates, whose husband is trying to find a place for his kidney dialysis treatment; I hope she takes care of herself during these exhausting days spent running around trying to get treatment for her husband.

FEBRUARY 15, 2020

Wuhan, tonight I care not about the boneheads,
I care only about you.

It is only when you are living amid a time of emergency that all the good and evil of human nature comes to the surface. It is only from that experience that you begin to notice things that you never imagined you would ever see. You are left shocked, saddened, and angry, and eventually you get used to it.

The snow is falling. Last night the wind was howling and there was a thunderstorm and today it began to snow. It is quite rare to see such a heavy snow in Wuhan. I heard that the wind ripped open a part of the roof at Leishenshan Hospital last night, which shows just how fierce the storm was. I hope the patients there who were affected are able to be safely transferred to different rooms; it is yet another small crisis for them amid a much larger calamity.

I'm in a really terrible mood today. Sometime during the early a.m. hours I discovered that there was someone on Weibo who goes by the name "Xiang Ligang[20] from CCTIME.COM" who ran a photo of cellphones for sale at a secondhand market alongside one of my posts that mentioned cellphones discarded next to a crematorium. He then sent out a message claiming that I was the one who uploaded the photo and accused me of spreading online rumors! My diary posts are always pure text and I never upload accompanying photos. One reader posted a comment directed at Mr. Xiang to point this out, but he didn't respond. But there are quite a few of these arrogant and nasty people out there trying to cause trouble for other people. This guy is a big middle-aged man who has a verified user account and over 1.1 million followers on Weibo. I'd like to curse him as a brain-dead idiot, but who would believe me? The fact that he would take advantage of the fact that I am stuck here in this quarantined city, unable to leave my own home, and even my Weibo account has been suspended, preventing me from speaking out—it really speaks to how low this man has gone. He should have saved that image and waited to post it after my account was restored, then we could settle things— that is, if he had any decency. Am I wrong? Instead, all I can do is post my thoughts on WeChat. One of my friends recommended a lawyer to me today, but what is that going to do? When you are living in a city that is so tightly sealed off, you can't even get to the post office to send off a letter to an attorney. Then before I was even able to get the lawyer to notarize my letter of complaint, Mr. Xiang suddenly deleted all his posts. The fact that he deleted everything was a clear sign that he was scared of a lawsuit. Hard to believe that there are people in the world like this!

There are actually quite a lot of people out there like "Xiang Ligang." I've seen plenty of them, but it's best not to heed them. That said, it is really a shame that such a person has over a million followers. What can they learn from someone like him? But as one might expect, his fol- lowers seem to have no basic sense of decency, either; they started curs- ing my online posts and sending me nasty private messages. Several of them were so out of control that you would think that our families had some kind of multigenerational blood feud, when in reality most of them probably never even read a single entry from my online diary. One young man named Xu Haodong, a self-described photographer from Wuhan, sent me a particularly long message filled with profani- ties and even threatened to come to my home and beat me up. What is it that could make him have such deep-seated hatred toward someone whom he never met and has absolutely no understanding of? Perhaps people like this are raised in an environment of hatred and animosity instead of truth and goodness? Or perhaps people like this are simply brainless.

Today the bad news just keeps on coming. A nurse named Liu Fan[21] was still working on the second day of the Lunar New Year [January 26] without wearing a face mask and she ended up getting infected. Later her parents and her younger brother all fell ill. Her parents passed away first, and yesterday she died. Her younger brother was the only one still hanging on. This afternoon my doctor friend told me that her brother just died. Just like that, the virus swallowed up an entire family. I'm devastated, but I also wonder if the virus was the only thing that swallowed them up.

What is making me even more depressed is that my middle school classmate whom I shared a desk with for many years also died yesterday. She was one year younger than me; I always thought she was so elegant and cultured. She had a soft and gentle voice, a great figure, and was quite stunning. We were in the school orchestra together. I played the *yangqin* [a Chinese-style dulcimer], and she played the *pipa* [a plucked lute]. We were the only two girls in the orchestra; we were in the same class and shared a desk. We stayed close all the way through high school. In mid-January, she went to the market twice to buy some things for the Chinese New Year and unfortunately ended up getting infected. It had been extremely difficult for her to finally get admitted to a hospital, but I heard that she was recovering nicely, then her family got the shocking news that she had suddenly passed away. All my old middle school classmates are crying for her today. All those classmates who are usually singing praises to our current "age of prosperity" are today saying things like: "The only thing that will quell the people's anger is the extermination of those evil monsters who caused us this pain!"

I also learned a new term today: "rogue virus." There was a specialist who said that this virus is quite strange and difficult to get a handle on. During the early stages of infection, there are often no symptoms, which has led to a group of "asymptomatic carriers." Once you are infected and recover, it seems as if the virus has been completely eradicated, but it may very well just be hidden away deep in your body. Once you feel as though you can finally get back to your daily routine, it suddenly bursts out. Thinking about it like that, it truly is a "rogue." Actually, the virus isn't the only one behaving like a rogue. Those politicians who act without regard for the lives of everyday people, not caring whether people live or die; those people who accept donated supplies and then resell them online for a profit; those people who intentionally spit in the elevators or wipe their saliva on their neighbor's front door; those people who steal packages of emergency medical supplies that hospitals have ordered before they even arrive; and of course those people who go around spreading all kinds of vicious rumors that harm people. Common sense tells us that as long as people exist, disease will always coexist with us. And the same holds true for our social lives—as long as there are people, there will always be those diseased people (what I mean is those ethically corrupt boneheads) living among us.

During times of stability, our lives are ordinary and routine, and the peace and quiet of the monotonous everyday gradually conceals the great kindness and the horrific evil that humans are capable of. Sometimes people spend their entire lives under the cover of the everyday; but when we find ourselves in a time of unrest, during a war or a terrible tragedy, those acts of great kindness and horrific evil all begin to reveal themselves. You begin to see things you never imagined humans were capable of. That experience allows you to witness things that were once unimaginable. You are left shocked, saddened, and angry, and eventually you get used to it. The cycle goes on like this, again and again. Thankfully, as evil raises its ugly head, the face of good rises up even higher. That is what allows us to witness those who are selfless and fearless, those who are willing to sacrifice themselves for others, those we call heroes. They are those angels in white that we see here today.

But let me say more about what is happening in Wuhan now, since that is what people are most interested in. A doctor friend of mine told me that before February 20, Wuhan must open up a new hospital wing with a thousand beds and have enough supplies for 100,000 patients. This means that the early estimate by specialists that there would be 100,000 people infected in Wuhan wasn't crazy talk, after all. As for those people infected, Wuhan should be able to offer care to all those who need it. Even though there are an incredibly high number of people infected, it still hasn't gotten worse than what some early projections indicated. Based on his clinical experience, my doctor friend believes:

1. The toxicity of the virus has shown a clear abatement as compared with the early cases;
2. After recovery there do not seem to be any lingering side effects, and there does not seem to be evidence of fibrosis in the lungs of those who have recovered;
3. Newly infected patients are all third- or fourth-generation infections and seem to mostly be mild cases that are easily treated;
4. As long as victims with more serious symptoms are able to get through an initial period of acute respiratory distress, most of them are able to be saved.

In the end, however, the number of deaths we are seeing each day doesn't seem to be diminishing, but that seems to be a consequence of early cases that were improperly treated. Once those cases got to a critical stage, it was already too late to save them. As I'm writing, my oldest brother just sent me a text: Professor Duan Zhengcheng[22] of Huazhong University of Science and Technology just died from novel coronavirus. This is a terrible loss for the university.

Besides this, my doctor friend made a special request for me to say: Currently in Wuhan there are only three hospitals in the entire city that are accepting non-novel coronavirus patients: They are Tongji Hospital, Wuhan Union Hospital, and Hubei People's Hospital. All other hospitals in the city are being used in the fight against the coronavirus. In order for patients to be able to conveniently pick up their prescription medications, 10 special pharmacies have opened across the city and patients can pick up their prescriptions with their insurance cards and certificate of diagnosis. Of the three hospitals that are open to non-coronavirus patients, two are in Hankou and one is in Wuchang; that means that, without any functioning public transportation, patients must rely on their local communities to help arrange transit.

The Order No. 2 for a complete lockdown of the city just came down. Whenever things happened in the Provincial Literary and Arts Federation housing complex building where I live, the orders used to come down to us from our work unit, but now the families living here have established their own management team. The team contacts people from the local community government to arrange for us to purchase food and supplies. We each have a number and when we are called we go down to the front gate to pick the items up. It is a new way of life for us, and there is a new management system in place to make sure it runs smoothly. We are all very orderly and take our time, patiently waiting for the next opportunity to go downstairs and pick up some supplies.

All this suddenly makes me think of a line from Haizi's poetry, which I have slightly revised and posted here: "Wuhan, tonight I care not about the boneheads, I care only about you."[23]

FEBRUARY 16, 2020

> *There is no peace when living amid a calamity . . .*
> *and "being-toward-death" is just a luxury of the survivors.*

I can't remember how many days it has been since the quarantine began. The weather today is so beautiful that it may as well be spring. All the snow from yesterday has melted away without a trace. I looked outside the window from the second floor and could even see the leaves outside reflecting the sunlight.

Although I'm in a much calmer state of mind as compared to yesterday, those internet attacks from the capital just keep coming. It is hard to understand what it is that could be driving such hatred. These people must be going through life every day just brimming with bottled-up anger. There are so many people they despise, so many things they hate. They have no regard for what their targets might be going through; they just stubbornly push forward with their campaign of hatred. The funny thing is that I'm the target of their hatred, yet we have never met and I have absolutely no connection to them.

It was just yesterday that "Xiang Ligang from CCTIME.COM" was rushing to delete his slanderous posts, but now he has posted a new essay where he writes: "Where did you get that photograph? You are stuck at home making up stories to incite panic by implying that there are large numbers of people dying from illness and no one is doing anything about it! Do you even have a conscience?" How can I even respond to such a ridiculous question? This guy supposedly works in the communications and media industry, yet he poses such an immature question. We live in an age when unmanned drones can precisely take out human targets from the air, yet somehow I'm unable to access online photographs from my home? I'm not able to understand what is happening right here in my own city? No one else who reads my diary is in a panic, but somehow you are? I'm here in this epidemic-stricken zone, quarantined to my apartment, keeping up with what is happening via the internet and conversations with my friends and colleagues, documenting what I see and hear each day, impatiently waiting for some kind of turning point. And there you are, free as a bird in Beijing, using all your precious time to launch daily attacks at me. And you dare talk about having a conscience? Well, I can tell you that most people who click on my posts tell me that they feel more at ease after reading them.

But there is another Weibo user by the name of "Pansuo" who commented: "Anyway when you see Fang Fang post things online like 'a doctor friend sent me a photo,' 'my classmate passed away,' or 'this or that happened to my neighbor,' she never uses people's full names, all she is doing is trying to spread fear. Reading her recent posts, I feel like she has created more than her fair share of 'anonymous characters,' it is quite a literary achievement!" So there you have it, another bonehead with no common sense. These suffering patients just passed away and their families are still in the grip of suffering; you think these families need to suffer the additional blow of having their loved ones' names all over the media? You think they would want everyone to know how they suffered? I live in Wuhan and was educated here; my classmates and neighbors all live in this city. My writings about this outbreak are completely open; don't you think the people around me would call me out if I was making all of this up? Hasn't "Pansuo" seen the official death toll numbers released by the government? There are more than 1,000 casualties in Wuhan alone. And my diary has only referenced a small fraction of those deaths! Just to make it perfectly clear, I will not be disclosing the names of any deceased individuals unless they have already been reported in official media coverage.

Chang Kai,[24] who was a film director with the Hubei Film Studio, was recently taken from us by the novel coronavirus. His entire family was also wiped out by this disease. Today one of Chang Kai's classmates published a memorial essay that has been flooding the internet. Chang Kai wrote a heartbreaking final testament before he died; reading it is enough to tear you apart. I wonder if those people who insist on only getting their news from CCTV and the *People's Daily* will also believe that Chang Kai's final words were also an attempt to spread panic. Just two days ago I wrote about a painter friend of mine who donated 100,000 yuan to fight this outbreak; well, today I just learned that his brother died from the coronavirus. I wonder if Xiang Ligang and people like him will also say that this was just another rumor.

Speaking of "my doctor friend," I should make it clear that I have more than one. I should also tell Xiang Ligang and his cronies that these doctors are professionals at the very top of their fields; so I am certainly not going to publicly reveal their names. The reason I insist on withholding their names is precisely because dregs like you exist. Our mindless government might buy your one-sided stories, but I will never let my friends become your victims. This afternoon another doctor friend (a leading expert in his field, but, again, I cannot reveal his name) called me. It has been a long time since we were last in touch, and we talked about my *Wuhan Diary*. He said that whenever his friends from outside Hubei Province call to ask him what is going on with the outbreak in Wuhan, he always recommends that they start reading my diary. He tells them that they can find some truth in my writing. Of course, we also talked about the coronavirus. My doctor friend thinks the outbreak should be more or less under control now. The toxicity level seems to be waning, but the level of contagiousness seems to be growing stronger. Among the current group of patients being treated, most of them have mild cases, with a high rate of recovery. The reason we are not seeing a dramatic change in the overall number of deaths is that there are still so many serious cases of infection from the early stages of the outbreak and many of those patients are passing away. These are all things I have written about before; the serious infections are all holdovers from the early stage of the outbreak. So it seems like doctors from different hospitals all have basically the same observations about where things stand right now. There are a few things contributing to the improvement of the overall situation:

1. The toxicity level of the virus seems to be diminishing;
2. Because there has been an influx of medical workers coming to Wuhan to provide support, the medical professionals can work more effectively;
3. There is no longer a shortage of medical supplies, and people are better educated on how to protect themselves;
4. After many days of clinical treatment, doctors now have more experience with what treatments and medications are most effective.

Director Wang from Leishenshan Hospital even told the media: "We have reached a true turning point in the evolution of this outbreak." From the new cases coming in, they have noticed that the number of patients with high fevers has decreased and has continued to steadily go down; moreover, there are not a lot of cases of the fever recurring. Director Wang emphasized that he had great confidence that things were improving.

Isn't this the news we have all been waiting to hear?

Later in the afternoon my doctor friend sent me a video. The video was of a young man delivering a popular science–style lecture about the coronavirus. In the video he kept repeating: "Don't go shooting off your mouth about things you don't understand!" I couldn't agree more.

When it comes to things beyond the scope of your educational background or ability to understand, try to observe and reflect before jumping to conclusions. And one should certainly avoid launching into these unfounded attacks against people; this is especially true for bone-heads like Xiang Ligang. One of them just left a comment criticizing me by asking: "Don't tell me that none of the victims' family members went to the crematorium? No one from the deceased person's family came to collect their personal belongings?" What can one say in re-sponse to comments like that? If they apply their everyday logic of how people behave during normal times to a period of utter calamity, there is no way they will ever understand what is happening here.

Right now Wuhan is in the middle of a calamity. What is a calamity, you ask? A calamity is having to wear a face mask, being quarantined at home, or having to show an official permit to access certain areas. A ca-lamity is when the hospital is going through an entire folder of death cer-tificates in just a few days, which in normal times can last several months. A calamity is when the hearse that brings bodies to the crematorium goes from delivering a single body in a coffin to delivering an entire truckload of bodies stuffed into bags. A calamity is not when you suffer a death in the family, it is when your entire family is wiped out in the course of just a few days or weeks. A calamity is when you drag your sick body out on a cold and rainy day and go from hospital to hospital looking for somewhere that can admit you and offer you a bed, but there are none. A calamity is when you go to the hospital first thing in the morning to see a doctor and don't get seen until the middle of the night the following day—that is, if you don't collapse waiting. A calamity is when you sit at home waiting for the hospital to inform you that they have a bed for you, but by the time that happens you are already dead. A calamity is when a gravely ill patient comes to the ER and if that person later dies, his fam-ily will never see him again or have a chance to say a proper goodbye.

You think that in times like this there are still family members who are accompanying their deceased relatives to the crematorium? You think there is an avenue for relatives to collect their family member's personal items and belongings? You think that the dead are still able to die with dignity? No, I'm afraid not. When you are dead, you are dead. They drag your body away and burn it immediately. During the early period of the outbreak, there was a great shortage of professional healthcare providers, hospital beds, and protective gear for medical workers. All this contributed to the widespread transmission early on. There was also a shortage of undertakers at the crematoriums, a shortage of hearses to transport the bodies, and the crematory ovens were far too few to keep up. Moreover, because the bodies coming in were infected, there was a need to quickly dispose of them. Do you know any of this? It is simply not the case of people not doing their jobs; we are facing a calamity! Everyone is doing the best that they can do, they are all overworked, yet still they don't seem able to meet the standards expected by those scumbags online. There is no peace when living amid a calamity; there is only regret for those patients who succumb to the illness; there is only the feeling of heartbreak when you see what your family is going through; and "being-toward-death" is just a luxury of the survivors.

The chaos from the early phase of the outbreak has passed. From what I have learned, specialists are now drafting a report on how to ensure that victims of novel coronavirus and their families are treated in a more dignified manner. This means creating measures through which the final articles of the deceased, such as their cellphones, will be saved for their family members. The current suggestion is to collect those items together in a secure place and disinfect them once this outbreak has passed. Then the telecommunications company will attempt to use the cellphone numbers to contact family members. At the very least, these phones will serve as an item to commemorate those who died.

If no family members are able to be contacted and the phones can no longer be stored, perhaps they can serve as an exhibit to bear witness to the history that played out here in Wuhan.

The reason I still have faith in this world is owing to those kind-hearted and rational people who are still busy working hard for something good.

FEBRUARY 17, 2020

You aren't the only one suffering and facing difficulties,
there are a lot of ways to live.

Another clear day; if it had been any other time, there would certainly be a lot of people outside sitting in the sun. A shame that no one will be able to enjoy a scene like this for a while. But it is understandable; after all, these are unusual times. I suppose that we should be happy that we can at least enjoy the sunlight and foliage through the window.

The strictest government order on the quarantine has just been issued: Everyone is now required to remain inside their homes at all times. Exceptions will only be made for those who are still required to report to work or carry out official business during the quarantine, but even they will be required to carry a special permit. I heard that if you are caught outside without a permit you will be put in strict quarantine for 14 days, but I'm not sure if that is true. One of those witty online jokesters posted that he thought the people of Wuhan actually had it pretty good. If they had been in Huanggang they would have also been forced to take the Huanggang Secret Edition Second Grade Math Exam while under quarantine, which more than half of the adults couldn't even complete! Those online jokesters have been fairly quiet these past few days; this is one of the better jokes I have seen from them. I hope they can step up their game—after being locked up at home for 20 days now, the people of Wuhan could use some comic relief that they can forward to their friends.

For someone like me, staying at home is a fairly simple task. My dog can just run around in my courtyard, so I don't need to take him out for walks. It is a good thing that he is so old; a few laps around the courtyard and he is ready to come back into the laundry room to take a nap. After I bought him his own little heating pad, he is even more reluctant to ever leave his little dog bed. This year it is really as if I had some second sense or something. Back in mid-January as we were preparing for the Chinese New Year, I suddenly had the impulse to buy a new heating boiler. The heating company came to install it on their last day of work before the New Year holiday. The old heater still worked, but it was getting old and, after using it for so many years, I was afraid it might not be safe to continue using it. The new heater is indeed much more powerful than the old one; you can set it so that the room temperature will stay between 22 and 25 Celsius and I don't have to worry about any safety issues with it. Earlier it warmed up a bit outside and the temperature in my apartment got up to over 25 degrees; I even started to feel hot!

With the strict prohibition of going outside now fully in force, those online grocery delivery groups have really been taking off while all the other traditional e-commerce sites have also been tweaking their sales methods. Had it not been for those e-commerce sites, I really don't know how we would have gotten through these days we have been stuck at home. Without the help of those websites, just feeding a typical family would have been challenging for most households. Now that those community grocery delivery groups have been popping up everywhere, the e-commerce companies are also getting on board. Their sales model allows them to make flexible adjustments based on the on-the-ground situation. They are now offering all kinds of meals available for "contact-free delivery"; residents can register through their grocery shopping group and the e-commerce companies take care of the purchasing and shipping. The manager of the online group can also better organize how the group functions in response to the adjustments made by the e-commerce companies. Compared to those idiotic actions taken by those stubborn old petrified bureaucrats who just stamp forms all day, these capable people from the private sector really put them to shame! This is what it looks like when your working method is informed by practical and realistic goals; the government should really take some notes from them and learn to appreciate this method of getting things done. To speak completely frankly, if it hadn't been for their stubborn old work model, repeated delays at multiple levels, and various mistakes, the outbreak would have never gotten to where it is today. My old classmate Lao Geng knows that I don't want to personally join any of those online grocery groups, so he just forwards me the lists of what they have available for purchase. The day before yesterday I ordered a Kengee Bread Set Meal. It was humongous—there was enough food for three people! It was really too much for just me; I'm afraid I'll be eating this for the next 10 days.

Today I also reached out to one of my doctor friends to get a sense of where things currently stand with the outbreak. Mostly it was just me asking questions and him answering them. I could sum up our conversation with the following points:

1. Regarding the comments about the "turning point" having already arrived, which were made by the Director of Leishenshan Hospital: My friend said that Director Wang's use of the term "turning point" was referring to something else. In medical circles, the term "turn-

ing point" has a different meaning. To put it plainly, it refers to when the number of infected patients reaches a peak. From this perspective, we still have yet to reach this turning point. This means that the number of infected patients is still expected to further climb. But my doctor friend thinks that by late February or early March we should see a true turning point. That means we still have at least two more weeks to go.

2. Regarding the large number of medical professionals who have been infected or even sacrificed their lives, I wanted to know how they have been doing. According to my friend, more than 3,000 medical professionals have been infected. The vast majority of them should be able to make a full recovery, but because this disease takes a long time to run its full course, the majority of them have yet to be released from the hospital. This figure of 3,000 is an official statistic provided by the government, but I suspect that the actual number might be a bit higher. Most of these individuals were infected either early on before doctors and nurses were wearing proper protective gear or later during that period when hospitals were running out of supplies. But right now very few healthcare professionals are getting infected.

3. As to whether hospitals in Wuhan have been using traditional Chinese medicine to treat coronavirus patients: My doctor friend responded that 75 percent of the patients have been treated with traditional Chinese medicine, which has shown clear signs of being effective. When I asked him why that other 25 percent of patients were not treated with Chinese medicine, he said that was because they were all undergoing intubation, so those other treatments were not able to be administered. All those patients being intubated were clearly the more severe cases, which I found to be a pretty terrifying percentage.

4. What percentage of the patients are considered to be critical, and what is the recovery rate for them? My friend said that previously in Wuhan the number of critical cases was around 38 percent; but that is because a lot of these patients were originally just staying at home and only came to the hospitals when things got serious. Now that we have added more sickbeds, patients are now able to come into our hospitals and get treatment in a timelier fashion, which has helped us get the percentage of critical patients down to around 18 percent. The rate of recovery for them is also much higher than it was earlier on. I figure that when you have close to 60,000 confirmed patients, you are still going to be facing some really high numbers. I'm afraid that the death rate will not be coming down anytime soon.

A reader online posed a question to me about why I just record these little details of everyday life and not important things like the People's Liberation Army entering the city, the support that people from all over China have shown to Wuhan, the miraculous construction of the Huoshenshan and Leishenshan Hospitals, and all those heroic and selfless individuals who have been rushing to Hubei to offer aid. How should I go about answering this question? When it comes to recording things, everyone has a different role to play; do you want to hear about this? When we eat we divide our meal up into main courses and appetizers, no? Throughout China there are so many official government news organizations and independent internet news organizations; every day they are all recording those things you asked for. They provide a macro-perspective on the big trends concerning the direction the outbreak is heading, their reports are often filled with heroic narratives and imbued with the hot-blooded passion of youth, etc., etc. There are so many articles out there written in that style that I can barely keep track of them.

I, on the other hand, as an independent writer, only have my own tiny perspective on things. The only things I can pay attention to and experience are those little details that are happening around me and those real people I encounter in my life. And so that's all I can write—I provide a record of those trivial things happening around me; I write about my feelings and reflections in real time as things happen in order to leave a record for myself of this life experience.

Moreover, my profession is that of a writer. In the past when I would share my thoughts on writing fiction, I would always say that novelists are often closely tied to those losers, misanthropes, and loners. We walk together hand in hand and often go out of our way to help each other. Fiction has the ability to express a broader means of embracing the world of human emotions. Sometimes I feel like an old hen assigned to protect those people and things that have been abandoned by history and those lives that have been ignored by society as it advances forward. My job is to spend time with them, give them warmth, and encourage them. Or perhaps my fiction can reveal an atmosphere that shares the same fate as these individuals and I will need their company, warmth, and encouragement. The powerful people of this world, the so-called victors, often don't really care about literature; for them, literature is just a flowery adornment. But for the weak and dispossessed, literature is often a bright light that shines through one's life, it is a wreath of straw you can cling to for support while floating down the river, it is that savior you can turn to when you are reaching the end. That is because, in times like that, it is only literature that can tell you that it's okay if you are behind, there are a lot of other people just like you. You're not the only one who is lonely, you are not the only one who is alone. You are not the only one suffering or in pain, you are not the only one feeling anxious and weak. There are a lot of ways to live. Of course it is great to be successful, but not succeeding isn't always a bad thing.

Look at me—a novelist documenting all these trivial daily occurrences here in this diary, and yet I somehow follow the direction of my literature to observe, to reflect, to experience, and, ultimately, to set my pen down to paper and write. Don't tell me this is a mistake?

Yesterday's post on WeChat was deleted again. Besides helplessness there is only helplessness. *Where can I share this record of my life in this besieged city? Mooring on the misty bank the messenger is filled with sorrow.* To observe, to reflect, to experience, and, ultimately, to set my pen down to paper and write. Don't tell me this is a mistake?

FEBRUARY 18, 2020

Amid the outbreak the people weep . . .
why do we need to push one another?

Today the weather remains clear and beautiful; it is enough to make one feel as if there are new possibilities for life everywhere. The clouds today have a lot of character. I was even discussing the clouds with my neighbor who lives next to my place out in the suburbs; I wondered what kind of weather could form clouds like that. They looked like what you call "fish scale clouds," but my neighbor said that's not what they were. Last year I spent almost the whole year out there in the suburbs writing; I only returned to my apartment at the Literary and Arts Federation building in Wuchang just before the Lunar New Year last year. My neighbor told me that they still didn't have a single case of infection out there in the suburbs. Oh my, I wonder when I'll be able to go back there. The flowers outside my front door and in the courtyard are probably all dead by now. That said, I never had much of a green thumb; almost every flower that ends up in my hands usually ends up facing a rather tragic fate. Either they grow for a while and then wither away or they simply stop blooming.

It has been almost a month since the quarantine began. When I first saw the lockdown order I had absolutely no idea that it would last this long. It is obvious that these severe quarantine restrictions that have been put in place have helped Wuhan emerge from its darkest days. By now people seem to have finally begun to grow accustomed to this new form of sheltered life. Even those spirited little kids bursting with energy have somehow managed to put up with this. Life's ability to adapt and tolerate changes is really something.

Those frantic pleas from those people desperate to get treatment have completely disappeared from the internet. Nowadays all the discussion you see online is information about how to order vegetables and groceries. Now that people are spending all their time paying attention to life matters, our days are looking more and more like the weather today, filled with new possibilities for life. All the large supermarkets have begun to roll out meal plan delivery services; each delivery carefully denotes the name of the district and drop-off site as well as the name and cellphone number of the contact person. This has made things endlessly more convenient for the manager of each grocery delivery group. I heard that the delivery group started by the Literary and Arts Federation has been a big hit; quite a few people from the nearby neighborhoods have also joined. The only issue is that there are tightly enforced restrictions when it comes to going from one neighborhood to another; I'm not sure how those people from nearby neighborhoods are able to pick up their deliveries. Just as I was wondering about this, I suddenly discovered that some of my colleagues had ordered groceries online and they were hoisting them up with a rope! The fact that they came up with this is quite amazing, but I suspect that there are a lot of other people doing similar things.

The order that my old classmate Lao Geng (his wife manages the grocery group and he helps her run it) put in for me arrived and, besides the different types of bread that it said it would include, it also included some fresh green vegetables. There is not much pleasure in cooking when you are home alone, so I usually just take the easy route and cook a bowl of noodles or boil some shredded potatoes. But the range of dishes waiting for us when this all ends is actually quite something. Today Pan Xiangli[25] sent me a WeChat message; she tried to console me by promising that she would treat me to a proper Shanghainese feast next time I was in town. "We'll pig out for three meals straight!" she promised. Okay then, it's a date! Others who have written to try to cheer me up have also repeatedly brought up the topic of food. Wuhan people love discussing which restaurant makes the best food in town, and that is even more the case now than ever. I'm not a member of too many WeChat groups, but the largest one I am a member of is a group made up of my former college classmates. For the past month or so the discussion has been dominated by talk of the coronavirus. While most of the members of the group are from Hubei, there are also quite a few members who are from Hunan. Normally there are a lot of jokes within the group that attempt to mimic the accent of those Hunanese classmates by referring to them as "Fulanese," which is how they sound when they say "Hunanese" in their local dialect. First thing this morning one of my classmates clicked "like" on a post about the "Fulanese"; it said that there were no new cases of infection reported in the Huagang region where the Fulanese have been providing medical support. I didn't carefully review all the data, but I had heard that the Fulanese had sent a lot of aid to Huagang some time ago. The recovery rate in Huagang is also the highest in all of Hubei Province, and the recovery rate in "Fulan" is the highest nationwide. Although my daughter was born in Wuhan, her residence card still lists her official hometown as being "Fulan." The relationship between Hubei and Hunan has always been particularly close. I'm reporting these comments about Hunan here but, in all fairness, places all over China have really been doing their best to help out with the situation in Wuhan. Those backup forces have allowed Hubei, which has been under siege, to finally heave a sigh of relief. The fact that things are now really starting to improve has a lot to do with the support and contributions we are receiving from other provinces.

Today one of my doctor friends called and we spoke for a very long time; he probably had a lot of bottled-up things he needed to get off his chest. He talked about how difficult it was for medical professionals early on when the outbreak first began. He talked about the incredible amount of energy that goes into saving even a single patient. After engaging in lifesaving intervention with a seriously ill patient, the biosuits worn by doctors and nurses will be covered with dangerous germs and need to be taken off immediately. But early on during the outbreak, when they were short of staff and supplies, they had no choice but to watch helplessly as patients died right before their eyes, yet there was nothing they could do. People dying in hospitals is a common thing, but seeing a patient who is clearly capable of being saved and yet you are unable to do anything because you are so utterly exhausted so you simply no longer have the strength to save another person or because you have run out of all the necessary medical supplies—now, that is something different. "You'll never be able to understand what that feels like," he said. "Doctors usually stay focused on their own area of specialization, but this time we all just put everything out there and worked together to save these people." I completely get what he was trying to express to me. During this outbreak we all saw images of doctors sacrificing everything to save these patients. Some of them even went online to scream about how terrible the situation was. It was those cries that finally exposed a lot of the problems and started to allow for donated medical supplies to start getting funneled directly into the hospitals that needed them most. A lot of peoples' lives were saved by those doctors' public cries for help—it was only because they spoke out that some of those patients were able to survive. My friend said that the temporary hospitals were constructed very well. If they had been built even sooner and more patients had been quickly quarantined, they would have been able to reduce the number of mild cases that later turned critical; that would have also saved a lot of lives. I suppose that a professional like him must know what he is talking about. It was precisely the quarantine policy that was able to put a halt to the rapid spread of the disease that we had been seeing. But now the people of Wuhan are much calmer than before. We are all starting to shop for food and get back to our lives a bit, but still we patiently await a true turning point.

A few days ago I wrote about a nurse named Liu Fan and her family who died from the coronavirus. (My apologies, I initially wrote her name with the wrong Chinese character. When the news was first breaking there was some confusion about her name and I went with the version provided by a doctor I know.) Well, it now seems that someone else online is claiming that story was nothing more than a "fabricated rumor"! What can I say? Sometimes those people who appear to be the defenders of truth online turn out to be the greatest fabricators of them all! Chang Kai, the film director from the Hubei Film Studio who died, was actually Liu Fan's little brother. I believe this already has been reported in the media. Chang Kai's last will and testament is an extremely reserved document. But I guarantee you that there is no one out there who can read it without feeling his deep pain. My doctor friend told me that the two siblings each assumed the surname of one of their parents—that's why one had the last name Liu and the other Chang. Their parents both worked in the medical field. Members of each of their families also seem to have been infected by the coronavirus, but so far they all seem to be doing okay. The people of Wuhan will never forget the tragedy that befell this family. I wonder after writing all this whether or not those people who are always attacking me online will start accusing *me* of spreading rumors? Actually, these people who have been attacking me are the same group of people who criticized my novel *A Soft Burial*[26] a few years ago. I wonder if they will seek out some high-ranking officials to provide them with protection like they did a few years back. Whether they do or not, I'll first make it clear right here: If they come after me I'll be here to fight back, just like I did before. I'll also make sure that their names are dragged through the mud, just like that earlier group who came after me.

Today there is something I want to get off my chest that has been weighing on me for a long time: Those ultra-leftists[27] in China are responsible for causing irreparable harm to the nation and the people. All they want to do is return to the good old days of the Cultural Revolution and reverse all the Reform Era policies. Anyone with an opinion that differs from their own is regarded as their enemy. They behave like a pack of thugs, attacking anyone who fails to cooperate with them, launching wave after wave of attacks. They spray the world with their violent, hate-filled language and often resort to even more despicable tactics, so base that it almost defies understanding. But what I really just don't understand is: How is it that they are able to publish these ridiculous things online and repeatedly turn the truth upside down, yet their posts somehow never get censored or deleted and no one ever stops their flagrant actions? Maybe they have relatives working in the internet censorship office?

These past few days I have been utterly exhausted and have a bad headache. An online reader left a message on one of my WeChat posts yesterday, saying that s/he could sense my exhaustion from my writing. His/her intuition is really spot-on. I need to start reducing the amount of time I spend writing and take more time to get adequate rest. I'll stop here for today.

But in closing, I wanted to respond to Huanggang XYM's post by saying: Here in this quarantined city the people are anxious, amid the outbreak the people weep. We are all facing similar difficulties, why do we need to push one another?

FEBRUARY 19, 2020

The specter of death continues to haunt the city of Wuhan.

It isn't as sunny as yesterday, but the sky is still quite bright. It started to turn a bit overcast by the afternoon, but it isn't too cold. According to the weather forecast, the next few days will be relatively warm.

Before I even got out of bed I received a phone call from my painter friend in New York who just donated 100,000 yuan a few days ago (I certainly hope no one accuses him of "colluding with the enemy" since he is living in the US!). He told me that another Chinese painter living in Germany with the surname of Su also committed to donating 100,000! He told me that this painter from Germany said that he knows me and had actually visited my apartment once! "These past few days he has been reading your *Wuhan Diary*, and his wife decided that they should do something for the people of Wuhan," he told me. Since they have faith in my friend's philanthropic plans, they decided to toss money his way. My friend had been quite anxious about raising enough money for a shipment of medical supplies that was about to arrive and was ecstatic when he heard this news. This Su family also originally hails from Wuhan and they have been extremely concerned about the situation here. For a lot of people originally from Wuhan, no matter how far they wander and no matter how long they have been away, Wuhan will always be their spiritual home. Special thanks to Mr. and Mrs. Su.

I mentioned I had a headache yesterday, so today one of my colleagues had her husband bring me over a bottle of essential balm. Her husband's job requires him to be out and about every day to help out around the city. When he got home last night, he dropped off the essential balm and some other traditional Chinese herbal medicine. When I went down to the main gate of the Literary and Arts Federation building, I was surprised to see quite a few people out. I haven't seen that many people out in public since the Lunar New Year.

I asked what was going on and learned that the orders for the grocery delivery group had just arrived. These people were all volunteers helping to unload everything. At first I thought that all the volunteers worked at the Federation, but I was surprised to learn from my neighbor that even her daughter was volunteering. Her daughter had studied in France and since coming back had opened up her own company here in Wuhan. She has been stuck at home like everyone else and thought it would be a good idea to volunteer to help out. According to the United Nations, the definition of a volunteer is: "Anyone who willingly participates in public serve beneficial to society without receiving any form of incentive or benefit, monetary or otherwise. Sometimes referred to as charity workers." These volunteer organizations are really incredible and it is great to see so many good-hearted young people supporting them. Through this volunteer work not only can they contribute their own abilities, but it is also a great way for them to observe society, understand something about life, and nurture their own abilities and knowledge. During the outbreak in Wuhan, there have been tens of thousands of volunteers contributing to all aspects of society. If not for them, we would have only had the mechanical government offices to rely on and I am sure that things would have been much worse.

Besides all those people delivering food, there were also several large bundles of celery piled up near the front gate. Standing beside the celery piles was a man who looked like a community worker. As I passed by, he said: "Please feel free to take some celery home." I told him that I already had enough vegetables back at my apartment so I didn't need any. He replied by insisting, "We got tons here, please take as much as you like! All this is designated for residents of the Literary and Arts Federation complex." I gave in and took a few sticks of celery, which was more than enough. Mr. Wang the security guard immediately rushed over and helped me grab a bunch more, saying, "There's plenty! It all came in from Shandong!" I was a bit confused and asked the worker standing there; he explained that all this celery was donated from Shandong Province. Two tons of celery was allocated to our district, which is actually way too much. We gave some to various government offices and took some for ourselves and distributed it to various families. The worker explained, "They aren't the freshest, but the heart portion of the celery is still quite good."

Seeing that pile of celery made me think back to that first shipment of vegetables that Shouguang city in Shandong Province donated to Wuhan. Somehow, some government department ended up having the vegetables delivered to supermarkets to be sold! That elicited a public outcry. Someone even circulated a telephone recording of some of the accusations made against the city government online. Actually, if you ask me, I think unless those vegetables were specifically earmarked to be donated directly to hospital cafeterias or to an organization with storage facilities, probably the most effective thing would indeed be to distribute the food to supermarkets where it could be sold at a discount price to citizens. At the very least, those supermarkets have storage facilities and delivery options; there are channels through which they can distribute the food to the people. Perhaps they could then donate whatever proceeds they generate to nonprofit charity groups in the name of the original donor. Or they could even refund the money and continue selling the vegetables at that discounted price for the local Wuhan market. That would be one way for everyone to benefit. At least the outcome would be better than just delivering the food directly to local communities like this. Ever since the coronavirus outbreak began, community workers have faced a particularly difficult situation; to request them to divide up donations and distribute them to all the different communities is a very challenging task. So I figure even though these items were donated, the whole process could still be handled in a much more practical way. If those donated items should go to waste, it would also be a waste of the donors' kindness and goodwill, not to mention their money.

I saw a video on my phone today of people crying as Dr. Liu Zhiming's[28] funeral car drove away; Dr. Liu had been the Director of Wuchang Hospital. There wasn't a dry eye among the people lined up to see him off one last time. He was an honest and talented professional who had established a solid platform to do good work for the medical community. Who knows how many people he saved over the course of his career? But these days the bad news just keeps on coming. Wuhan University just lost one of its PhDs to the virus, Huazhong University of Science and Technology just lost a professor. . . . The specter of death continues to haunt the city of Wuhan.

Currently the confirmed cases of novel coronavirus in Hubei Province have already exceeded 70,000 people. This isn't far off from my doctor friend's early estimate. Each day there are roughly 1,500 new confirmed cases. The numbers seem huge but in reality the rate of increase is continuing to slow down. The number that still hasn't begun to decrease is the number of deaths, which is currently just over 2,000, according to the official government statistics. There are also some people who died who were never confirmed to have contracted coronavirus and others who passed away at home before ever making it to a hospital; I suspect none of them are included in those numbers. So I'm afraid that we still don't have a completely accurate tally of just how many victims there really are. Once this outbreak has passed, various government departments will have to work together in order to come to a more accurate number of just how many people died during this tragedy.

The overall situation continues to be quite serious. Currently there are still nearly 10,000 critical patients being treated at Huoshenshan Hospital, Leishenshan Hospital, and other facilities around the city, many of whom are still undergoing lifesaving procedures. These are all patients who were infected during the early stages of the outbreak. Many of them did not receive immediate care, and these delays led to the worsening of their condition. How many of them will end up losing the battle? This weighs heavily on us, as it certainly does their families.

When we talk about a turning point, it is always framed by the grave situation we faced early on. At that time, you would turn on your phone and all you saw were videos of patients begging for help; all the hospitals were inundated with sick people trying to get treatment. At least now all patients are able to be received at the hospitals; even if a patient refuses treatment, the hospitals force them to be admitted. Once admitted everyone is guaranteed medical treatment. My doctor friend told me that most of these new patients only have mild symptoms and most should be able to fully recover. The turning point is within sight.

I also saw some news that said that Wuhan was going to switch over to a new system. They were gearing up to establish four groups: a group that will ensure that patients all have access to hospital beds; an outbreak control group; a group responsible for coordinating things for medical volunteers arriving in Wuhan; and a CCP assessment group. These four groups will oversee these various tasks and, while overall they seem to have been designed with practicality in mind, I do feel that it would have been better to have a "division of supervision and assessment" rather than a "CCP assessment group." That would have been a sign from the government that the people's lives are what is most important, and not the responsibilities of the Chinese Communist Party. After all, this war against the coronavirus affects everyone in society; there are many nonparty members who are on the front lines fighting and they shouldn't be seen as outsiders.

By the way, those ultra-leftists attacking me seem to be gaining in numbers. It has really become a case of "one's abilities falling short of one's reputation." I'm the kind of person who likes to talk about common sense, something I have mentioned quite a few times these past few days. Someone asked me what I mean by "common sense," well, let me give you an example. If a dog runs over to bite you, you should pick up a stick to hit him. But then what do you do when that dog runs home and comes back with a large pack that includes some big scary dogs and even some rabid ones? Common sense will tell you to run the hell away! Just let those dogs have their turf back. Let them bark like mad for a while and before long they will eventually start to snap at each other, fighting over who has the loudest bark or who has the biggest bone. By then you will be back at home enjoying a book over a hot cup of tea. Just like you quarantine yourself during an outbreak, you need to quarantine yourself from those rabid dogs. This is what you call common sense.

FEBRUARY 20, 2020

> *We have actually held out for a long time already;*
> *we can't allow those people who have been fighting for us*
> *to have fought in vain and, for those of us who have been*
> *patiently holding on, we can't just throw all that away.*

It is another clear day; the sky is crystal clear and I can imagine what that warm sun looks like shining down on those empty streets, a deserted Zhongshan park, Liberation Park, and East Lake Garden Lane; such a shame there is no one outside to enjoy any of that.

I really miss those days when I used to be able to go for bike rides down East Lake Garden Lane with my colleagues. I used to go there almost every week. We would ride out toward the more deserted side of Luoyan Island, riding up the hill and over the bridge; the entire trip would take about three hours. On the way, we would usually find a quiet place beside the lake to sit down and chat before stopping at one of those off-the-beaten-path vendors on the way home to pick some farm-fresh vegetables. I don't think we would qualify as "brave and fearless revolutionary warriors" by any stretch of the imagination; in fact we normally try to fully enjoy the lives we have built for ourselves. But now I discover that my two primary biking partners (they are both colleagues as well) are both dealing with serious illnesses: One of them is sick herself and the other one has a family member who has fallen ill. Neither case seems to be the coronavirus, but they are both the kind of serious illnesses that make people give an awkward look when you mention it. They have it much more difficult than I do. But how many other people here in Wuhan suffering from all kinds of illnesses are left with no choice but to simply wait things out? They are still waiting.

Today's news about the coronavirus triggered a lot of discussion among my classmates. Everyone was quite shocked by how dramatically the number of new cases has fallen. What is going on? Did we today suddenly arrive at the turning point we have been hoping for? First thing this morning one of my doctor friends sent me a text; he was ecstatic: "We've got it under control! It's a miracle!" He went on: "We don't need to worry about adding any new sickbeds; we just need to focus on taking care of the patients we already have." But not long after that he sent another text that seemed to reveal a more cautious tone: "Perhaps it's too soon? But it really is amazing! I just have trouble believing it." But an hour later his tone had completely changed: "I took a closer look at the figures and realized that the dramatic drop has to do with the fact that Wuhan has tweaked their standards for evaluation again. . . . We'll have to wait and see what tomorrow's numbers reveal."

When I saw his messages in the afternoon I couldn't help but ask a few more questions about the situation. My doctor friend clarified: "Based on the figures released today, we cannot make any clear-cut conclusions that there have been any fundamental changes in the spread of the disease. Just like the sudden leap we saw a few days ago, today's sudden drop should be looked at in a similar fashion. But the overall trend does seem to indicate some improvement." When I asked him again about the time frame for a true breakthrough, he confidently responded: "We should see that coming within the next week."

One more week before we see a turning point? I certainly hope so, but I'm also hoping that we don't end up disappointed again.

At the same time, I also saw a post online from a specialist who said that even though things might be improving a bit, we need to continue being vigilant and keep our guard up. It has been nearly a month since the quarantine began, and most people I know can barely take it anymore. I've heard several people say that they are on the verge of just bust-ing out of their homes. They all think that as long as they wear proper protective gear, they will be able to protect themselves from being infected. But in reality they might end up getting infected and not even realize it. They could go home and then infect their entire family and by then it will be too late for regrets. If everyone decided to rush out into the streets there would certainly be interpersonal contact and transmission that takes place. If that happens, all our patience and hard work will have been in vain. The single most devious trick the novel coronavirus has up its sleeve is its incredibly high rate of contagiousness. Now that its power is on the decline, what it most craves is for more people to start venturing outside, which would give it the opportunity to regain its strength. Do you really want to help facilitate its rebirth? We have actually held out for a long time already; we can't allow those people who have been fighting for us to have fought in vain and, for those of us who have been patiently holding on, we can't just throw all that away.

Today in my neighbors group chat I saw an essay posted entitled "I Give My Thanks, And I Pray" by Mr. Xiang Xinran,[29] the architect who came up with the plans to rebuild Yellow Crane Tower. The essay was his attempt to express thanks to those classmates of his who have been expressing their concern during the current outbreak. The essay was dated today. Mr. Xiang is nearly 80 years old; he is actually a close friend of my neighbor Tang Xiaohe. I have met him a few times over the years but we were never close. But today when I read this venerable old man's essay I was truly moved and quite sad. With his permission, I would like to share his entire essay with you:

My name is Xiang Xinran and I am currently reading yesterday's edition of my local community publication *Coronavirus Report*. "In accordance with the blanket recommendations issued by the municipal government, the district has already identified 15 individuals who

fall into the four categories of: confirmed coronavirus patients, suspected coronavirus patients, patients with a fever, and those in close
contact with confirmed patients. We have provided these individuals
with treatment as needed and they have all now been removed from
our residence community."

According to the municipal zoning, the district in which I live
is considered to be at highest risk for novel coronavirus infections.
There have already been six local residents who have already passed
away after contracting the coronavirus. Most of them were not admitted to the hospital before they died. Although there is a hospital
designated as a coronavirus treatment center just next to our community, it is extremely difficult to get a bed there. Patients who have
already tested positive for coronavirus line up outside the hospital all
night just hoping to get in. The line of patients stretches all the way to
the entrance of my neighborhood. (Our complex quickly sealed our
back gate to keep the patients from coming in.) This is what Wuhan
was like during the early stages of the outbreak.

Because our community is mostly made up of people formerly
affiliated with the old Design School, everyone knows each other
here; we are all former coworkers and longtime neighbors, so seeing
so many of our friends suddenly taken away is just too difficult to face
and has left us in a state of fear. As this dark cloud descends on our
city, elderly residents living by themselves like my wife and me are left
completely helpless!!

It was at that moment that I received a message over WeChat
from an old classmate: "Since we know you are in Wuhan, we are
even more concerned about the fight against the coronavirus that is
currently raging there and we want to express our support!" That's
right. I graduated in 1963 and was assigned to Wuhan to work at
Southcentral Architecture and Design Institute. There were three of

us from my graduating class who got sent to Wuhan, and I was the only one who stayed here all these years.

Gradually other classmates also started to send their thoughts and prayers for me online. Even more of them just picked up the phone to express their concern and lend an encouraging voice. One of my old classmates who now lives in the United States started chatting with me online. . . . All these friends have been treating me more like family than a friend in the way that they have been expressing their concern; this has provided my wife and me with warmth and strength. I will always be forever thankful for these expressions of concern.

I was especially moved by one classmate who passed on a message from one of our teachers; he told me to: "take care of yourself, drink plenty of water, and be sure to have some smoked Asian wormwood. . . ."

I'm actually not at all afraid of death. I have, after all, already made it past the average life span in China; it is only a matter of time before death comes, which is natural. However, if I die from this virus, that would, without question, be considered a form of "murder." I'm not going to stand for that!

It has already been more than a month since I have gone downstairs and left my building. I often stand on my fifth-floor balcony staring blankly at the dead-silent world that surrounds me below.

I used to see a lot of posts suggesting that elderly people shouldn't worry too much; they should just try to eat well and enjoy themselves. There is some logic to that because even if we do worry there isn't much we can do to change things! After all, at this stage in life, what are we capable of doing that might actually affect the world? But then again there is that old saying: *If by morning you have grasped the moral path, even if death should come that very evening you shall have no regret!* And so I have no choice but to worry about what is happening and to express my concern.

During these days as the disease runs rampant through our society and we remain cloistered inside our homes, I keep wondering why the Chinese people have been destined to face such a cruel fate! Why have our people continued to face calamity after calamity? When I think of all this, I feel like the only thing left to do is pray. And so I pray that after this calamity has passed, China will face a world of peace and prosperity . . . at least, that is my hope.

Each word, every sentence, is backed up with genuine feelings. When he writes "if I die from this virus, that would, without question, be considered a form of 'murder.' I'm not going to stand for that!" I wonder how many people in Wuhan share those thoughts?

There are a lot of old-timers living alone here in Wuhan just like Mr. Xiang. During normal times there would often be caregivers or hourly helpers who would be around to help people like Mr. Xiang, but since the outbreak occurred during the Chinese New Year, most of those workers all went back to their homes in the countryside, leaving the elderly alone to fend for themselves. For a while I was worried that Chancellor Liu Daoyu[30] might also be alone at home without any help, because he normally has a helper who probably also went home for the New Year. I sent him a text over WeChat and was relieved to learn that his son and daughter-in-law had come home for the holidays and now they were all stuck at home together. My old classmate Lao Dao's parents are both 96 years old and they are also quarantined where they live; their daughter isn't even allowed to go there to help them out. At least they are both in good health and able to take care of themselves. They not only try not to be a burden on society, but they also do their best not to let their daughter unnecessarily worry; like so many other residents of this city, they too are trying to be optimistic and wait out this terrible outbreak.

To think about it from another angle: I'm afraid that many of these elderly residents need to expend a huge amount of energy just to take care of everyday things and live a normal life. Many of these older residents need to summon up all their strength just to carry out basic tasks. We all know that just taking care of everyday household chores like cooking, cleaning, washing clothes, and straightening up is a big job when you put everything together. I'm not sure if local communities have people responsible for checking in on their elderly residents to make sure everything at home is okay and to help them out when needed.

The dark clouds of death continue to circle the sky above the city of Wuhan. Today one of those clouds floated past me: A famous editorial writer for the *Hubei Daily* just got infected, along with his entire family. They requested to be admitted to the hospital two weeks ago, but never got a call back. By the time they were finally admitted, his condition had already deteriorated. He died today. And today there is one more shattered family added to this world.

FEBRUARY 21, 2020

I donate my body to the nation; what about my wife?

Thirty days now since the quarantine was first imposed. My goodness, it has been so long. Today is sunny and warm; the weather is so nice that you have the urge to go outside and take a walk. Back in another era, those old-time residents of Hankou would pack a wicker picnic basket full of snacks and hire a rickshaw to take them down by the lake for a stroll. Today the lakeside areas in all three of the major urban districts around Wuhan have been turned into parks; you can take a stroll almost anywhere. When spring arrives each year the wetlands in Huanghualao are always filled with people taking photos and flying kites. And then in the East Lake area there is a garden bursting with plum blossoms; but this year they are all blooming in vain. I'm afraid that by now all the plum blossoms have already shed their petals in desolation and loneliness. And so here I express my nostalgia for those flowers that no one will see.

Everyone is just about at the point where they can no longer take it anymore (I feel really bad for those small children who still want to go outside to play every day!); we all want to get out. But there is nothing we can do; in order to stay safe, in order to survive, in order to plan for the future, we must just close our doors, stay inside, and wait. If there is one thing we can do to help during this outbreak, that is it.

Yesterday's statistics revealed a dramatic drop in the number of new infections, triggering widespread debate and discussion online. But my doctor friend already told me that it was actually a shift in the way they calculated their statistics that resulted in that number. I'm sure they revised their counting method in order to make the numbers look a bit better to the public. It came as a surprise then when today the government immediately corrected the error and readjusted the figures back to where they should be. It is clear that fudging the numbers has no effect when you are fighting a disease. But I wonder if the speed with which they corrected their mistakes speaks to a larger change in how the government will be operating moving forward. Because when it comes down to it, the only way we are going to get a handle on this outbreak is if we speak the truth, correct mistakes in a timely fashion, and immediately fill the holes when we find them.

A new group of government leaders to spearhead the fight against the outbreak in Hubei has arrived, and they have begun to correct the feeble and sluggish response of their predecessors. The power of the coronavirus has been brazen, but things are clearly starting to turn around. The strategies we have employed seem to be working. A quick response is essential in trying to get ahead of the disease instead of being dragged under by it. This is especially the case with Wuhan where for the past few days we have appropriated a strategy that is quick and efficient. People have been able to clearly see this shift from various reports and videos that have been circulating online.

But sometimes I also feel that there is no reason for our leaders to be so sharp with their words. As long as the people have faith in their government, they will give them time; but the leaders also need to give those people under them ample time to carry out the policies they set in place. I'm afraid that no policy will be effective if it is rushed. Let's take, for instance, the government's policy of "drawing in the net," which has been very important for the city of Wuhan to investigate all the cases. Through this process the city has been able to accurately identify everyone in the city who has tested positive, is a suspected carrier, is running a fever, or had close contact with confirmed patients. However, I'm not sure if it is realistic to push this widespread tracking to be done in just three days. It is simply a question of what is realistic and practical. Wuhan is a large city with a complex system divided into several districts; there are a lot of residents who don't strictly fall into any of those official residential communities; there is also a lot of disorganization when it comes to those areas between the city and the surrounding rural areas. It will be almost impossible for those investigators to cover the entire city in just three short days, let alone carry out any kind of conclusive investigation. And what happens if they break their necks for three days but fail to produce a report? It'll be the District Head's job on the line. He, in turn, will probably try to fire all those lower-level officials under him to save his own skin.

Today I saw a video of an old man who was one stubborn old devil: no matter what people did to convince him to self-quarantine, he just flat-out refused. Wuhan's development is tied to its history as a port city; that means that there have always been a lot of people who have grown accustomed to a rather carefree and undisciplined lifestyle, many of whom can be quite unruly at times. I wouldn't necessarily call this old man "unruly," but he was certainly stubborn. I think we have a lot more stubborn old men like him in this city than unruly people. In the video, the police did their best to persuade him to self-quarantine, but in the end they had no choice but to carry him away by force. Think of how much time is wasted each time the police have to go through this process and multiply that by all the people out there like him. And you think three days will be enough time to cover the entire city? I'm really worried about those District Heads; once these three days are up, I wonder if a single one of them will still have a job. I really hope that the leaders in charge are just trying to beat their drums to stir things up a bit, but hopefully they won't go all the way down this perilous cliff.

As we arrive at today, the bad news just keeps on coming. I'm sorry, but I'm not the kind of person who is able to just focus on the positive and ignore the negative things happening. The bad news is, naturally, about death. The god of death has continued to wander among us; every day you can see his shadow moving closer. Yesterday Dr. Peng Yinhua passed away; he was only 29 years old. He was originally supposed to get married on Day Eight of the Lunar New Year, but with the outbreak he had to push his wedding back and he instead went to the front lines to battle the coronavirus. Dr. Peng unfortunately ended up getting infected and passed away; he'll never be able to walk down the aisle with his new wife. So young and full of promise for the future; it is just a terrible shame. But there is even worse news concerning new cases of widespread infection. I saw a meme a few days ago that was attached to a photo that said, "Prison is the safest place to be right now." But today came the news that several prisoners in jails all over the country have already tested positive for the coronavirus; they were all infected by prison guards. This is horrendous news! There are some inmates with a strong tendency toward antisocial behavior, which will make treating them even more challenging. I asked a doctor I know on WeChat about this and he confirmed that this was indeed a challenging development. I then asked him if the overall picture was getting better or worse. His response: "Things are improving, but it is very slow."

Another item that I want to be sure to put on the record: A patient here in Wuhan named Xiao Xianyou just died. Just before he passed away he left behind a final testament that was just two lines long and consisted of 11 Chinese characters. However, when the newspaper ran a story about his death, they used the following headline: "Seven Final Words That Left Everyone in Tears." Those seven words that left the newspaper editors in tears were: *I donate my body to the nation*, but in reality there were another four words that appeared after that: *what about my wife?* I'm sure that even more people cried when they read those last four words. Of course, it is a moving gesture to donate one's body to science, but that last breath before he died was reserved for an expression of how much he will miss his wife, which is every bit as moving. So why didn't the newspaper just title its article "Eleven Final Words That Left Everyone in Tears"? Why did they take special pains to remove those last four words? Perhaps the editor thinks that love for one's nation is a sublime love, whereas love for one's wife has lesser value? Perhaps the newspaper felt that endorsing this lesser form of love is beneath them? I chatted online with a young reader about this today, and he had a lot to say; he was very unhappy with the media's way of handling this. I'm really glad that young people like him are learning to be critical of what they are reading in the media. I told him that the government loves that first line he wrote, but the people love that second line; the media only cares about the issues, but everyday citizens care most about human life; these represent two different value systems.

I can't help but think about those aid groups who have volunteered to come to Wuhan; before they set out to leave, some local leaders delivered some speeches to send them off. The political leaders who gave speeches mostly focused on three points. The leader of one group summed them up as: "Our first task is to preserve the honor of our group, our second task is to do whatever we can to save the sick, and our third task is to protect ourselves in the process!" A different group leader put it in these terms: "Number one is to save the sick, number two is to protect ourselves, and number three is to preserve the honor of our group." These are both political leaders and there is a perfect overlap in terms of the content; however, from the way they list their priorities you can tell a lot about the value system of these organizations.

Let me say a bit about what has been going on in my own life lately. While I usually sleep in every day, my middle brother tends to always be an early riser. But last night my brother was up late; he even sent me a text: "You stay up writing your diary, I stay up doing online shopping!" I wondered why he was up so late doing that. He told me that if you don't act quickly, all those products get sold out within minutes, so you need to stay up and order as soon as items are restocked. After being stuck at home for 31 days, he has eaten almost all the food he had at home. He said that these past few days he was starting to get anxious. Since they shut down the city, people have been buying up everything at the supermarket across the street from him and you have to fight the crowds just to get your hands on anything. Those online vendors list their new stock of items for the next day at 11:30 p.m. and people instantly start snapping them up right away. My brother already filled his online shopping cart with items and was ready to hit the purchase button as soon as it was 11:30, but the system was frozen. By the time he got logged back in, everything in his cart was already sold out. He and my sister-in-law were going crazy last night. At least a few days ago he was able to order some rice, noodles, cooking oil, vegetables, and medicine, some of which have already been delivered, and a few other items he is still waiting for. I told him not to worry too much: "They're not going to let us starve! Things aren't that bad in China yet!" His neighborhood is the single most dangerous area for coronavirus infections; it has been listed as the area with the highest number of infections for quite a while now. He is also not in very good health so if he were to catch the coronavirus, the results could be really scary. So everyone in the family keeps insisting that he had better not take a single step outside his door. But we all know that it is really difficult being stuck in a small apartment like that for over 30 days.

I'm fortunate to have a much better setup than my brother, as I have had a bunch of colleagues and neighbors helping me out ever since this thing started. Yesterday one of my colleagues sent her husband over to bring me a few cans of chicken soup; I wasn't expecting that at all but accepted this gift with a smile. However, there was a catch: In exchange for the chicken soup, she insisted that I send her a copy of my diary each day the second I finish each installment. For me it feels like I'm making an unfair profit! I naturally agreed to her deal. Everyone at the Writers Association has been really good to me; I've basically watched a lot of them grow up. This colleague is one of them. When she first joined the Writers Association, she was probably not even 20 years old; she was so cute and stubborn back then. Now in the blink of an eye, she is almost 50.

Just as I got to this point, someone posted in my classmates' forum: "Wuhan plans to construct an additional 19 temporary hospitals." Seeing this news reminds me of a message that Mr. Liu from the Wuhan

Botanical Garden put up on Weibo. Let me copy Mr. Liu's suggestion here: "If the novel coronavirus outbreak is not a short-term setback, an extended lockdown in Wuhan will affect the economic national recovery; moreover, the impact of a long-term quarantine will also have a severe psychological impact on the citizens. Instead I would like to propose a 'River Isle Quarantine Model.' This is what it would look like: By utilizing the islet areas of Baishazhou, Tianxingzhou, and all those decommissioned passenger ships, we could house 10,000 patients there. Besides this, Tianxingzhou is roughly 22 square kilometers, which is actually two square meters larger than Macau. Macau has a population of 600,000 people. Based on this, it should be no problem to build a massive hospital in Tianxingzhou that could accommodate 150,000 patients. And then there is still Baishazhou and those decommissioned passenger ships. If we can move all the patients in Wuhan to these sites on the river, we will be able to keep the virus off the mainland. Then we can gradually, one at a time, start lifting the quarantines in Wuhan, Wuchang, Hankou, and Hanyang. If people are afraid it will take too long to construct a large hospital, we can start with 100,000 medical tents where patients can be treated. In short, a long-term quarantine is not a long-term solution; the nation won't be able to handle that, nor will the people."

I find Mr. Liu's suggestion to be quite bold and interesting. However, there would still be a lot of issues that would need to be resolved, such as how to deal with all the sewage waste produced there, and I'm afraid that it would be too cold for patients to live in medical tents during this time of year. I'm not an expert in these matters, but perhaps various specialists will have ways of getting around these problems?

People are now starting to discuss more about the timeline for economic recovery, even more than the outbreak itself. A lot of industries are on the verge of collapse and countless individuals who are just hanging on without any source of income are facing the question of how they are going to get by if this continues. All these issues have a direct bearing on our social stability. As we quarantined our sick, we have also locked up the healthy. As more time goes by, the damage this causes begins to multiply. I've already begun to hear a lot of people make the appeal that healthy people need to get on with their lives, too.

But I don't have any answers; all I do is record things as I see them.

FEBRUARY 22, 2020

The spread is so difficult to contain, which is indeed a challenge.

The weather remains clear and warm, yet here I am, lying in bed looking at my phone.

The first thing I encountered online was an audio recording of a woman from Wuhan criticizing her district. She went on and on in her crisp and sharp Wuhan dialect. She didn't use many profanities, but she littered her speech with all kinds of idioms, which made a lot of people laugh and want to follow her online. Listening to her speak also gave me quite a kick. I'm only all too familiar with that accent of hers; she must be from the area around 27th Street in Jiang'an District, where I spent several years when I was a teenager. It isn't really the most typical Wuhan dialect; it is a bit off when you compare it to the standard Wuhan dialect spoken in downtown Hankou. But she still speaks it better than me. Several friends all sent me links to this recording today. I asked them if they really understood Wuhan women; she rarely used any profanities, and what she said actually made a lot of sense; I guess you could consider the way she spoke an elegant way to curse someone.

Beautiful weather paired with some good old-fashioned elegant Wuhan cursing really put me in a good mood and helped get this day started off right.

One month into the quarantine and today I did another interview with Xia Chunping, Assistant Editor from China News Agency. We did the interview portion online and then in the afternoon he and his crew came over to take some photos, at which time we chatted a bit more. The guards on duty at the front gate were quite meticulous about following all the rules when Xia arrived. Although Xia Chunping and his crew all had proper press credentials, the guards still made them all officially register and took everyone's temperature before letting them in. I joked and said it was a good thing they didn't just show up unannounced. During his visit Xia Chunping not only brought me some additional face masks, he also brought over some milk and yogurt. When I got back to my apartment I also discovered that he had also snuck a box of chocolates into the bag! When I saw the chocolates I immediately called my colleague and told him to pick them up for his daughter next time he was around. Whenever people give me chocolate I usually pass it on to my colleague's daughter. One day when I saw that little girl she said: "Grandma Fang Fang, you are like a real-life Lei Feng!" After I heard that, I was even more eager to give her chocolate; after all, now I had a theoretical foundation for my actions!

Less than half an hour after Xia Chunping left, I received a text from a friend in the United States who had just read the interview I did with him! The link even included the photos he had just taken of me! The speed at which the internet can spread news is really shocking; it is truly hard to believe. Almost everyone in my family is in engineering and the sciences, and that has heavily influenced me; I suppose that I too have become fairly well acquainted with technology; I gave up writing by hand and started using a computer back in 1990. But I still have trouble keeping up with all the latest technological advances and often find myself blown away by the newest capabilities out there. The news organization Headlines Today (Jinri Toutiao) featured me on its site and I uploaded an installment from my diary onto its "Micro Headlines" page; within one day it had been read by 20 million users, and a few days later it was up to 30 million views. For a writer like me who is used to a very small circle of readers, those numbers are terrifying. It just feels unnatural to me, so much so that I almost wanted to give up writing this diary. It was only after several old classmates encouraged me to continue that I decided to stick with it.

I'm quite familiar with how official government media organizations function in China. When they interview you, they ask a ton of questions, but usually only a small portion of your answers actually make it into print. But because I understand how they work, I usually still try to provide detailed responses to their questions as much as possible so that the editors will have plenty of material to choose from. The good thing is that when they add additional material without my permission, I always take a stand and they understandably agree to take that material out; they always do their best to respect my wishes. Overall, China News Agency has a relatively relaxed standard that they go by, while of course remaining fairly prudent when it comes to certain topics. They are certainly not as free and open as some of the social media and independent media platforms that I publish on. Comparatively speaking, Sina Weibo remains the platform with the most liberal policies for expression in China. I'm also quite fond of writing short posts in those little boxes; I pop out a post in a single breath, which always feels good. It is, however, a shame that they can't stop those ultra-leftist groups from continually reporting my posts, which has resulted in my account being suspended. I left a message for them, saying: "I really love you guys at Weibo, but you have really let me down!"

First thing this morning my doctor friend sent me a note with his latest thoughts on the coronavirus outbreak. I also followed up with him in the afternoon to get a better sense of where things stand. I would summarize his thoughts as follows: According to statistics from the past three days, the overall trend is improving, but there has yet to be a fundamental change. The spread of the coronavirus has yet to be fully contained. The number of presumed cases is still quite high. The only good thing is that there is less pressure than before to provide additional hospital beds. There are two reasons why the shortage of beds is not as bad as before: The first is that many patients have now been discharged, and the second is that a lot of patients have died. Every day there are nearly 100 patients who die.

This news is all quite sad. While Wuhan's ability to investigate cases of infection within the city is quite impressive, there are a lot of citizens who are not entirely happy with the way things are being handled. At the same time, it is still quite difficult to control the spread of the virus; perhaps it is precisely because of this that Wuhan is now constructing an additional 19 temporary hospitals. The plan is to increase the number of sickbeds to the point that there will always be open beds there waiting for new patients; that will help significantly cut down the number of mild cases that turn critical. My doctor friend reiterated what he told me before: There are still nearly 10,000 patients who were infected early on who are now still in serious or critical condition. That alone makes it hard to reduce the number of patients who are dying. Critical patients with breathing problems are put on oxygen or respirators to help alleviate their symptoms. That reminded me of a report I read yesterday by a Caixin Media reporter that was about how people's lives were on the line, dependent on the availability of a single breathing tube. During my conversation with my doctor friend, he said: "We are now seeing a certain degree of effectiveness with the use of traditional

Chinese medicine." This reminded me of a question posted online about whether or not Chinese medicine was at all effective against the coronavirus. I passed this question on to my doctor friend, since he is trained in Western medicine. I really wanted to know how doctors who specialize in Western medicine look at the use of Chinese medicine for treating coronavirus patients.

According to my doctor friend: "Right now there are many hospitals in which the entire treatment ward is managed by doctors who practice Chinese medicine, and they have achieved very positive results. Of course, those traditional Chinese medicine doctors also employ some Western medicine and Western medical treatment practices. This mixture of Chinese and Western medicine has yielded very positive results and has also won a high level of approval with state-level medical agencies. At first a lot of doctors trained in Western medicine were extremely resistant to this approach and even mocked it. However, now that it has yielded positive results, most of those early critics have all quieted down. I suspect that once this outbreak has passed, the state will lend a good deal of support to further develop the field of traditional Chinese medicine. After all, over the course of this battle against the coronavirus, traditional Chinese medicine has really shined as an effective treatment method and everyone has taken notice; even practitioners of Western medicine have to admit that. Traditional Chinese medicine treatment is also much more affordable than Western medicine. I have never really understood the principles of Chinese medicine, but I also never looked down on it. After all, traditional Chinese medicine has been with us throughout 5,000 years of Chinese history, whereas Western medicine has only been in widespread use in China for a few decades. There are certainly ailments for which Chinese medicine is quite effective." The previous passage was pasted together from several texts that my doctor friend sent me. I restructured it a bit, but the content is entirely taken from his comments.

I have a college classmate who now teaches at the Institute of Chinese Medicine (he was a graduate of the Chinese department; I wonder if he teaches students how to read classical Chinese medicinal texts? I never asked him that). Ever since the coronavirus outbreak began, he has been confident that traditional Chinese medicine would prove to be an extremely effective treatment. Moreover, he has stood by this belief and wholeheartedly promoted it over the past few months. He even got angry that Wuhan wasn't utilizing even more traditional Chinese medicine in its treatment of coronavirus patients. I posted some of the things my doctor friend said in my college classmates group chat. One former classmate who works in the media said that, in some respects, you could even say that the coronavirus has saved traditional Chinese medicine. I find that comment somewhat frightening.

Then my classmate from the Institute of Chinese Medicine replied: "We should thank the coronavirus for allowing traditional Chinese medicine to finally show its face! The basic approach of Chinese medicine is completely different from that of Western medicine: 'Chinese medicine always leaves the virus with a way out; it politely sees the virus to the door, but whether it lives or dies depends (usually the virus dies off).' But Western medicine tries to completely eradicate the virus, but when it fails there are no incantations left to cast." I found his viewpoint interesting, but a bit biased. His understanding of traditional Chinese medicine has a philosophical twist, yet his understanding of Western medicine seems just plain twisted.

This evening the discussion of traditional Chinese medicine continued on my group chat. Apparently, there are quite a few old classmates of mine who are totally against traditional Chinese medicine. Then my classmate from the Institute of Chinese Medicine jumped in again to further discuss his viewpoint: "Strictly speaking, there is no such thing as a true synthesis between Chinese and Western medicine. They are each theoretically incompatible, like two cars driving on completely different roads. When we talk about a synthesis between Chinese and Western medicine, what we are usually talking about is using Chinese medicine as the basis, while employing some Western medical equipment, supplies, and therapies in the treatment plan, depending on effectiveness. But actually there are a lot of problems with this approach; in fact, these two traditions are often in conflict with one another." I'm really not well versed in the various debates between Chinese and Western medicine. Usually when I go to the doctor I seek out specialists trained in Western medicine. However, when it comes to everyday health maintenance issues, I usually turn to Chinese medicine. For instance, every winter I tend to start drinking a lot of hot water infused with Chinese herbal medicine. I even introduced this method to my colleague Chu Feng, and she said she felt like a new person after she started drinking it.

I just noticed a report online that the various stories about Wuhan people getting fed up and cursing the system were starting to be taken seriously by various government offices. Various District Heads and the Commission for Inspecting Discipline have all begun to take notice, and Zhongbai Supermarket has already begun to adopt some changes; I guess speaking out can lead to some good results. One of my friends told me that an English-language version of these "Wuhan curses" has already come out online. I'm sure that will give me another good laugh.

These Wuhan curses have also had an impact on several related topics. To be honest, after all the time that has gone by, basic things like getting enough food have become a pronounced issue for many people in Wuhan. Over time, the group-buying model has also revealed its shortcomings. Every day at pickup time there are crowds of people showing up to pick up their groceries at the entrance to each development. And all the items rarely arrive at the same time, so people often have to go down several times to pick up their entire order. It started out with us only having to go out once a day to pick everything up, but now we have to go out several times just to pick up a single order. At the same time, some residents are getting a bit unreasonable; instead of just ordering daily necessities, they are ordering entire cases of beer and other things that they don't really need. That really puts an unreasonable burden on the volunteers, who are already past the point of exhaustion. But what are we to do? Management is a science, but never mind daily necessities; the big question is how to better manage this coronavirus outbreak. A novelist like me surely isn't the right person to ask.

I saw an interesting post online that summed up where things stand: The first group of people with the coronavirus were infected before the Lunar New Year; the second group of people infected all flooded the hospitals; the third group of people infected flooded the supermarkets; the fourth group of people infected started to blindly sign up for online shopping groups.

According to my doctor friend, the spread is extremely difficult to contain, which is indeed our greatest challenge.

FEBRUARY 23, 2020

You need to be brave and accept the
consequences of your decisions.

Today is another bright, clear day. I'm reminded of a book from my childhood, called *Bright Clear Day*, although I can't remember what it was about anymore. A few days ago I thought that the plum blossoms must have all shed their petals by now, but yesterday I surprisingly discovered that all the crimson plum blossoms in our courtyard had broken out in a riotous bloom. In all the years past, I have never seen them blooming like that—gloriously announcing their presence amid a flurry of beauty and color.

Within the blink of an eye, the first month of the Lunar New Year has passed and we are no longer even bothering to count how many days it has been since the quarantine began. It doesn't really matter anymore, because I just stay quietly at home, patiently waiting while trying to remain as calm as I can be. I'm not waiting for a turning point anymore; I'm just waiting for the day when I can go outside again. As far as I can tell, the turning point doesn't really matter anymore. It has, after all, proved to be elusive, so what's the point of just waiting in vain? Who knows; perhaps, as Director Wang of the Leishenshan Hospital said, the turning point has already come and gone? Indeed, the darkest, most tragic and painful days that Wuhan has faced during this outbreak are already behind us. Right now the coronavirus might be slow-moving and difficult to get through, but the situation is still much better than it was before. That said, we have yet to escape from the clutches of death. This morning a young doctor was taken by the coronavirus; just like Dr. Peng Yinhua, who passed away two days ago, she was only 29 years old. Her name was Xia Sisi. She leaves behind a two-year-old child. Last night another male doctor died; he had only just turned 40; his name was Huang Wenjun. We sigh and we cry; there are a lot of people sighing and crying these days. And then we silently forward these bits of news to one another. Is it a total of nine doctors who have died fighting the coronavirus now? It is difficult to keep track anymore.

Today I was thinking about the fact that they keep saying that people with preexisting health conditions are more susceptible to the virus. And don't they say that if you don't receive treatment early you are more likely to end up with more serious symptoms or even risk death? These doctors were all between the ages of 29 and 40 and don't seem to fit into any of these categories; they were all healthy and received treatment early on, so how come none of them made it? I decided to bring these questions to my doctor friend. He said: "That's right, elderly people with underlying health conditions are more likely to succumb to this disease. And when medical professionals get infected, they indeed have access to excellent quality medical care. The reason these doctors ended up dying has to do with inherent differences in the patients' constitutions. Each person has a different level of sensitivity when it comes to how the body reacts to an infection." He didn't explain it that clearly to me, but he did reiterate what he had told me before: "This is a very strange virus. Yesterday I saw a news report about a 97-year-old who had completely recovered and was just released from the hospital. When I saw that, I also began to wonder if there was perhaps some other reason to account for the high death rate among healthcare professionals."[31]

Today in my classmates group chat, my former Group Leader from college, Lao Yang, posted some very complimentary things about another classmate named Lao Xia. Although Lao Yang later went to Beijing, where he assumed a senior government post, since we all started out together in the same group in college, we still consider him our "little Group Leader." Almost everyone in our college class has already retired; there are only a few of us born in the early 1960s who are still working; Lao Xia is one of them. When Lao Xia went to college in 1978 he was only 17 or 18 years old, but his baby face made him look more like he was 14 or 15! So I'm not sure why, but ever since then, we started calling him Lao Xia, or "Old Xia."

Lao Xia has worked in media ever since graduation; he has never switched fields. According to Lao Xia, "Ever since the outbreak started, the entire editorial office has been like a war room. Reporters have been rushing to the front lines, following the story wherever it takes them. Besides reporting, they have also dived into community work." Lao Xia is actually responsible for four districts; he is committed to standing by those areas and providing services to the residents there, like helping them get food and medicine. It is really a tough job. Among all my former classmates, Lao Xia is the only one I know of who is out there on the front lines fighting this virus. He jokingly said: "I'm out there contributing to the effort on behalf of Dorm Eight!" Dorm Eight is the building we all lived in at Wuhan University when we were all in school together. One former classmate suggested we recognize him as this year's Dorm Eight Person of the Year!

Speaking of people who work in the media, from what I know there are 300 journalists who have come to Wuhan to cover the coronavirus outbreak. I'm sure there are a lot more than that if you also include all the freelance journalists and reporters working for various websites. It is their tireless efforts running all over town to conduct painstaking interviews that have allowed us to really get a sense of what is happening through their in-depth coverage. Among them there are several investigative journalists who have delved very deeply into the details of what has been occurring. They have been covering every major stage of this outbreak, which has helped shine a light on all the problems and obstructions that they have witnessed; even more important is that they have introduced us to countless heroic figures and incidents that otherwise would have gone unnoticed.

Wuhan is very different than what Wenchuan was like in 2008 after the earthquake; this is an area with an infectious disease still raging. Since the virus is invisible, you often have no idea which places are dangerous. You often have no way of knowing whether or not the person you are interviewing is infected. Then there are also many cases where you know the person you are talking to *is* infected, yet you still push forward with the interview because you know you have to get the story out there. I'm told that many of the reporters out there are quite young and have a very strong work ethic; they work hard and they're not afraid of the risks involved. When I was younger, I worked at a television station for a while, so I have firsthand experience of just how exhausting and difficult those types of on-location assignments can be.

But today I saw an essay that was quite sharp; it really pained me to have to read it. I would like to share an excerpt for later reflection: "I have absolutely no respect for those media bosses in Hubei and Wuhan. Of course some of those government officials should take responsibility for what is happening! Don't you dare try to convince me that you have a clear conscience on this! Are your own career and salary really more important than the safety of tens of millions of citizens? You've all received extended professional training; how can you not know just how dangerous this virus is? Why don't you do something to fight it and start reporting the truth for a change?"[32]

What he wrote was quite heavy-handed, but at the same time it is worth reflecting on. I'd like to ask the author of that essay if he really thinks there are any senior leaders left in the field of media who still have common sense, professionalism, and a strong work ethic? Over time the most talented get weeded out and those inferior managers rise to the top; meanwhile the most innovative and talented people in the field find jobs elsewhere. When you are too good, you call too much attention to yourself and get weeded out. There must be a lot of people working in media who simply use their power to get ahead. Those people would never commit the flagrant error of speaking out for the people during the Chinese New Year, of all times! What is it, then, that they should be doing during the start of the Chinese New Year? Everyone in the media knows this! The people are nothing in their eyes; all they need to worry about is making their superiors happy, because they are the only ones who can protect their status—but that has absolutely nothing to do with the needs of the people.

But when it comes to brave professional journalists in Hubei and Wuhan, there are still a lot of them out there. Didn't Zhang Ouya publicly call for the leaders supervising the fight against the coronavirus to be replaced?[33] Unfortunately, his boss was much more upset about this outcry than he was about the actual coronavirus! They tend to immediately clamp down on those people who speak out while neglecting to take this monstrous disease seriously. With the exception of patients and health workers, the journalists are the ones who are forced to get closest to this virus. They are able to fearlessly stand in the face of this virus now, yet when the outbreak first began, they all chose to remain silent. This is a tragedy. At the same time, those people working in the media are also in a difficult position. They get it from both sides. Their superiors don't allow them to speak the truth, while their readers demand that they do speak the truth. They are often left with no real options. More often than not, they end up siding with their superiors. With that being the case, when the public curses them for their inaction, they have no choice but just to bear up and take it. I have always felt that once you make a decision you need to be brave and accept the consequences of that decision.

It seems like they disinfected the area around my front door again today. Staying at home all day, you tend not to notice what is happening outside, but when I went out to dump the trash I saw a flyer notifying residents that disinfectant had been used in the area. In the evening I received a text from Xiao Zhou, who is responsible for managing this area; it said, "There are some donated vegetables outside your door." I opened the door to take a look and saw two large bags of bok choy; they looked really fresh and tasty. I'm not sure who donated them, but it is exactly what I needed.

FEBRUARY 24, 2020

> *There is only one true test, and that is how you treat*
> *the weakest and most vulnerable members of your society.*

Day Two of the Second Month of the Lunar New Year, the dragon has raised its head. Normally, I suppose that the spring plowing should begin today? But it is unclear if there are any farmers out in the fields today. The clear weather continues and it is quite warm; it feels as if the large, bright sun might even be able to bake the virus out and kill it. The Chinese roses in my courtyard have begun to sprout; I haven't really taken care of them, yet they continue to grow vigorously.

In normal times I like to order Kengee's "craftsman bread." Today the store manager, Mr. Lu, had a box sent over for me. I really don't know how to thank him. My colleague Dao Bo was on duty at the main entrance and saw me approaching from far way; when I arrived, she said, "I could tell it was you!" I take big broad steps when I walk, whereas Dao Bo always takes her time in her pointy high-heel shoes. We went on a few work trips together and she could never keep up with me. Dao Bo helped me bring the box of bread back to my apartment, and I let her keep some as a way of expressing my thanks. We often share goodies with one another; I give her oolong tea and she brings me samples of her home-cooked dishes. I can't even remember how many years we have been doing this for, but her fried lotus roots and pearl meatballs are some of my all-time favorite dishes. One of the best things about living in a big community like this is that you never go hungry.

An old classmate from Beijing posted a question in our online group chat asking what was going on with the 18th Command issued by the Wuhan Outbreak Prevention Control Center. Someone who understood the situation immediately responded by explaining that the

17th Command had been a mistake and now they were correcting it. The 18th Command was sent out to supersede the 17th Command. The old saying "bad news travels fast" is spot-on. In barely any time at all I saw a professor posting his interpretation of what happened, using the old idiom "Issue an order at dawn and rescind it at dusk." He even said that this wasn't even a true case of "issuing an order at dawn and rescinding it at dusk," it was "issuing an order at dawn and rescinding it before noon!" My god, the whole country has their eyes on Wuhan and yet we keep insisting on making silly mistakes; it can be so frustrating.

Doctors are still doing everything they can to save those patients infected early on whose condition has now turned quite serious; however, the mortality rate for these patients is still quite high. From this you can see that once the coronavirus reaches a critical stage it becomes extremely hard to treat; whether one lives or dies is completely dependent on the patient's ability to fight the virus. Medical practitioners are doing a much better job of preventing mild cases from taking a turn for the worse. I heard that some of the patients admitted to the temporary hospitals don't want to leave even after they have recovered! Those temporary hospitals are extremely spacious, they provide excellent food, and even have entertainment areas so patients can sing and dance! So the patients love being there for the social benefits. The hospital takes care of everything for you while you are there and, most importantly, it's all free. So a lot of people would prefer to stay there than being cooped up alone at home. The whole thing is so strange that it almost sounds like a bad joke.

The main task at hand is to control the outbreak so it does not spread any further; it is also the most difficult task we are facing. Although the new political leaders who are overseeing things here in Wuhan have ordered a thorough census to get a better sense of where things stand, even that is a complicated and challenging task in a large sprawling city with more than nine million residents. You need to mobilize community workers, local cadres, and even university teachers and each one has to go door-to-door to dozens, hundreds, in some cases even a thousand households to conduct surveys and collect information, all the while running the risk of getting infected themselves. And they have absolutely no recourse when they encounter residents who are resistant or refuse to open the door for them. They can't call the police to intervene; the police are already stretched too thin. It is hard enough for these community workers and public officials to get their hands on enough face masks, let alone protective biosuits. A few days ago one of my colleagues from the Hubei Writers Association called to see if I knew anyone who might be able to help him get a biosuit. It is extremely difficult to guarantee the safety of these workers and volunteers when they go into those districts with extremely high infection rates. If they get infected and then go home and spread the virus to their own families, it will be even worse. But it will be even far worse if we don't find everyone who falls into those four categories and ensure that they are all either properly quarantined or receiving treatment. The city will never be able to reopen until we do that. And in order to prevent the further spread of this disease, it is of the highest priority that we go door-to-door to every household in Wuhan.

This afternoon one of my old classmates from Beijing sent a recommendation from Zhang AD who graduated from the same department as me in 1977. According to AD, the massive numbers of asymptomatic carriers has created a huge hurdle for the country when it comes to managing this outbreak and preventing further spread. He grew extremely anxious thinking about this today and came up with a recommendation that he was hoping I could share with my readers. After reading it, I thought it might be useful, so I am including his comments below:

My recommendation: Have the state mobilize China's three largest telecommunications companies (China Telecom, China Mobile, and China Unicom) to contact every cellphone user in the country and send out a notification establishing a National Emergency Response Network. Similar to the QR Code Health System already employed in cities like Hangzhou and Shenzhen, every person will be required to do a daily health check-in. Besides the three big telecommunication companies, we will also need the two largest private e-pay companies (WeChat Pay and Alipay) to sign on. Through the network created by these five companies we can cover the vast majority of China's 1.4 billion residents. Those people without cellphones or without an e-pay account are highly unlikely to be living in areas where mass outbreaks are occurring. Elderly people can be contacted through their family members. If we add the Shenzhen company DJI and other top drone companies into the mix (employing them under the National Emergency Response Network), we can use their drones to patrol virus zones. These drones can also deliver announcements, send out broadcasts, and conduct surveillance while minimizing human contact. They can also increase work efficiency when it comes to quickly identifying all potential cases. This must be implemented as soon as possible.

Another important benefit of using WeChat Pay and Alipay is that we can not only pinpoint the whereabouts of carriers, but we can also track down everyone they had close contact with during a given time frame (from November 1, 2019, until now). We will be able to track everyone using this system!

I copied the above text directly from AD; I'm not sure if it is practical, but I'm putting it out there for specialists to consider. AD's father is actually the lyricist of the famous song *Yellow River Cantata*, Zhang

Guangnian.[34] (As a matter of coincidence, my colleague Dao Bo, whom I wrote about before, has an aunt who is the composer of *Yellow River Cantata*, Xian Xinghai.) Back when I served as editor of *Celebrities Today* magazine, I once serialized several selections from Zhang Guangnian's diary. Later, when he published his diary as a book, he sent me a copy. Inside the book was a letter in which he mentioned the fact that his son AD was actually my classmate. Since Mr. Zhang is such a senior figure I didn't think it would be appropriate for me to directly respond to his letter, so I never wrote back. At the time I was quite young and had very high expectations for myself; I didn't want to be perceived as someone taking advantage of the fact that I was editing a magazine about celebrities to try to get close to them. Instead, I always tried to keep a respectful distance from the famous people we featured. But later when I learned that Mr. Zhang had passed away I really regretted never having written back to him.

This afternoon I read a report by a journalist with Caixin Media about the situation that many retirement homes and nursing homes are dealing with amid this coronavirus outbreak. Even without the outbreak, the elderly are already in a particularly weak and marginalized place in society. I suspect that a lot of them live in circumstances that are already well below the average, compared with most people in China today. But once this virus started hitting many healthy young people, you can only imagine what it is doing to the elderly.

It was probably around 10 days ago that I heard about a string of deaths at a state-run retirement facility. I never mentioned it in my posts because I was not able to further authenticate the accuracy of the story. I need to be careful, with so many people just waiting for the opportunity to tear me down, not to mention the constant threat of censorship hanging over my head. But now that I have read the reporter's meticulous interviews, which include locations, times, and actual names of people featured all clearly laid out, I don't see any reason to continue avoiding this issue. Saying things like "I don't have any tears left to cry" doesn't even come close to doing justice to the true pain I have been feeling inside when I see these stories.

The Caixin Media reporter's essay stated: "Yesterday some family members received a telephone call from the retirement home where their relatives live to inform them that some of the elderly residents needed to be quarantined. The family members responded with a flurry of questions: 'Where should we bring them to be quarantined? Who will take care of them there while under quarantine? What are the standards that qualify someone to be quarantined or receive treatment? Have other patients in the retirement home also been infected? Will they receive effective treatment? Can you share their test results with us? Will the management at the retirement home be willing to share all information with us in a timely manner? Will the government be willing to increase staffing for those retirement homes, including nurse support and medical resources?'" Family members were extremely upset and worried as they anxiously awaited the retirement home's response to their inquiries. As I see it, since the government has already agreed to take care of these people, they will naturally see things through and make sure these elderly patients are not neglected; the people running things are, after all, human too.

But what really needs to be said is that the true test of a country's level of civility has nothing to do with building the tallest skyscraper or driving the fastest car, nor does it matter how advanced your weapons system is or how powerful your military might be; it is also not about how advanced your technology is or even your artistic achievements, and it is especially not related to how lavish your official government meetings are or how splendid your firework displays are, or even how many rich Chinese tourists you have buying up different parts of the world. There is only one true test, and that is how you treat the weakest and most vulnerable members of your society.

There is one final thing I want to talk about today: A few days ago, they finally unfroze my Weibo account. At first I was reluctant to go back on Weibo; I guess you could say I was disappointed in them. There are also a lot of bastards out there on Weibo, and several of my classmates suggested I stay away from that site in order to protect myself from getting hurt. But after thinking it through, I decided to start using my account again. I heard a recording a few days ago that ended with the following words: "Don't leave the world in the hands of the bastards!" It is for that same reason that I decided not to leave my beloved Weibo in the hands of those bastards. At least Weibo has a way of blacklisting people who don't follow proper online etiquette, so I can report each and every one of those people who come after me. That blacklist is a biosuit, it is my N95 face mask that I use to quarantine those infectious bastards!

FEBRUARY 25, 2020

Once the music has ended, we will seek out a cure.

The weather is remarkably beautiful; it must have gotten up to around 20 degrees Celsius in the afternoon. With the heat on in my apartment it actually started to feel hot. But with nightfall, it began to suddenly rain, a strange and unexpected turn of events. Not that it really matters, though, since we can't go outside anyway; instead, staring at my cellphone has become my required homework each day.

First thing this morning I saw a few videos that I really need to say something about. The videos I saw fall into two categories: The first category was videos documenting the disastrous results of several vegetable donations from other provinces coming into Hubei. There were videos of deliveries being confiscated on the road, entire bags of vegetables being thrown in the trash, and other footage of vegetables just rotting away in storage facilities. There was an entire series of videos about this. The other set of videos was of citizens complaining about the price gouging going on in those grocery delivery services for vegetables. A lot of people right now are being especially thrifty with their money. Even during normal times, they are often very careful when they go shopping. When they drop the price for soy sauce by 2 fen, there is a line wrapping around the block to get in on this great deal! You ask "why?" Because in their minds they have only just enough cash to get by, so people save any way they can. Most people feel those grocery delivery groups are quite expensive for vegetables of mixed quality that you can't even pick out yourself. How can you expect people not to complain? Moreover, after being stuck at home for so long, everyone is more irritable than normal.

These videos were all sent to me by friends, so I can't confirm their authenticity. But no matter whether they are real or fake, I still feel that there has to be a more suitable way to distribute all the donated vegetables that have been coming into Wuhan. Right now we have a situation where the donated vegetables aren't getting into the hands of the right people, while the vegetables being sold in stores are way overpriced. Somehow, we are failing on both ends. Moreover, it is a real insult to those kindhearted people who have been making these donations. I really can't think of a better option than donating all those vegetables to a vegetables wholesaler that can evenly distribute them to all the major supermarkets. They can require supermarkets to sell them to the public at a deeply reduced rate; whatever profit is made can then be refunded, donated, or used to subsidize other food items. This would allow the public the opportunity to purchase affordable vegetables while, at the same time, freeing up community workers so they aren't spending all their time transporting these donations. Of course, those work units or districts that have arranged for their own direct donations are a separate matter. The weather is warming up and it is becoming increasingly difficult to preserve all these fresh food donations. We should keep everything as practical as possible.

Let me get back to the coronavirus. This morning one of my doctor friends sent me a message saying that, besides Wuhan, outbreaks in most other cities in China are now more or less under control. Wuhan is the only city where the virus has continued to spread and is still not under control. The stress on hospitals that had too few beds is now finally starting to ease up, but the reason the virus continues to spread is not something I fully understand. Wuhan has been under quarantine now for more than a full month, which means that, assuming the coronavirus has an incubation period of up to 24 days, everyone infected should have already started showing symptoms by now. With everyone locked up in their homes, there should be very few, if not zero, new infections by now. So then why are there still so many new cases of infection that keep popping up? My doctor friend was also confused by this, and he really couldn't explain the reason behind these new confirmed and suspected cases. What is the source of all these new infections? This is something that needs to be investigated; they need to do research on how these new patients are getting infected and then enact new prevention measures based on what they find. Although we have paid a huge price, the end result of this long period of quarantine has fallen short of our initial hopes. My doctor friend again used the word "strange" to describe this novel coronavirus. He even said that we need to hold our ground against this disease; but we should be prepared for its lasting even longer than we thought.

If what he said is true, that means we will need to be prepared to remain quarantined at home even longer. I'm afraid that at this point no one really knows exactly for how long all this will last. It has been one long and bitter quarantine. Even those comedians and meme writers have fallen silent. It has been really hard on the people of Wuhan. First we had to go through that initial period of fear and anxiety, which was quickly followed by a period of unprecedented sadness, pain, and helplessness. And now, although we are no longer living in terror and the sadness has dissipated a bit, we must face an indescribable boredom and restlessness, along with endless waiting. But there is nothing else we can do. All I can do is tell everyone, as well as myself, that we need to hang in there and wait. It is something we simply have no control over. We have already hung on so long, I'm sure we can get through the remaining days ahead. I'm sure it won't be too long now. The entire world knows that we are making this sacrifice for them; we have closed our doors so that everyone else can continue on with their lives. Just put on the loudest and most vulgar TV show that you can find to pass the time, something like *Sunny Piggy*, that sappy adaptation of *Journey to the West*. What else can we do?

This morning I saw another video of a woman who insisted on going outside even though she wasn't wearing a face mask. No matter what people said, she refused to go back in and insisted on talking to people without putting her face mask on. Community workers and public officials are all left in a tough place when they encounter people like this. Then there was a video of a small street filled with people and all the shops were still open; it was bustling as usual, as if there were not even an outbreak. The person shooting the video kept narrating as he walked down the street, saying: "Look at how free everyone looks! It doesn't look at all like Wuhan!" I saw some people I knew in the video and even recognized the street where he was filming. With people behaving like this, it feels like this entire quarantine doesn't really mean anything! Most of those people feel like the coronavirus has nothing to do with them; however, the difficulties we are seeing in controlling this outbreak and the fact that we have all been forced to remain quarantined for so long have everything to do with the behavior of people like that!

Yesterday I forwarded a suggestion made by AD, and quite a few people posted responses online. A lot of them thought that his suggestion was completely impractical because it would be too big of an infringement on people's privacy. There were a lot of people who saw it like that. I sent some of those comments to AD, and he responded as follows: "That's how things are. Of course an individual's movements are part of their private information, but when it comes to the suppression of this coronavirus, some of those lines become a bit hazy; under this National Emergency Response System we need to utilize whatever means necessary to steer us out of this situation!"

I actually thought of that very issue when I first posted his initial suggestion yesterday. The issue really hit home when I read the last sentence of his original post: "We will be able to track everyone using this system!" After reading that, I even hesitated for a few seconds, but in the end I still decided to send it out. That's because I'm here in Wuhan and what I know is that the lives of nine million people are more important than their privacy. Right now our primary concern is a matter of survival. What is privacy when compared with the cost of a human life? Those patients lying on the operating table with a doctor working on them won't give a second thought to things like privacy. If technology can create happiness and assume a heretical guise, it is only natural for us to harness it to expel evil. In Chinese martial arts novels, you always read about those evil villains who have mastered the art of poisoning their enemies—but they always have an antidote hidden up their sleeve. Right now privacy isn't what's most important for the people of Wuhan; survival is.

Right now the god of the underworld is still playing his death fugue. Once the music has ended, we will seek out a cure.

Today one of my classmates told me that he was getting ready to go outside when his three-year-old granddaughter pleaded with him: "Grandpa, please don't go out. There is a disease outside!" I also saw a video online of a child, also around three years old, who wanted to go outside and asked her daddy for the key. She said that she just wanted to look around at Wal-Mart. But the most heartbreaking story is the grandfather who was dead for days, but his grandchild was afraid to go outside because of the coronavirus, so he just lived on crackers for several days. There are all too many stories like that. There are so many children who won't dare go outside because their parents keep scaring them by saying: "You'll get sick if you go out! You'll get sick!" The virus has already found its way into their hearts, living like a devil inside them. I wonder if when the day comes that they can finally go outside whether or not there will be children too scared to go out. Who knows how long the dark cloud of this will linger on inside them? These children have never committed any crimes against this earth, yet they too have to endure this suffering along with the adults. This afternoon a few colleagues and I chatted online, and we each reflected a bit on what we were doing in our lives before January 20th; we ended up all cursing those people we felt were the biggest culprits behind all of this, which made us all feel a bit better. We have all been traumatized by this in different ways; looking back, none of us feel lucky—we just feel like survivors.

This afternoon, Headlines Today had an article that tried to cover up for the *Yangtze Daily*; it was highly likely that it was the work of one of those "sophisticated critics" who specialize in saying nasty things in nice ways. The article quoted some lines from a *Yangtze Daily* reporter who had attacked and mocked Professor Dai Jianye[35] and me, calling us "internet trolls." I'm not going to even bother engaging with the devious motives of this "sophisticated critic." But that reporter from the *Yangtze Daily* is really in a weak position; she lacks even the most basic understanding and judgment. When I discussed the article "Seven Final Words That Left Everyone in Tears," I just focused on one small aspect of the story; I thought it should have been titled "Eleven Final Words That Left Everyone in Tears." It would have been a great article if they had just changed that number. And I doubt that it was even the reporter's fault; based on my experience, I would bet that it was actually an editor behind a desk somewhere who came up with that headline. All I did was raise a few questions about the article from the perspective of a reader, and now that suddenly makes me an "internet troll"! Frankly speaking, I have always had a good impression of the *Yangtze Daily*. When I was a teenager I actually wrote several articles for the former editor with whom I actually collaborated on some stories. For many years now, the paper has managed to maintain a very high editorial standard and level of reporting. Did its high level of professionalism and quality reporting ever before result in such an embarrassing spectacle as we are seeing today? The fact that it is now being targeted for criticism is something for which they have only themselves to blame. The good reputation the paper had was destroyed by those people who keep writing articles that fawn over what the officials are doing, the people who ignored the second half of those "final words," and those other "sophisticated critics." We should all reflect on this together. As I get to this point, I feel that I might as well do some "trolling." But on second thought, forget it. Some of my classmates work in the newspaper industry; I'd hate to embarrass them.

Finally, there are a few bits of news I want to record here:

1. Twenty-six medical professionals have now died in the fight against the coronavirus. I hope they rest in peace. The reason we take care of ourselves and stay locked up is so that their sacrifice will not be in vain.

2. I heard from a professor friend that representatives from the World Health Organization in Beijing said that, to date, the only medicine proven to be effective in fighting the novel coronavirus seems to be remdesivir.

3. There are more than two million face masks coming into Wuhan every day. Every morning starting at 10:00 a.m. you can reserve masks using your ID card or other forms of identification. You can search for the details on how to purchase them online.

FEBRUARY 26, 2020

Shouting slogans like "by any means necessary"
is not based on good science.

Today it is cloudy and overcast but not too cold. Outside my window you can see signs of spring everywhere. I let my dog out to play in the courtyard; it has been a full month since he had a bath and is starting to get stinky. Unfortunately, the corner of his dog tub is cracked, so it can't hold water anymore and the pet store is still closed so I can't buy a new one. It is another annoying little item that I'll have to deal with in the next couple of days.

My doctor friends keep sending me updates about the situation with the coronavirus. I decided to summarize what they told me, along with some reflections based on my own understanding of the main issues, into seven points:

1. The number of patients in Wuhan who have made a full recovery and been discharged from hospitals continues to increase. It is clear that as long as infections don't turn critical, there is a very high rate of recovery. One of my classmates was just discharged from the hospital yesterday and has now checked into a hotel for a 14-day quarantine period. She is clearly feeling much better about her situation than before.

2. The number of people dying from the coronavirus is clearly starting to decline. This is excellent news. Humans are quite tough, after all. One girl I know who used to live across the street told me that her uncle just died. Before that, her aunt had also been taken by the coronavirus. That's another two people in one family. I basically watched her grow up when she used to live by me. She told me that her aunt and uncle went to the hospital on the 30th, but since there were no cars or public transport available, they were forced to walk all the way there. Just thinking about that scene is almost too much to bear. At first she was too scared to tell her parents, since she knew how close her mother was to her uncle; she didn't know how to break it to them. My god, after hearing so many stories like this, I'm really at a loss as to what I can say to console her. All the doctors are working so hard; they are really doing everything in their power, but we need to urge them to keep going in order to spare the world from even more heartbreak and pain.

3. For the past week the number of newly confirmed patients and suspected new cases has continued to fluctuate. I checked the numbers and yesterday there were 401 new confirmed cases of

coronavirus in Wuhan. But the total number of new cases in Hubei Province, not counting Wuhan, was less than 40. Outside of Hubei Province, there were less than 10 new cases reported nationwide. That is to say, right now the coronavirus is more or less under control all over the country, with the exception of Wuhan. This brings me to something that I am still rather confused about. Everyone in Wuhan has been quarantined at home for the past month, so where are all these new patients coming from? I asked another one of my doctor friends for her take on this phenomenon. She feels that there are still some blind spots where there are even more unreported cases. For instance, no one anticipated there would be a huge spike in infections inside the prison system, nor did anyone anticipate the large number of infections in nursing homes. These are all places that were initially overlooked during the early stages of the outbreak. Moreover, both nursing homes and prisons have robust numbers of staff and workers, so when they go home each day, how many people are those staff members in contact with? I'm afraid that these may be sources for many of the infections. Besides this, there is also a floating population, and I'm sure that some of them must also be infected, but no one knows just how many. All these people are somewhat marginalized vis-à-vis mainstream society; however, when you add them all up, the total numbers are not at all insignificant. And then there is that fact that when the elderly get infected, unless they have severe symptoms, they cannot be admitted to those temporary hospitals (there is an age restriction), so that many of them never get into the hospital system. This is also a problem. The only thing to celebrate right now is the fact that almost all the new infections are mild cases, and they tend to have a very high recovery rate.

4. The availability of hospital beds has continued to improve. When I followed up about the issue of older patients' being unable to get admitted into hospitals, my doctor friend said that now things have finally eased up and elderly patients with minor symptoms are now allowed to be admitted. Actually, I have heard from other sources that there are a lot of patients and their families who have been particularly picky about which hospitals they go to; there are only certain hospitals that they will even agree to be admitted to. Often they decide not to be admitted if they can't get into the hospital of their choice. I figure that amid this novel coronavirus outbreak, the treatment you receive in all these hospitals must be fairly consistent? You should just get in where you can and start getting treatment first. If you put off treatment, you will have a much greater chance of getting worse; if you wait for a bed at your preferred hospital, you might not even be alive by the time you get in! So for all those people out there being picky about which hospital to go to, I would recommend just focusing on getting into *any* hospital you can get into; after all, it is your life at stake.

5. The outbreak in Wuhan is still not yet under control. (There are some people who don't agree with this doctor's views and think it is under control. But my doctor friend refuted that by asking, "Then where do you think these hundreds of new patients a day are coming from?") Up until now, it has been very difficult to get to where we need to be. My doctor friend said that after several government officials were fired in Huanggang, their disease prevention measures have markedly improved and good measures are now properly in place. Huanggang is a poor region with a high population; due to its close proximity to Wuhan, medical personnel are able to go back and forth quickly, and they have been able to swiftly get a handle on the outbreak in Huanggang. Overall, Huanggang has done an ex-

cellent job in managing this outbreak. The national forces that were called in to provide support for Huanggang have already left the area for Luotian Hot Springs, which is basically announcing that they have emerged victorious against the coronavirus in Huanggang. This reminds me of a text I received this morning about Liu Xuerong's "Five Firsts": He was the first to expel the Municipal Director of the National Health Commission from office; he was the first to close districts, villages, and roads; he was the first to require all residents to have mandatory temperature checks; he was the first to have the police line up to salute and welcome medical teams and supplies that were coming into the city; and he was the first to send exhausted medical teams to Luotian Hot Springs Hotel and Resort for a much-needed two-week vacation to reward them for all their hard work. The name Liu Xuerong sounded quite familiar, but I couldn't remember who he was. I searched him online and realized that he is a graduate of the Huazhong University of Science and Technology electrical engineering program and currently serves as the Huanggang Party Secretary.

6. After having the city of Wuhan under quarantine for such a long period of time, the people have been forced to put up with all kinds of inconveniences, which have really pushed us to the very limit. Yet the results have still been far from ideal. We need to immediately start trying to figure out just how those hundreds of new cases got infected. There is no way they have all been in incubation for a full month and suddenly now just started to show symptoms—they must have newly contracted the disease somewhere. A hundred new infections a day is not a small number; we should be paying a lot of attention to this! Further extending the lockdown long-term isn't a solution, as it will lead to a chain reaction of other serious problems. We need to get to the bottom of these new infections and

start quarantining people with laser-like precision. If we are able to quarantine everyone who falls into the four categories (confirmed cases, suspected cases, patients with a high fever, and close contacts of patients), everyone else should be safe and we can start restoring society to its normal functioning order. This entire section consists of comments from my doctor friend, relayed here, almost verbatim.

7. The first group of medical volunteers from outside Hubei has been working hard for more than a month, and many of them have already reached their breaking point; they are now in desperate need of rest and reorganization. But where are the backup troops? There is no way the country will be able to send another 30,000 medical workers to relieve them! If we don't get this outbreak under control soon, things will start to turn very dangerous. These are also comments taken word-for-word from my doctor friend.

I read a really interesting interview in *Caijing* magazine with Professor Wang Liming from Zhejiang University. Many of the ideas that Professor Wang expressed in this interview were quite smart and helped me understand some of the things I had been confused about. These are a few highlights from the interview:

1. As a scientist, it seems that conspiracy theories are taking over, to the point that they are now becoming a regular part of our world. The modern world is becoming increasingly complicated, and science and technology are becoming increasingly specialized and non-intuitive; it is getting to the point that your average person can no longer find their way in this confusing modern world.

2. Ever since the Enlightenment, humankind has felt that everything in the world is able to be understood through the existing framework of human knowledge. Of course, you can see this as the tri-

umph of human knowledge, but it can also be seen as a sign of human arrogance.

3. When attempting to control this public health threat, we must first respect science and the opinion of specialists in the field; we must not let political motivations displace the guidance of specialists.

4. I want to again emphasize that, while it is wonderful that the nation has been funneling all its energy and resources to fight this outbreak, in the process of determining the problems that need to be addressed, and as we adjust our focus over the course of this struggle against the coronavirus, we must respect the principles of basic science. Shouting slogans like "by any means necessary" is not based on good science.

5. I think that at this stage of the outbreak, what we really need are infectious disease specialists who can help us analyze the unique characteristics of the novel coronavirus. We need them to look at how this virus differs from other infectious diseases and then make scientifically based predictions about how this virus will likely behave, moving forward, so that we can adjust our strategies for future containment. Our strategy for controlling this outbreak cannot be guided by haphazard decisions.

6. Since the outbreak of the novel coronavirus, tens of thousands of people have been infected, several thousand patients have died, and with that we have suffered economic losses totaling several hundred million yuan. During this time, we have not seen a single responsible party stand up and accept any of the blame for what has happened; no one has accepted even a portion of the blame, and no one has apologized to the people. It is as if everyone has silently accepted the fact that no one is to blame for any of this. During this period of struggle against the coronavirus, we need to be brave, and we need "positive strength." Of course, it is correct that we shouldn't

only focus on the negative aspects of this, but we should also not forget where the responsibility falls and should use this to improve our system.

Today one of my classmates sent me a message, hoping that I might respond to a post online imploring the physician-husband of the recently deceased Dr. Xia Sisi to step back and stop treating patients on the front lines of the outbreak. According to my classmate: "We want to try to do something like they did in *Saving Private Ryan*. Someone responded by suggesting that we should establish something like the Sole Survivor Policy that the United States enacted after the five Sullivan brothers were all killed in action during World War II. Perhaps if you can say something about this in your diary, you can help prevent other doctor families from suffering multiple losses on the front lines of this epidemic."

I completely understand the thoughtfulness and kindness behind this request; however, I'm not entirely in favor of this appeal. First, I feel we need to respect the wishes of Xia Sisi's husband; only he can decide whether or not he wants to go to the front lines; second, Xia Sisi was infected early on, before we knew that the novel coronavirus was contagious and before medical personnel were wearing proper protective gear. Back then, many doctors were, in fact, not taking *any* special precautions when dealing with patients. Things are very different now; medical personnel are fully equipped with protective gear, and there is now a very low rate of infection among doctors and nurses; and third, there isn't a hospital out there that is not part of the front line. Although that is not to say that everyone needs to have direct contact with coronavirus patients. And so I feel that perhaps it is best if Xia Sisi's husband tries to carry on with his normal routine, whether that means going to work at the hospital or taking some time off to deal with his loss.

FEBRUARY 27, 2020

That's right; there is nothing better than staying alive.

Overcast again with a chill in the air, although it really isn't that cold. If you were to go outside and look up, you'd discover that the absence of the sun leaves the sky feeling dark and gloomy.

The diary post that I uploaded yesterday on WeChat got deleted again. It was also blocked on Weibo. I thought my account might be completely blocked, but I tested it and figured out that they had only blocked that one entry, but I was still able to send out other messages. I suppose I should be happy about that. My god, I have grown so apprehensive that I'm not even sure what to say anymore. It feels like I can't say anything. Fighting the coronavirus is the most important task before us; we should all be doing everything in our power to cooperate with the government and follow its lead. Do I really need to shake my first in the air and swear my allegiance to the cause? Will that be enough?

Here we are still locked up in our homes, unable even to set foot outside the door, yet others have already begun to chant victory songs about how we vanquished this outbreak! I even saw an image of a book cover of a new publication about how we emerged victorious over the coronavirus (I'm not sure if that cover was real or a parody)! What can the people of Wuhan say? No matter how anxious or restless we may be, we have no choice but to bear it, no? Victory will be shared by all. Today I saw another meme online: *When you hear people say, "We will sacrifice everything at any cost," don't misunderstand "we" as meaning "us"—you are actually the "cost."*

What's the point of saying anything else? We just have to wait. We need to try to remain calm and steady and just wait. To borrow my big brother's way of describing it in simple language: "It's boring as hell, but you have no choice but just stay home and binge-watch TV miniseries to help pass the time."

Today my doctor friend told me that quite a few patients have just been released from the hospitals. So far, more than 2,000 patients have recovered; mild cases are fairly easy to treat. There are now quite a few hospital beds available. The number of patients dying has also dropped considerably. I looked up the figures and discovered that during the previous couple of days there were around a hundred deaths each day, but yesterday that number dropped to 29. How I hope we can get that number down to zero soon! Then all those anxious and worried families will finally be able to rest easy again. As long as we can stay alive, everything else can be figured out later. If it takes longer to treat people, it's okay; take your time, we can handle the wait. I just watched an episode of *Southern City News* that profiled the process of a doctor trying to save a coronavirus patient. The episode included interview footage with both the doctor and the patient, and it was quite moving. The patient who survived said that he needed to rely on his own willpower, along with the faith his doctor had in him to get through it. Another patient said that after surviving this entire journey he feels that he will now treasure each and every day that lies ahead. That's right; there is nothing better than staying alive.

What continues to stump people is the continuing high numbers of new infections that we are still seeing, which has left Wuhan in something of a stalemate position with the virus. Just yesterday the number of new and probable infections was up to 900. This is not the result we have been looking for. All these people must have gotten infected after the citywide quarantine went into effect. We need to know who these people are, where they live, the circumstances of how they got infected; it would be good if the coronavirus report that comes out every day could include more details like this. If some of these details were made public, perhaps others would be better able to protect themselves. Also, based on location, perhaps the government could start relaxing the quarantine for areas located far away from the hot spots. Another doctor friend of mine feels that the coronavirus outbreak is already under control; almost all the new cases are confined to jails and nursing homes. If that's the case, then how come so many people still need to be quarantined to their homes? Perhaps we'll be getting some good news soon? But that is just a hopeful guess!

From the perspective of infectious diseases, 900 is a fairly large number, but when you look at it in relation to a population of tens of millions of people who live in Hubei Province, it is just a tiny fraction. But this tiny fraction of the population is holding tens of millions of healthy people hostage in their own homes; when you think about it like that, who wouldn't be upset? And what will those healthy people be facing down the road? Will the price they have to pay be even greater? I can't say for sure.

And then there are those five million people from Wuhan who are stuck outside the city unable to return home; I wonder how they have been getting through all this. They faced a lot of prejudice early on; I wonder if that has improved at all? There are also those people from other provinces working in Wuhan who are stuck here and unable to get out of the city. I saw a report the other day about some of them who don't have enough money for a hotel or simply couldn't find a hotel and ended up sleeping in the train station. Others don't have enough to eat and end up going through the garbage and eating other people's leftovers. Those people in change of steering the ship often neglect these small details; those in charge of looking after the majority often overlook those more marginalized individuals. One good bit of news was that I did later see a report about a "help hotline for individuals from out of town stuck in Wuhan during the coronavirus outbreak." Each district has its own hotline for people to call. I just don't know if when you call, those hotline operators really have the power to help these people out. I know that a lot of those types of hotlines are only set up as a show to make the political leaders look good. If you actually call these numbers, you'll find they are basically useless. Just give it a try. If you call, you'll just get the runaround, but no real help; in the end you'll just waste the price of the phone call. The world of officialdom is filled with people who have never learned a damn thing in their entire lives, but one thing they have mastered is the art of putting on a show; and they have ways to deal with you that you would have never imagined even existed. Their ability to shirk responsibility is also second to none; if they didn't have a good foundation in all these worthless skills, this outbreak would have never grown into the large-scale calamity that it is today.

From the first cases of the coronavirus in Wuhan to the point when the quarantine was imposed, there was a delay of more than 20 days; this is an undisputed fact. But what was the main reason for this delay? Who, exactly, caused this delay that would give the coronavirus time and space to spread, leading to the unprecedented lockdown of the entire city of Wuhan? Quarantining nearly nine million people to their homes is a strange and rare situation, but certainly not one to be proud of. There must be an investigation to get to the root cause behind this delay.

There are a lot of reporters in China who kiss up to the government, but we still have never had a shortage of brave journalists who dare to speak up. These past few days I have witnessed a group of journalists who have been relentlessly digging to get the real stories out there. In the internet age we need to rely on journalists to carry out in-depth investigative research, and we need netizens everywhere to do their part by helping to shed light on those critical events in order to gradually expose all those secrets that have been hidden away and covered up.

No matter what happens, there is a process we need to go through to get to the bottom of what has happened. For instance, there were three groups of specialists that came to Wuhan. We need to know things like: Who were the members of each group? Who led each group? Who was the host organization in Wuhan that received them? Which hospitals did they visit? How many departments did they visit? How many meetings did they hold? Who spoke at those meetings? Which doctors did they question? What kind of information did they get from those doctors? What kind of records did they review? What did they learn from the materials they reviewed? What conclusions did they come to? Who had the final say in the groups' decisions? These are the questions we need to be asking. After all, those eight words, "Not Contagious Between People, It's Controllable and Preventable," resulted in untold suffering for the Wuhan people; there needs to be some accountability. If we dig deeply enough, we can certainly figure out who have been the liars through all this. We need to figure out who lied and why they lied, under whose orders did they decide to skirt the truth; did they know these were blatant lies, or was someone intentionally spreading false information and they just chose to believe it; did they feel they had no choice but to accept these deceptions? Did these lies come from the government or from those teams of specialists? Through careful investigation we should be able to get to the bottom of all of this. For a catastrophe of this scale, simply firing a few officials is not enough to settle this matter. The people of Wuhan will settle for nothing less than full accountability for all those who had a part in orchestrating these lies and carrying out the damaging policies that followed. More than 2,000 "murdered" souls (I'm sure there are even more who have not been counted in the official numbers) and their family members have died and suffered, medical professionals have been struggling day and night to save critically ill patients, nine million Wuhan residents have been forced to self-quarantine, five million Wuhan residents have been stuck outside the city, unable to return home—all of us want an explanation; all of us want some kind of closure.

But all we have gotten is endless waiting—waiting for the city to reopen, waiting for an explanation.

FEBRUARY 28, 2020

The period we refer to as Early Spring
always seems to have a few days like this.

The weather is still overcast and it is starting to get colder. Dusk is coming earlier than before; if you don't turn on your lights by 4:00 p.m. it will already be quite dark inside. The period we refer to as Early Spring always seems to have a few days like this.

I noticed that someone had forwarded a video on Weibo of former Chinese Premier Zhu Rongji[36] doing a self-introduction in Shanghai. There was one sentence he said in his speech that I really liked: "The core of my philosophy boils down to independent thinking." That is also my belief. I participated in a literary conference right after graduating from college and heard the veteran writer Jiang Hong say it this way: "We have to make sure that our heads are firmly supported by *our own* shoulders!" That quote left a deep impression on me. I thought, that's right, our heads, our thoughts, shouldn't be resting on the shoulders of our teachers, or the newspapers we read, and especially not on the documents passed out at government meetings; they need to be sitting firmly on our own shoulders. My brain only has value if I use it to foster independent thought. So it doesn't matter if the ultra-leftists curse me or the ultra-rightists criticize me; none of them can change my view of the world, nor can they shake my views on society and human nature. Yesterday I was chatting with my classmate Yi Zhongtian[37] and I told him that I thought, at their core, those ultra-leftists and ultra-rightists were essentially the same. He wholeheartedly agreed with me. The reason I say these two radical groups are the same is simply because neither one of them is capable of accepting anyone with views different than their own. As Yi Zhongtian described it: "They are like two sides of the same coin; neither one is able to embrace a pluralistic environment; both of them want a world that only accepts one type of voice, one type of viewpoint."

Every day I record the little things happening around me and add a few thoughts and feelings that I find interesting. This is a purely individual record written in diary form. It isn't intended as a vessel for grand narratives, nor can it record all the details surrounding the coronavirus outbreak, and I certainly try to avoid the impassioned language of those idealistic young writers. Instead I try to write freely, getting my emotions down on paper. This isn't a news chronicle, and it certainly isn't a novel. At the same time, the emotions I express are often very different from those of other people, nor are they always in line with what other people expect. But an individual record is never supposed to fit into a standardized package. Isn't that common sense? But there are some people who have expended boundless energy working up their anger toward me, all because of this diary. They waste what should be time spent doing enjoyable things to curse me. It's a real shame. Of course, if they really derive so much pleasure from these hateful acts, perhaps I should just allow them to get their kicks.

I read an essay today that said Fang Fang shouldn't be hiding out at home writing her diary based on gossip she hears; she should get out there in the field where everything is happening! How can I even respond to that? It isn't a question of wanting to get out there in the field; I'm living *in* the field! The entire city of Wuhan is where this is happening! I am one of the nine million victims of this epidemic. My neighbors, classmates, coworkers are all locked down here in Wuhan; we all are. When they go online and share their experiences and what they have witnessed, why shouldn't I be documenting all of that? Don't tell me that only the sites where these doctors, police officers, and public service people are working qualify as "the field"! I'm here in the field recording what I hear and see, but if you insist on calling that gossip, there is nothing I can say; do as you wish.

Forget it, let's not talk about this stuff.

In last night's diary entry I raised the question of where all these new patients are coming from. Not long after that, a friend sent me a data spreadsheet of all the newly diagnosed patients in Wuhan. This allowed me to see that the new cases are not concentrated in one area; they are spread out all over the city. This means the idea of gradually starting to open up a few districts that are less heavily affected by the new coronavirus cases is simply not practical. Today one of my doctor friends sent a message to tell me "the coronavirus is now spreading in clusters"; these new cases are dispersed throughout all 13 administrative districts in the city. Right now the entire country has the coronavirus under control; the only task ahead is caring for those patients already infected. The only trouble spot is Wuhan, where the novel coronavirus has still not been able to be controlled; we need to remain vigilant.

The good news is that more and more people are being released from the hospitals. I looked up some government statements and it seems that after careful monitoring, there have been no observed cases of recovered coronavirus patients spreading the disease to others. Moreover, most of the new cases have turned out to be patients who were previously in the "suspected cases" category; the ratio seems to be as high as 80 or 90 percent. These government sources are much more optimistic than what I am hearing from my doctor friends. They have already reached their target of having hospital beds available at all times. It wasn't long ago that hospital beds were so tight that the temporary hospitals were forced to admit some of the more serious cases. Now all those patients in critical condition have been removed from the temporary hospitals and transferred to the main hospitals. My doctor friend said that actually the "serious cases" we are seeing right now cannot compare to what we were dealing with just a few weeks ago.

The death rate has dramatically declined. There are a lot of people posting stories online stating that recent autopsies of deceased coronavirus patients have discovered an issue with built-up phlegm in many of the victims. That led to new treatment measures, which have cut the number of deaths in half. My doctor friend said that "the decline in deaths should be attributed to a multitude of factors: All our medical resources have been replenished, medical caregivers can now deliver better and more specialized care thanks to an increase in abilities, energy, and resources; but it is certainly much more than just the result of some discoveries made during recent autopsies. Once patients take a turn for the worse, Acute Respiratory Distress Syndrome (ARDS) sets in and large amounts of fluid begin to collect in the pulmonary alveoli and it is common for large amounts of sticky mucus to form. In many instances, the first thing that doctors do once a breathing tube is inserted is to extract the excess mucus either via a suction tube or through a bronchoscopy. However, because the sticky phlegm builds up and congeals inside the bronchus and pulmonary alveoli, it cannot be sucked out, which is a common sign of ARDS. This is precisely why the lungs are unable to function normally; even if the patient receives pure oxygen, it still isn't enough to compensate for dangerously low blood oxygen levels." Those were the doctor's exact words. I was only able to get a basic understanding of some of the technical points, so I naturally cannot comment on how accurate this assessment is. But with my doctor friend's permission, I have included what he wrote above as part of the record.

I also want to record what Professor Liu Liang and his team have been doing; under the most difficult conditions, they have been conducting autopsies on novel coronavirus victims in order to further research this disease. I saw a video interview with Professor Liu that really opened my eyes to the challenges that he and his team are facing each day. I really have the utmost respect for the work that he is doing. I'm sure that his efforts will greatly benefit our future treatment and preventive strategies for this virus moving forward. I'm especially moved by those family members who have selflessly agreed to let their loved one's bodies be donated for research. Without their sacrifice, Professor Liu's team would be unable to achieve any new breakthroughs in our understanding of the novel coronavirus. Human knowledge is always long eclipsed by the broad expanse of the unknown; in order to expand our understanding by just a tiny bit, we need to rely on the strenuous efforts of many people. But for a literary person like me, all I can do is keep a record of the things I see and hear.

Right now there are still quite a few new suspected cases of coronavirus in Wuhan. Who are these people? Where did they get infected? I got a private message from someone online telling me that some of them are volunteers and another portion of them are community workers. That sounds like it makes sense. Those volunteers have been out and about all over the city providing all kinds of services; those

community workers have also been incredibly busy during this unusual time. The higher-ups are always giving them pressure to carry
out all kinds of tasks, and the citizens down below go to them for almost everything. Some of these people can be very difficult with their
requests, and everyone is waiting for them to deliver results; but it is
still hard to say who the ones getting infected really are. Their protective gear is not nearly as good as what medical professionals have; in
fact, some of them only have disposable face masks. But then one of
my friends told me that there were a lot of infections among the volunteers and community workers early on, but right now there are close
to none. She said: "During the early stage of the outbreak, things were
fairly stable at all the retirement homes, prisons, and mental hospitals.
More recently there has been more testing being done at these types of
facilities, and that has resulted in some new cases being added to the
numbers." Everyone seems to have their own interpretation to explain
the spike in numbers.

The people of Wuhan seem to be quite calm these days. Of course,
they might just be weary and depressed. In order to prevent multiple
exposures, people are no longer allowed to crowd around the main
gate to pick up their online grocery deliveries. But everyone is stuck
inside and they still need to eat, so they came up with an alternate
method: Everyone now ties a rope to a bucket and slowly lowers it
down from their balconies, then community workers fill up their buckets with their groceries and hoist them back up. Some of them hoist
their buckets all the way up as high as the sixth floor! It is a technical
feat, but most people are adapting quickly. I watched a two-minute
video of some people hoisting their groceries up and couldn't help but
feel a strange sadness. The challenges and difficulties that the people
of Wuhan and all these community workers are experiencing are really
quite out of the ordinary.

FEBRUARY 29, 2020

The silence of the collective is always the most terrifying thing.

It is clear again today. That's how the weather has been going lately: clear then overcast, clear then overcast; it's kind of like my *Wuhan Diary*—first they allow it, then they crack down on it, then they allow it, then they crack down on it again. I've been cooped up at home for so long, I wonder how I'll adapt once we are allowed to go outside again. I even wonder if I'll be *willing* to go back outside. Today my neighbor Tang Xiaohe sent me a series of recent photos of East Lake; they look like they were taken by a drone. The lake is empty and quiet, the red and white plum blossoms along the lake are in full bloom; it is truly gorgeous beyond description. I forwarded the photo to another colleague and she said that staring at the photo, she felt like she was going to cry. My goodness, "how I lament the disappearance of spring. Crimson apricot flowers. Red begonias. I gaze on the delicate branches, and silently curse the lord in heaven."[38] These lines of poetry really fit my mood right now.

I have a very strong sense that most people in Wuhan are feeling a bit depressed these days. Even my most vibrant and outgoing colleagues have all fallen silent. Barely anyone in my family sends texts to our group chat anymore. Is everyone just sitting at home binge-watching TV shows? I certainly hope that's the case. It is a real test of will to remain quarantined and idle for this long. Everyone in the city of Wuhan is living with this strange, unspeakable stress; I'm afraid people outside the city have no way to truly understand what we are going through. There are no words strong enough to capture the sacrifices that the people of Wuhan have had to make during this outbreak. We will continue to hold on; we will continue to listen to the government and follow the instructions they give us. Today is already the 38th day of the quarantine.

With the exception of Wuhan, the coronavirus is now under control, with zero new cases reported outside of Hubei. The situation in Wuhan is also looking better. My doctor friend told me that there were nearly 40,000 people who fall into the category of having had close contact with confirmed patients; he wondered if all the new suspected cases were from this same pool of people. If they are, then these new confirmed cases are also mostly from that pool of suspected patients. Assuming that is true, then we indeed have a much clearer picture of the outbreak and its pattern. We just need to screen those 40,000 patients to confirm this. From this perspective, the outbreak in Wuhan could be considered to be under control. However, my doctor friend remains cautious about getting too optimistic; he feels that the published government statistics need to be a bit more detailed before he is ready to make any conclusions. But I'm already starting to feel more optimistic. Although there are still some people from those four categories who have fallen through the net and remain among the general population of nine million residents, I'm sure that with our current screening capabilities and methods we will be able to locate everyone quickly.

Today one of my friends sent me a video from Shandong Province; it was of the people in Zibo welcoming the Blue Sky Aid Team back home after returning from their humanitarian aid trip to Wuhan. Everyone was in tears to see the group safely returning home. After watching the video, I was in tears too. It is hard to imagine what things would have looked like in Wuhan if we didn't have support from all those aid teams that came in from all over China. So many people were crying because they all understood the dangers involved in coming to Wuhan to offer help; returning home in one piece is indeed a blessing. I have heard that in Wuhan, besides the high rate of infections among medical professionals, the police have also been hit hard. I was somewhat surprised to learn this, so I searched online and, indeed, nearly 400 police officers in Hubei Province have been infected with the novel coronavirus. I never imagined it was so many.

I decided to write to a police officer friend of mine to find out what the situation was like with him and his fellow officers. He responded by saying that he and his colleagues have consistently been on the front lines of this outbreak. He personally has not taken a single day off since the outbreak began. They needed to ensure that all the basic transportation networks in the city were still functioning for deliveries and so that medical personnel could still get to where they needed to be, yet at the same time they also had to control pedestrians and private cars that shouldn't be out on the streets; somehow they needed to be able to differentiate between these two groups. A lot of police officers have been helping drive patients to and from the hospitals; there simply were not enough EMTs and medical workers to transport all those patients. Moreover, all the roads in and out of the city need to have officers on guard 24 hours a day in order to ensure that medical aid workers can pass, while making sure that other traffic is prohibited. Besides this, a police presence is also needed at each hospital, quarantine location, and various public service locations in order to maintain order, direct traffic, and help resolve conflicts between doctors and unruly patients. Since the police have so much contact with patients, their risk for infection is also quite high. So it is not strange at all to hear that so many police officers have been infected. My friend encouraged me on: "Please write about what the police are going through; we really have been working nonstop!"

The people of Wuhan have a popular saying: "When you're busy, you work yourself to death; when you're idle, you bore yourself to death!"

But now it seems clear: When you are idle it is the psychological stress that gets you; when you are busy it is the physical stress that gets you. We all need to grit our teeth and get through this together.

For the past few days, reporters have been investigating why there was an almost 20-day lag in responding to the initial outbreak. They have been chasing this story with great tenacity and the deeper they dig, the clearer the picture is becoming. It is hard not to admire what they are doing. A lot of great journalists may have left the field, but there are still some amazing reporters out there doing good work. One reporter rolled out a timeline that clearly shows that for some reason the Wuhan Municipal Health Commission waited several days before making a report.

One investigative reporter interviewed a specialist who claimed that he didn't know what had been happening. He was even suspicious about whether there were any doctors who had really been infected, so he called to ask, but everyone denied it. I decided to check with one of my doctor friends, so I asked him: "I heard that there were some specialists who called the hospital to ask about the virus early on?" My friend responded: "There is no way they could call us at the hospital." So I followed up, "But couldn't they have called and spoken to one of the hospital administrators?" My friend said he wasn't sure. I then called another doctor friend to get her perspective on this. She was extremely direct in her answers: "They all came down here to the hospital; how is it possible that they didn't know?" But according to the specialists, it is a big hospital and there was no way for them to check everything. The officials just said that they were following the advice of the specialists. I told my doctor friend what those officials and specialists had said and she replied: "Actually, all the doctors knew that there was human-to-human transmission going on with this virus; we all reported it. But no one informed the public, at least not until Zhong

Nanshan arrived in Wuhan and made a public statement about it." Another doctor I know told me: "The silence of the collective is always the most terrifying thing." But then who is actually included among this "collective"? I didn't ask him that question; I didn't want to make things complicated; after all, I'm not a reporter. But someone online summed things up perfectly when he said: "The blame game contest has officially begun!"

Let me share a few quotes from an interview with Dr. Peng Zhiyong, director of Zhongnan Hospital of Wuhan University:

This virus indeed spread extremely quickly. On January 10, our 16 ICU beds were already full. When I saw how serious things were, I immediately went to the hospital administrators and said that we need to report what is happening. They also thought the situation was grave and sent a report to the Wuhan Municipal Health Commission. On January 12 the Wuhan Municipal Health Commission sent a three-person team of specialists to Zhongnan Hospital to investigate. Based on their clinical observations, the specialists thought that the virus somewhat resembled SARS; however, they insisted on sticking to standard diagnostic protocols. During the next few days, our hospital administrators followed up several times with the Health Commission, and I know that other hospitals did as well.

Just before this, the National Health Commission had already sent a team of specialists to Jinyintan Hospital to investigate. They came up with a set of standards for diagnosis, such as having visited the Huanan Seafood Market, fever, and a positive test result for the presence of the virus; only when all three of these criteria were met could a patient be confirmed as positive. They were especially strict about that third criteria, even when in reality very few people were actually tested.

Based on my past knowledge and clinical observations treating patients, I deemed this illness to be a strong contagious virus that should require the highest level of protective measures. Viruses don't bend to the will of man; we need to respect the spirit of science and move forward based on what the scientific evidence tells us. Responding to my requests, Zhongnan Hospital's ICU adopted strict quarantine measures, and our department only had two medical workers who were infected with the novel coronavirus. As of January 28, hospital-wide there were only 40 medical workers who were infected, a number much lower than at other hospitals.

From the previous three paragraphs, you can see that the situation was quite dire before January 10th. In the end, doctors needed to individually take action to protect themselves. And even at Zhongnan Hospital where they took aggressive protective actions early on, they still had 40 medical workers who were infected, which is a very low rate of infection as compared to other hospitals. If you think about it, the whip of collective silence struck down on all of us. This is something that all hospitals will need to reflect on once the epidemic has passed.

In the afternoon I spent a long time talking to a friend about how the coronavirus has been affecting children. This virus has torn so many families apart; but in some ways the children have been affected even worse than the elderly. How many children have been orphaned over the course of this outbreak? I'm not sure if anyone has even calculated that figure yet. Just among the doctors who have died that we know about, there are already four: two infants and two unborn children whose fathers have already died. My friend told me that there is an entire group of around two dozen children who have lost both parents to the coronavirus; then there are many others who have had both of their parents ordered into hospital quarantine or have lost one of their parents. The government has already made arrangements for these children to be taken care of together in a group home. They are all minors; some of the young ones are just four or five years old. According to my friend, many of them are terrified by the sight of people wearing biosuits and face masks. At that tender age they probably don't even know how to express their fears and share their feelings with anyone. Sure, their basic essentials are now all being taken care of, but what about the psychological scars inside them? This is especially important in the case of those newly orphaned children. Those big, strong trees that once sheltered them from the wind and rain have now been toppled and they have no one left to rely on; many of them will never know unconditional parental love again. I wonder if there is anyone there to help them through this pain? As my friend always says, the earlier they receive psychological intervention, the better.

I keep hearing these recordings online of a child somewhere crying and screaming: "Mommy, don't leave me! I love you so much, Mommy. . . ." As a mother, anytime I hear such a voice, I can't help but feel a cold shiver run through my entire body.

MARCH

We still have many more tears left to cry.

As we move further and further away from the Lunar New Year, I have decided to start using the Western calendar instead of the lunar calendar to date all my entries.[1]

The weather continues to fluctuate back and forth between clear and cloudy, which makes a lot of people even more stressed out. I only now suddenly realize that today is Sunday. When you are cooped up at home all the time, one of the biggest problems is that you completely lose track of time. I usually have no idea what the date is and have even more trouble remembering what day of the week it is. When can I go outside? When can the city open back up? These are the questions that are weighing most heavily on us these days. Everyone can now clearly see that things are improving with the coronavirus. Everyone in China is pitching in to help Wuhan get through this difficult period. We *will* get past this; everyone in Wuhan has the self-confidence to get us through this. It's just that we still don't know *when* we will be able to go outside again or *when* the city will finally reopen. In private, this is all that anyone is talking about.

It has now been a full 42 days since my middle brother has stepped even one foot outside his apartment. At least I can go out to my court-yard if I need some fresh air or want to walk around a bit. At least the courtyard area is safe. Today my daughter showed off some photos of her cooking skills in our family group chat. Although she always complains about how annoying it is to cook, she is still trying her best to maintain a certain quality of life. The pork braised in brown sauce that she just cooked really looked like the real deal! The other day she said that she felt like she had lost some weight, but I'm sure she'll put those pounds right back on after she gobbles that pork down! Her dad responded to the photo of her dish with a flurry of wild compliments. It is sometimes hard for us to imagine that the younger generation could be this capable. My daughter said that she has already saved a bunch of online cooking recipes. I guess she doesn't need her parents to teach her how to cook; they've got their own way and there are a lot of great teachers online for them!

But as time rolls by, sadder things keep happening. This catastrophe has truly shattered us. It doesn't take much to make us cry anymore. A colleague sent me a video that was taken in the community where she lives. A citizen was expressing his thanks to a local cadre and that male cadre was crying like a baby. One of the comments posted below the video said: "The people of Wuhan have shed a decade worth of tears this month." There is a lot truth behind that comment. These tears are not just tears of sadness; they are mixed with a hundred different emotions. But don't expect the people crying these tears to advance forward singing songs of triumph or to summon up their energy and announce to the world that they have emerged victorious—we still have many more tears left to cry.

This morning at 5:00 a.m., Director Jiang Xueqing[2] of the Wuhan Central Hospital, where Li Wenliang worked, passed away. He was 55 years old and at the prime of his career. I previously mentioned the fact that I know a lot of people in Wuhan and often run into people I know on the street; I may never have met Director Jiang, but the wife of one of my college classmates knew him very well. She sent me a message this morning, describing Dr. Jiang by saying: "He may not have been a whistleblower, but he was always a kind man with strong principles. His patients all trusted him and he always made time for his friends. He helped me get countless friends in to be seen and would always say: 'Whenever you ask me for a favor, I always do my very best to take care of it!' Over the years so many patients sought him out because of his stellar reputation, and he always treated them with kindness when they came in for their appointments or needed surgery. . . . I tried not to send too many of my friends to see him, but he would always say that patient recommendations were the most important endorsement for a doctor." Since she knew him so well, my classmate's wife was really crushed by this loss; she regretted the fact that she hadn't done more to support him when he was alive.

One of my doctor friends also sent me a message about Dr. Jiang Xueqing, saying that he was the only breast and thyroid cancer specialist in China to have received the prestigious "Chinese Physician Prize." Too many medical professionals have tragically sacrificed their lives during this epidemic. In private, someone shared with me the story behind Dr. Jiang Xueqing's death, and it was really too appalling for words. The tragic nature of what happened isn't just about the loss of his life, but also concerns those aspects of his story that we are not permitted to talk about. So . . . I won't talk about them.

With much difficulty and great sluggishness, the outbreak in Wuhan is finally starting to take a turn for the better. There are still several hundred new confirmed and suspected cases that continue to appear on our radar each day. One of my doctor friends was a bit dejected by the numbers he was seeing, based on which he made a prediction: "I think we still need another 10 days before we will see a fundamental change, but we are still probably another month away from really having it under control; then we will still need another two months before we can completely eradicate this virus." As far as we are concerned, all these time frames—whether it is one month or two months away—are all too long. I really hope my friend's prediction is wrong. The spring sunshine today is boundless; I really can't bear for the virus to be the only one that gets to enjoy this beautiful sunny weather; we are all longing to get outside again.

I've been receiving a lot of messages about a healer named Li Yue-hua who everyone says can work wonders; they say that his method of providing injections along traditional Chinese acupuncture points is able to cure the novel coronavirus; moreover, he has been administering treatment without any protective gear and yet continues to be impervious to the virus. I had actually been hoping to write about him here in my diary. Actually, this record is just random sketches that I am jotting down; I don't really have a clear list of topics that I want to cover. But after getting so many letters from people suggesting that I introduce Dr. Li Yuehua to my readers—I have even received videos of him treating patients—I decided I should write about him. Some of the videos I saw were indeed quite something. I heard that he is very much willing to go to hospitals to treat novel coronavirus patients, but they have not approved him. Online, people have been arguing like mad about whether or not he should be allowed to treat patients. I reached out to my friend who teaches at the Institute of Chinese Medicine to get his opinion; he had three points to make:

1. Right now the crux of the issue isn't whether or not Li Yuehua has an official license to practice medicine; the real question is whether or not his method of treatment works. If it is effective, then we should let him start treating patients. After all, shouldn't we all be looking for practical solutions right now?

2. There are a lot of folk doctors whose ability to practice is hindered by the fact that they do not have an official medical license. As far as I know, right now there are two methods for capable folk doctors to attain a license: One is by going through an "apprentice training program," and the other route involves presenting "proof of specialty"; traditional Chinese doctors can go either route to attain the legal right to practice medicine.

3. There are some government offices responsible for granting licenses that actually go out of their way to ignore the empirical facts and instead they just want to clamp down on these folk healers. They do this in the name of fairness, but it is clear that a lot of them have an ulterior motive. But to step back for a moment, Li Yuehua is clearly an example of someone illegally practicing medicine. However, if his method of treatment is found to be beneficial to novel coronavirus patients, the relevant departments should treat this as a special case and make an exception for him to treat patients. They can worry about credentials and licenses later. But right now those government offices are caught up in the issue of Li Yuehua's legal credentials, and they don't seem willing to let that go. They have now pushed Li Yuehua into a corner (the documents I saw seem to indicate that they not only want to use procedural methods against him, but may also be planning on taking legal actions against him). On the surface, it looks like everything they are doing is by the book, but in reality it is quite cold-hearted. If Li Yuehua's method of treatment works, let's not get all tied up on the question of his medical credentials. Those patients he has successfully treated should have a say in this. It shouldn't be too difficult to determine the effectiveness of his treatment methods; all they have to do is conduct a simple investigation by looking at his former patients.

I think my classmate's comments make sense. I'm a layperson when it comes to these issues, so I won't add any additional commentary. Normally, I don't believe in any of those traveling healers. I once went to see a private Chinese medicine doctor about a problem I was having with my foot; the treatment he prescribed was incredibly expensive and, in the end, the medicine he gave me only made my condition worse! Finally, I just went to see a doctor trained in Western medicine to fix the problem.

Ever since then, I usually stick to Western medicine. But occasionally I still use some Chinese herbs for little everyday things. But like many others, I also feel that if Li Yuehua says he has a method that can treat the coronavirus, then what's all the fuss about? Let's at least let him give it a try? Didn't Deng Xiaoping have a famous saying: "It doesn't matter if a cat is black or white, as long as it catches mice it is a good cat." Let me use it here: "It doesn't matter if it is Chinese or Western medicine, if it can cure a patient it is good medicine." We need to be practical when treating patients, especially during an emergency situation like this one. There is nothing more important than saving human lives, so why don't we give this a chance? And if, in the process, he ends up getting exposed as a charlatan, all for the better; let's get it all out there in the open!

MARCH 2, 2020

People in the future will need to know
what everyone in Wuhan went through.

It is raining again and extremely overcast. It feels as cold as it was back during the Lunar New Year. One of my colleagues braved the rain to deliver some steamed buns, Mandarin rolls, and some other snacks to me. I have lived in the Literary and Arts Federation compound for 30 years now, and my neighbors and colleagues have always looked out for me, for which I am especially thankful. Tonight I will eat Mandarin rolls and a bowl of millet porridge. As I said before, cooking for one is never much fun.

These days I tend to stay up late each night and sleep in the next morning. By the time I saw the messages my doctor friend had sent me, it was already noon. In contrast to his rather sullen mood from yesterday, today my doctor friend seems rather excited. That is because he figured out the reason for yesterday's spike in new cases; most of them came from a group of 233 inmates who all tested positive. We also saw the Hubei government's swift response, which came in the form of several prison officials being fired. The speed with which the government responded was quite shocking. Then today, for the first time, the number of new cases dropped below 200; new suspected cases also fell to under 100. According to my doctor friend: "There is now hope that within two or three days we could be entering a new low rate period (meaning fewer than 100 new infections a day) in the trajectory of this virus." There is hope for the people of Wuhan yet. Does this mean that they might be able to reopen the city earlier than expected? That is precisely what the nine million residents of Wuhan are most hoping for. I asked my friend about that tonight and he said it still might be another two weeks. That would still be a bit ahead of schedule, but at least we won't have to continue on like this into April.

"Depressed" is still the word that I would use to describe my impression of Wuhan people these past few days. Today online I noticed quite a few people all using the words "city of sadness" to describe Wuhan. I don't know quite what to say; if you use the word "sadness" to describe what the city of Wuhan was going through during the Lunar New Year, I would argue that it doesn't even come close to describing the seriousness of the situation. Perhaps you could modify sadness with the word "bitter" and we might be getting a little closer to the reality. All you have to do is reread Chang Kai's last words and you will know what bitter sadness means. A few days ago there was an essay about what a medical worker from Guangdong experienced when he first came to Wuhan to provide aid. This description was included in the essay: "I remember on the second day of the Lunar New Year, I was assigned to the critical care unit around noon; within that first hour or two three patients already died. That night two more patients lost their fight with the coronavirus. There was one day when a patient came into the ER but died before we could even get him into a room. During those first few days there were simply too many patients; at the peak we were seeing between 1,500 and 1,600 patients a day coming in with a fever." And that is just the situation at a single hospital in Wuhan; now multiply that by all the other hospitals in the city. Just think about how many scenes like that are playing out simultaneously throughout the city. I hope that when they have time, some of those medical workers from all over China who came to Wuhan to provide support during this outbreak can get what they saw and experienced here down on paper. I'm sure that this is the kind of experience that will stay with them for the rest of their lives. But I hope they get it down on paper because people in the future will need to know what everyone in Wuhan went through.

This reminds me, I wonder if those reporters who had been review-ing what happened here in Wuhan are still doing their investigative reports? For those of us in the city, this is extremely important work. Now that things are starting to turn around, their investigations into what happened need to be on the agenda. Otherwise, time will slip by and all the pain and sadness we experienced will fade away with it. What I fear is that once people get back to their normal, happy lives, no one will be willing to revisit this painful moment; instead they will do everything they can to forget about those people like Chang Kai who died amid this tragedy. That also reminds me of a suggestion someone made about building a memorial to the victims of the coronavirus. I hope they leave space on that memorial to etch Chang Kai's final words into stone. When future generations read those words, they will be able to get a sense of the catastrophe we lived through in Wuhan during 2020. Everyone in Wuhan, including those medical practitioners who worked so hard to save their patients, should all fully support those journalists' investigations into what actually happened: Who was responsible for that 20-day delay? It was precisely those 20 days that cost more than 2,000 people their lives and caused many thousands more to be sick today, and it is still uncertain if they will be able to make it; nine million people ended up quarantined in their homes and five million people were trapped outside Wuhan, unable to return home. This isn't something we can let go. This is one buck that cannot be passed. I read an essay today entitled "The Story Behind Why Specialists Missed the Boat on Reporting an Unidentified Respiratory Disease," and there was a section that read: "As he was recounting what happened to *China News Weekly*, Zeng Guang banged the desk and asked, 'You really think I even heard of anyone named Li Wenliang or Zhang Jixian?'" My dear brave journalists, if you still have a conscience, please continue fighting the good fight! Please listen to the voices of the nine million Wuhan residents who stayed behind and the other five million who were left drifting. We all want to know who has been hiding the truth from us!

After 40 days of quarantine, people are reaching their psychological breaking point; this is something I have been very concerned about from the very beginning. I know that there are a lot of counseling and help hotlines you can find online, but I'm not sure if they are really addressing the real problems people are facing. Most happy families are quite similar, but unhappy families each suffer from their own set of misfortunes. I read an article entitled "Nine Million Different Kinds of Broken Hearts in Wuhan"—talk about a title! The article contains stories culled from dozens of posts by people from Wuhan who have been writing online about their difficult experiences. Letting your emotions out through talking or writing is an important psychological outlet for dealing with stress; this is actually part of why I keep this diary going every day. However, the label "positive energy"[3] keeps getting periodically thrust on those individuals who are just trying to find an outlet for release. It is a label that sounds completely appropriate and proper, the kind of label that a lot of people are eager to champion. But if you cry and make all your complaints public, they will claim that you are creating a panic, you are sabotaging the war against the coronavirus, and you've become part of the "negative energy." The destruction of negative energy is the incumbent duty of positive energy. My god, if people in this world use such a simpleminded perspective to understand and judge the things around them, then I suppose that I have been brought into this world in vain. If "positive energy" starts taking on this ignorant and arrogant guise, then I really have no idea what is so "positive" about it. Whoever said that after we cry and complain, we can't get back on our feet and continue moving forward?

Over the course of the past few days, there have been quite a few reporters who have interviewed me. One of them asked me a question that I thought was quite interesting: "Over the course of this outbreak, who are the people or things that have been overlooked?" Now that I have had some time to think about it, I feel that there are simply too many people and things that have been overlooked. When this thing first started, the citywide lockdown was imposed quite hastily; it was like trying to seal a large wooden bucket with a hundred holes and no bottom. All the while, the government was doing its best to try to stop the water flooding out of the bottom; meanwhile, there was no one left to stop the water leaking out of those hundred holes. We need to thank all those volunteers who stepped up to help seal off the city; these young volunteers were really amazing. They are the ones who noticed all those holes and sprang into action to fill them. There was Wang Yong, who helped organize transportation for the flood of medical personnel going in and out of Jinyintan District each day; during this first month of quarantine, Wu You supplied free medicine to the citizens of Wuhan but got in trouble for doing so; and then there was Liu Xian, who came all the way from Sichuan Province to provide free lunches for medical workers at Wuhan hospitals. There are many people out there like them. No one ordered them to do any of these things and when people saw them taking action, no one offered to help. Actually, each government department has administrative personnel who should have been taking care of these types of things once the quarantine went into effect; they are the ones who really should been taking responsibility for all these details. The worst part is that they seem to place themselves above the common people (or, to put it another way, their level of administrative competency is too low); unless they get a memo in writing ordering them to take action, they move in slow motion. The government should really step up and properly thank all those volunteers who sprang into action and filled all the gaping holes that were left unattended. If not for them, who knows how many more terrible things would have befallen Wuhan?

I learned another phrase today, "secondary disaster." The lockdown in Wuhan was something that we had no choice about, but after an extended period of quarantine you really need to have an overall plan in place. If you don't have an overall plan, the later consequences will be hard to imagine. If government officials fail to take the issue of the people's livelihoods seriously, if they don't put in practical measures to deal with the economic issues that many healthy people will be dealing with, if they aren't flexible enough to come up with thoughtful policies that will take care of these kinds of issues, I'm afraid that the problems awaiting us will result in another "epidemic." There are a lot of people who have been discussing these issues lately.

Last night one of my classmates forwarded me a letter of appeal that has been circulating widely on WeChat; the letter raises the issue of migrant workers, and I want to share it with you here:

The people are the core of the nation, the people require food to survive, the government is the people's government, the people support
the nation through their labor. As we fight this epidemic, we call on
various government agencies to establish a "Working Committee
for Migrant Worker Employment." Right now all people from Hubei
are unable to leave the province, companies outside of Hubei are
canceling their contracts with Hubei workers, and others are simply
being turned down for jobs from the get-go. In 30 days when restrictions begin to be lifted on districts in Hubei where the virus is under
control, we should have government buses or volunteers who can
take workers directly to a place of work in order to avoid their being
quarantined for an additional two weeks once they arrive. If the government does not pay attention to this issue, migrant workers from
Hubei will end up being replaced by workers from other provinces,
which will lead to widespread unemployment for Hubei workers. This
will be a massive side effect of the coronavirus outbreak, and it needs
to be addressed by the government. Take for instance those remote
mountain areas where there are few people; currently there are no
government-run job placement services for those areas. Because of
the coronavirus outbreak, many employers are scared as soon as they
hear that someone is from Hubei, which has led to a true employment
crisis for many people. If the Hubei government does not immediately take action to put measures in place to help get Hubei migrant
workers back to work in those remote mountain areas and other
areas unaffected by the virus, we will be facing an imminent wave
of unemployment. Many workers don't have any savings and they
have not been able to earn any wages this year due to the outbreak;
families need to eat. What are they to do? The government should
help promote the availability of Hubei workers to nonaffected areas
and encourage companies to hire Hubei workers. The government

needs to reassure them and help arrange employment opportunities while these various companies arrange transportation, quarantine facilities, and screenings before employment begins. These should all be reasonable requests; after all, not all people from Hubei have been infected. As the government fights the coronavirus, it needs to simultaneously take steps to ensure that the people's livelihood is being taken care of. For most migrant worker families, not working today means that they will be going hungry tomorrow! We hope that all the various government agencies in Hubei prioritize this request and fast-track it for discussion at upcoming meetings; the people's livelihood is an issue that affects everyone. Please forward this message.

What I have attached above is the complete letter of appeal, which I am passing on.

MARCH 3, 2020

You need to give us all an explanation.

It is still overcast and a bit cold and windy. This morning my neighbor out in the suburbs texted me a photograph. Under the photo was a message that said: "The begonias on your front porch are in bloom, but your WeChat seems to have been shut down." I'm used to my posts on WeChat being taken down. But knowing that my begonias are blooming is really something to be excited about. There was a big drought that lasted throughout the summer and autumn last year. All the leaves on the trees withered and fell. I was really concerned that the tree might die. But its will to live was so strong; in early spring it lit up with radiant flowers. Even through the screen of my phone I can feel the excitement of its full bloom.

There is again a mixture of both good news and bad news today. I spoke to one of my doctor friends about where things stand with the coronavirus epidemic, and he is now extremely optimistic about how things are going: "Everything is now looking much brighter concerning the coronavirus. Building off the foundation of the good news from two days ago, yesterday things continued to improve. The combined total of new confirmed and suspected cases added up to fewer than 200 people, which included a particularly large reduction of suspected cases. During the coming two days we should be entering a phase where new patient numbers are expected to drop below 100. According to these figures, controlling the spread of the coronavirus is now a goal within our sights! Building on the progress we have made, we will need to put everything into improving treatment results, further lowering the death rate, and shortening the period of hospitalization as much as possible."

That's right, it is absolutely essential to get the death rate down lower. A shame, then, that news of more deaths keeps coming in. One bit of news that shocked a lot of people today was the death of Dr. Mei Zhongming from Central Hospital. He was the assistant director of Dr. Li Wenliang's department. An extremely skilled ophthalmologist, he was only 57 years old. His specialty practice was extremely in-demand. Once news broke of his death, all his former patients started posting condolences and remembrances online. One of my former colleagues from the television station told me that they were neighbors. Tonight everyone in the community where he lived will be praying for Dr. Mei. I hope he is able to rest in peace.

I don't think there is a single hospital in all Wuhan that has been hit harder than Central Hospital. In terms of its location, Central Hospital is located very close to the Huanan Seafood Market, so it is the hospital that had the earliest contact with novel coronavirus patients. That first wave of patients with severe symptoms all came here for treatment. Back when people had absolutely no knowledge of this virus, the doctors at Central Hospital basically became a human first line of defense. It was only after, one after another, all these doctors began collapsing from the illness that they (and their administrators) finally woke up to the realization of just how horrific this new virus truly was. However, it was already too late.

My middle brother is a longtime patient at this hospital. He told me that Central Hospital is very well regarded; it used to be connected to the Wuhan No. 2 Hospital. He reminded me that his wife even had an operation there. As soon as he said that I realized that the No. 2 Hospital branch on Nanjing Road where I used to go for checkups when I was younger is actually Central Hospital; they just changed the name. No. 2 Hospital's earlier incarnation was the Hankou Catholic Hospital, which had a 140-year history. In my novel *Water Beneath Time*[4] I even wrote about this hospital being bombed by the Japanese during the war. The original No. 2 Hospital still stands at its original location; it is now a branch hospital of Central Hospital. I heard that more than 200 medical workers from Central Hospital have been infected by the coronavirus; many of them are suffering from severe symptoms. All of them are considered among the first wave of patients infected by the novel coronavirus. A while back there was a report that stated that after Li Wenliang was censured for speaking out, "Starting from January 2, the hospital requested that no hospital employees publicly discuss this illness; they were prohibited from posting any photos or written materials that could be later considered evidence of this virus. Only when changing shifts are medical employees permitted to verbally exchange patient information to fellow caregivers to provide for continuity of care. When patients came in for medical help, doctors were forced to remain completely silent about this possible outbreak."

Another news agency, Chutian New Media, also published an article about Central Hospital, which included some illustrated text, which read: "Wuhan Central Hospital has already become one of the hospitals with the highest number of infected workers. Currently there are more than 200 medical workers infected, including all three of the hospital's assistant directors, and the hospital's director of nursing care; the directors of several of their specialty clinics are currently relying on extracorporeal life support to keep them alive; numerous chief physicians are on respirators, and many of the front-line medical caregivers have severe symptoms that have left them teetering between life and death. The ER has been hit particularly hard; the Cancer Ward has lost 20 medical workers . . . the losses go on, but they are too many to enumerate. After suffering wave after wave of panic and heartbreak, we all know that one of us might be next." This report is a bit more detailed than the previous one. I have no way of going to Central Hospital in person to authenticate these numbers, but whether or not these figures are completely accurate, we do know without question that the human losses at Central Hospital have been particularly devastating.

During the early days of the outbreak, they experienced "the unbearable heaviness of being." I can't help but wonder: If these doctors knew the disease was infectious and many of them indeed became infected, then why didn't they take protective measures? Why let themselves be drawn in like moths to a flame? When a hospital experiences such devastating numbers of deaths, isn't there anyone who feels guilt or accepts any responsibility? You would expect those who made minor errors to resign out of shame and those who took major missteps to face some sort of punishment from their superiors. You can't just write everything off by simply hiding behind the fact that "this is a new virus so we didn't have enough knowledge about how to respond!" That is not an excuse. The Chinese people have always had trouble bringing themselves to repent; but when so many lives are dangling before you, we need people to stand up and take responsibility: You people, that's right, you! Stand up and repent! Today someone posted an appeal online that we should allow Central Hospital to temporarily shut down so all the employees there can take a break. They have lost so many of their own employees to this illness, and many more remain critically ill; the psychological trauma for those still on the job is simply too much for them to bear.

The toll of 20 days of delays, 20 days of lies, is much costlier than simply the number of deaths. The quarantine has now been in place for 40 days; the deadliest days are behind us, but the most difficult days may still be lying ahead.

The people of Wuhan continue to be quite depressed. Another doctor friend of mine said that all the sadness and depression have left people feeling uncertain about the future, causing people to easily slip into a state of psychological insecurity. Besides this, there is still the issue of people's livelihood; most people currently don't have any new income coming in, which has further contributed to their feeling of insecurity. They don't know when they'll be able to get back to work and have no idea when they will finally be able to go outside again, which has left everyone feeling lost. When someone is left fumbling in the dark and has no power to control their own fate, they end up losing their most fundamental sense of security. During times like these they need something to hold on to in order give them the sense that everything will be all right; for instance, they need to have an explanation. When the outbreak was at its worst, no one had the time or energy to carry out investigations or worry about who was responsible for what was happening; instead, everyone tried to be understanding and put all their reservations aside. Now that things are starting to ease up, all those questions we have been harboring inside are starting to come to the surface, and now people want answers. Then there are some aspects to all this that seem to have been addressed very quickly; for instance, that incident concerning the female inmate who went to Beijing after being released from prison, or the controversy surrounding Li Yuehua's practicing medicine without a license. These all occurred in the middle of this outbreak, yet the government was able to take swift action. However, what about those issues that the public really wants an answer to? Take, for example, the case of Dr. Li Wenliang: They have been investigating this for so long now, but where is the explanation we have been waiting for?

The case of Dr. Li Wenliang is indeed a knot that needs to be untangled. In actuality, the multitude of deaths suffered at Central Hospital is another knot. If we don't untangle these knots, how can the knots inside our hearts be unraveled? Over time these knots become tighter and more complicated, just as the scars deep inside our hearts expand and reach deeper. Psychological services experts say that it is only after you have removed yourself from a place of immediate danger that the true trauma begins to rise to the surface. To put it plainly: You need to offer an explanation about what happened to Dr. Li Wenliang. You need to give us an explanation about what went wrong at Central Hospital; all of us deserve to hear that.

MARCH 4, 2020

Online shopping, binge-watching, sleeping: This is our life now.

Today is truly a clear, bright day. The sunlight is brilliant and spring is in the air. All the colors—green, jade, red, and pink—seem to be contending to fill every space with a good dose of "positive energy." The Chinese roses in my courtyard are beginning to sprout new branches, even though I never tended to them because I spent all last year at my place in the suburbs working on a book. I never trimmed their branches, tied them to a pole, or gave them fertilizer; they just grew freely on their own without anyone's impeding them. Seeing them like that, I almost felt guilty when I tied some of their branches to the railing.

It is now a hard fact that the coronavirus is officially under control. As a longtime resident of Wuhan, I know how difficult it has been to get to this point. When you introduce the terror of an invisible virus that can be anywhere into a large sprawling city like Wuhan, which has a messy three-town structure[5] and a complex maze of traditional alleys and old lanes, it is indeed an incredible feat that we have been able to get the coronavirus under control in such a relatively short time span. Things were especially chaotic during the early stages of the outbreak because the situation overlapped with the Chinese Lunar New Year and the government made a series of mistakes. Once the government put a new set of leaders in charge and put an iron-clad policy in place for battling the coronavirus, we began to see clear results. Right now the head of this monster has been cut off and all that is left is its writhing tail; we have now freed ourselves up enough to start taking care of other matters, like those people from outside provinces who have been stuck in Wuhan during the quarantine, as well as those Wuhan residents who have been unable to return home. These issues should not be too difficult to resolve. Today my doctor friend told me that the situation is continuing to improve, and he expects that by tomorrow the city should be able to get back to an initial level of functionality. Finally, I feel like we are able to heave a sigh of relief.

This afternoon a friend sent me a long audio file. It was recorded by a hospital administrator who had come to Wuhan to provide aid; in the audio file he recounted his team's entire journey to Wuhan and the process of providing care to coronavirus patients. He originally sent this narrative to a friend and it is extremely logical, reserved, and objective. All he does is focus on the treatment process but he doesn't get into too many other details. But whenever he mentions Wuhan and the people here, he begins to lose it a bit and you can hear him start to choke up. Only those of us here in Wuhan realize what lies behind those moments when he loses it. We know that he personally witnessed the situation early on; he just can't get into those details, which is what kept causing him to uncontrollably choke up. You can tell that this doctor is a kind man with a good heart— someone who truly treats his patients with compassion and love. I want to again express my sincere hope that doctors like him who traveled to Wuhan to lend their aid and support will be able to record everything they saw here, especially during that early period, and get it out there. Those documents will become some of the most important testimonials to what happened during the fight against the coronavirus in 2020.

When I first began this diary, I didn't think at all about how many people might read it; I just wanted to jot down some reflections for myself. When I noticed some of the big-name verified users on WeChat using some shocking headlines to publish stories about me, I became quite uncomfortable. After all, I know that here in Wuhan there are a lot of people writing blogs like this, besides writers and poets. It's just that each of us uses a different method and focuses on different aspects of what is happening. But each of these records is extremely precious. When discussing fiction, I used to say that although literature is a form of individual expression, when countless individuals express themselves it collectively becomes a forum for national expression; and when many nations come together to express themselves, it becomes an expression of an entire era. By the same logic, one person's document is never enough; it can never capture the entire picture, but when you collect countless individual records together, you can begin to get a more complete picture that represents the truth of what happened.

Starting yesterday, they began a massive three-day project to clear and disinfect the Huanan Seafood Market, the site that became a focal point of the outbreak early on. The market was shut down back in early January and ever since then people have been coming every day to disinfect the area. But when they first shut the market down, their actions were rather rushed and many of the items in the various stores there were left behind. I suspect that no one ever thought the market would be shuttered for such a long time; and they certainly never imagined that the virus that emerged there would set in motion a catastrophe that would engulf all of China and later the world. After they shut off all power and water to the market and the temperature started to warm up, a lot of the seafood left behind started to emit a wretched stench. My middle brother said that people could probably smell that stench all the way down by the Vanke Building. There are more than a thousand vendors at that market, and the vast majority run legitimate businesses. Like everyone else in Wuhan, they too are victims here; moreover, many of them suffered much more than other people. During the process of disinfecting the market, I'm sure those storeowners had to dispose of everything in their shops. I wonder what the site of the market will become in the future. Some people have suggested turning it into a memorial hall dedicated to this calamity.

Today I'll just talk about shopping. Online group shopping has become increasingly flexible. There are really countless possibilities in the world of the internet. The way in which this program self-adapts to the market is really incredible; it can really do all kinds of tricks. My middle brother told me that his wife has also been recording everything that happens every day, all the details about how she does her shopping. My brother even sent me a few of the things she wrote, and I picked out a few passages about shopping in the age of coronavirus. I know that the internet censors won't bother deleting posts about grocery shopping.

What follows is a record of how my middle brother's family has been handling their shopping these past few days; you can look at it as a snapshot that reflects the experience of most people in Wuhan.

1. I actually already went downstairs once today to pick up some donated vegetables. Miss X called earlier to remind me to pick them up. At first we felt like those donations were only for low-income families and elderly people who need extra support; although we are both over 60 and don't have any children living with us, which fits the qualifications, we kept feeling like we shouldn't accept any donations since our overall situation isn't too bad. So the first few times that they called, we decided not to go down to pick any donations up. We didn't intend on picking up any today either, but then our building manager personally called to tell us there was already a bag for us waiting at the first-floor entrance. She told us to hurry down to pick it up. After hearing that, I bundled up with all my protective gear and went down to the first floor. There were two huge bags of vegetables and a stack of plastic bags so you could load up as much as you wanted. I took four heads of lettuce, just enough for two meals if I stir-fry them. I repeatedly thanked them, but didn't dare stay too long and quickly took the elevator back up to my apartment. Although four heads of lettuce doesn't amount to much in terms of cost, that feeling that someone is thinking of you and cares was worth so much more.

2. I still have to be careful when approaching this whole online shopping thing. This is, after all, an unusual period we are going through; sometimes even if you plan well, you can't keep up with all the changes to how they do things. All the pork was sold out so I quickly changed my order to add 30 eggs to take the place of the pork; anything to prevent me from making an extra trip outside. It

is a good thing that everyone infected, suspected, or in close contact with coronavirus in our community has already been taken away. When it was time to pick up my order, I put on a double layer of face masks; when I got there I made sure not to talk to anyone and quickly changed clothes and washed my hands when I got home.

3. This morning I received a notification from my Add More Group that my first order was ready for pickup, but the only item in our order that came in was two packages of chicken breast. I'm really annoyed at this method of online group shopping; there are too many people, so you have to wait for a long time before your pickup time comes and it is really hard to predict when deliveries will arrive. I've been waiting for my number to come up ever since the early afternoon; I checked the status an hour after I had dinner and they were only up to #60, but it seemed to be stuck there for a long time. But I still had to keep checking my phone, just in case they suddenly speeded up. I didn't want to risk losing my slot. When I checked the group chat again, I saw that someone had posted a message saying the boss went to dinner and it was unclear when he would return. Someone in the group had already said that it was normal for the deliveries to go on past 10:00 p.m. Our family was #114 and we didn't get a text to pick up our order until 10:56 p.m. There were still more than 60 orders behind me. The boss must be hungry and exhausted after doing this all day long; I hope he was able to have a good meal and take a breather; it must be damn hard on him! It's not easy for us either, but I know that he has it harder than us. Can you imagine having to run around the city all day and night like that; he is really working himself to death; even if he doesn't get infected, he'll end up collapsing out of sheer exhaustion.

4. For the past few days now, the most exercise I have been getting has been going to the south gate of our development to pick up our on-

line orders. Or perhaps I had better say that those little trips down to the south gate have given me a shot of adrenaline, as every time I go outside I tense up and can feel the anxiety kick in. I'm really not exaggerating; last night when I picked up our two bags of groceries (they weighed about 2 kg) I brought them in at around 11:00 p.m.; normally I would wash up, get into bed, watch a little TV, and then go to sleep, but last night I was still wide awake at 1:00 a.m.! This morning I slept in until 7:30 a.m., but I still feel exhausted from yesterday, but in order to keep myself on schedule I forced myself to get up and start my day. The good news is that another delivery service popped up today that allows you more control over the items you select. They had all kinds of items I have been looking for, like Angel yeast extract, tapioca, and Lao Gan Ma hot chili sauce—I immediately put in my order.

You can see that those community workers are really thoughtful; you can also see how hard that supermarket boss works overseeing all those grocery pickups. Online shopping, binge-watching, sleeping: This is our life now.

Today is day 42 of the lockdown.

MARCH 5, 2020

Common sense can sometimes be the most profound.

It is a clear sunny day; the sun is so bright that it almost dazzles the eyes. We have handed our roads, avenues, and parks over to the virus while we stayed at home, letting it roam the open city like a wandering ghost in search of victims. The sun at high noon is powerful enough to make you feel like it could burn the virus to death. According to the lunar calendar, today is the day the insects awaken from their winter sleep. It is day 43 of the quarantine. A few days ago I told a friend that I feel like I'm busier now than I am during normal times. I didn't watch a single TV miniseries and although I prepared a bunch of movies that I wanted to watch, I never got a chance to see a single one. My neighbor Tang Xiaohe was showing off a video of her granddaughter eating. The way she eats in that video is so adorable. One friend told me, "I spend my days watching videos of Xiaohe's granddaughter eating and my nights reading Fang Fang's diary; that's how I pass my time these days." Those videos and my friend's message brought me a lot of smiles.

Today is a really special day. There are three people who trigger a lot of memories for me on this date. The first one is Premier Zhou Enlai;[6] he is someone that anyone from my generation would be very familiar with. Back when I was growing up, just seeing his name in the newspaper would always give me a sense of comfort. March 5 is Zhou Enlai's birthday; I still remember the large-scale unrest set in motion after his death; it was referred to as the "April 5th Tiananmen Square Incident." I'm afraid that a lot of young people have never even heard of this incident. At the time, there was a poem that everyone was passing around to copy; even today I still remember that poem just like yesterday: "Melancholy approaches and I hear the demons howl, I cry as the wolves and jackals scowl. Shedding tears in tribute to a great man, I raise my eyebrows as swords melt away"[7] The second person, whom I'm sure many readers will be familiar with, is a man named Lei Feng. Ever since my childhood, the memory of Lei Feng has been there with me, and it has never faded. Lei Feng was a kindhearted soul who has been a companion to my entire generation as we grew up. Today is the day we commemorate Lei Feng. There was once a period of time that whenever March 5th arrived, young people nationwide would be mobilized to go do good deeds, like walking old ladies home—for a while there weren't enough old ladies to go around! How many people in China have grown up learning from Lei Feng? But there is one more person, someone that I'm afraid may have already been forgotten or many people never even knew existed—his name was Yu Luoke.[8] Fifty years ago today he was executed for things he had published. He was only 27 years old. For people of my generation who were the first group to take the college entrance exams after the Cultural Revolution, there is almost nobody who doesn't know his name. His fate is what prompted so many of us to start thinking about the fate of our people, the fate of our nation, and our own future. Some people feel that Yu Luoke's essays were not terribly profound; they claim that everything he said was common sense. That's right, that's exactly what it is. However, I often feel that people seem to be blinded by a misguided pursuit of "the profound." Common sense emerges from the deepest truths and those things most commonly put into practice. Common sense can sometimes be the most profound, like "all men are created equal." Bei Dao once wrote a poem to commemorate Yu Luoke; there was one line that kept getting quoted in articles for years: "In an age without heroes, I just want to be a man." Sometimes it isn't easy being a normal man who lives according to the principles of common sense.

Let me get back to the coronavirus; although things have taken a turn for the better, progress continues to be slow. The number of new patients continues to hover at just over 100, and we haven't yet entered the period when things can slowly start getting back to normal. If we can get the numbers down over the course of the next two days, we might be able to break through this stalemate period. A while back one of my doctor friends referred to the coronavirus as a "rogue virus"; the more time that goes on, the more it really resembles one. You really have no way of knowing where it might be hiding or who else it might infect, which could easily undo all our previous efforts.

A few days ago my friend Jiang, who is a film director, told me that her friend Li Liang, who had just been released from the hospital but was still under quarantine, had suddenly passed away. Jiang is a director with the Wuhan Municipal Bureau of Culture. She used to frequently visit Li Liang's clinic for treatment. Li Liang was a physical therapist. Just before the Lunar New Year, Li Liang went into Central Hospital to have a procedure done to his cervical vertebra. Li Liang came down with a fever on the 10th day of the Lunar New Year and was admitted to the temporary hospital in Hanyang. He had two tests for the coronavirus, but both came back negative so they transferred him from the hospital to a hotel for quarantine. Meanwhile he continued to feel terrible; at one point he even called his mentor and broke down in tears over the phone. In the end, he was unable to escape from the fate that was chasing him. Only 36 years old and he left us, leaving behind his young wife and their infant child.

Jiang and I discussed the question of just how accurate the coronavirus test is, over the phone. This is something I know very little about, but it reminded me of a report I recently read that stated there were quite a few patients who had been discharged from hospitals after testing negative, but then as they were under quarantine, they were retested and were positive. Jiang and I both wondered if there is perhaps some problem with the criteria hospitals have been using to decide when to release patients. Indeed, I quickly found an article online from an expert arguing that the criteria for releasing patients were much too lax. And then today there was just an announcement that went out: Starting tomorrow, all patients currently at the temporary hospitals or about to be released from other hospitals in Wuhan would need to have a blood test to check their antiviral antibodies before being released.

There was a video today that really blew up on the internet. Some leaders from the central government went to inspect one of the smaller districts in Wuhan. While they were there, someone in one of the high-rise apartment buildings shouted from their window: "It's fake! It's all a sham! You leaders only take a quick look around and leave!" A lot of people online were heatedly discussing the video, some of them saying that there were still some men with spines left in Wuhan after all. I can't say for sure if it was real or fake, but for many years now, inspection visits by government leaders have always been adorned with all kinds of formalities; that is something that everyone knows. Actually, you can't blame the local leaders for that; they put on these fake shows at every level of government—if those low-level leaders don't fall in line, they will never have a future career in politics. But don't tell me that Wuhan's current citywide quarantine is somehow just the result of government leaders wanting to put on a show! In the past I would always speak up at those government meetings, imploring everyone to just speak the truth. Even when carrying out official government directives, we need to seek truth from facts. Those directives are often imposed uniformly without taking practical conditions on the ground into consideration. But if we are seeking truth from facts, that leaves room for us to express to the higher-ups when something has been overlooked so we can fill the holes. But who is going to listen? Dealing in lies, sometimes even touting those lies out in the open, getting wrapped up in appearances to the point where you are just throwing away money to put on a show for the bureaucrats—these are the things that have long become the "coronavirus" of our society. Once this outbreak has passed, I wonder if we will find a cure for this disease.

The people of Wuhan were very lucky this time. A friend I trust assured me that the video I saw was authentic. Leaders from the central government had a meeting in the afternoon and decided to immediately address the issue regarding the public's outcry. Take a look, isn't this great? If those people hadn't shouted out from their windows, how would the leaders ever know the difficulties the people are going through? If they just remain silent and go along with the charade, aren't they the ones who will end up suffering? So if they have something to scream about, they should speak up! While it can be very difficult to find your own voice outside the majority, it is still important to foster those individual voices, no? That's why I so respect those Wuhan citizens who dared to shout out from their windows. The meaning of those cries is quite important. It might even make those leaders think twice the next time they try to put on another artificial display. Because they will never know whether or not there are citizens nearby who might be ready to speak truth to power. If we want social progress, we at the very least have to begin by putting an end to these pompous artificial displays.

Another interesting bit of news today involved the government recognizing a group of individuals and groups that have been instrumental in fighting the novel coronavirus. Two of the individuals that the government commended are particularly important to mention. One of them is Dr. Wang Guangfa, from Beijing. Dr. Wang was among the second group of specialists who came to Wuhan early on. I once described him as being a member of the first group on Weibo, but that was a mistake that I would like to apologize for. Dr. Wang left the people of Wuhan with four words: "It's Controllable and Preventable." Those four words combined with those other four words, "Not Contagious Between People," led the people of Wuhan down a path toward utter catastrophe. I'm sure that Dr. Wang has many achievements to be proud of, I'm sure that he is an exceptionally skilled doctor, and he might not even be the person who came up with the phrase "It's Controllable and Preventable." But, no matter what, he was the one who publicly uttered those words during a press conference. Standing before the suffering people of Wuhan, he should have at least a small sense of shame; at the very least he should apologize to the people of Wuhan. I carry no prejudice against Dr. Wang; but when I saw him emerge from the hospital and face an army of reporters, I didn't see an ounce of uneasiness, only smugness. That is what really disgusted me. I don't think it is appropriate for a doctor to behave like that. Dr. Wang may have been recognized by the government for his exemplary contributions, but he still owes a debt to the people of Wuhan. All members of those two teams of specialists owe us a debt. This debt must be repaid. Otherwise how will those nearly 3,000 wronged souls ever rest in peace?

The other person honored at the ceremony today was Dr. Li Wenliang. Li Wenliang was also recognized as an exemplary role model for his actions. I wonder if that is the end of his story? And I wonder if Li Wenliang was watching from the other side; if he could see what was happening, would he laugh or would he cry?

MARCH 6, 2020

How long can this deadlock last?

It is a dark and overcast day; my mood has also turned gloomy with the weather. There is a heavy feeling in the air; the sense of gloom seems to be everywhere. There is no big change with the outbreak compared to yesterday; still over 100 new cases, so I guess we are still at a deadlock. How long can this deadlock last? Will it be over by next week?

For the past few days I have been feeling like a lot of Wuhan residents: stressed out, depressed, and I have a headache. And I've become really annoyed with the telephone; I truly have no desire to speak with anyone. I'm just trying to live as simply as possible. And I don't feel like talking. I figure it is a good time to revisit my writing on what happened in Wuhan before the lockdown. At the time I jotted down some of my thoughts when I forwarded other people's posts online; I've collected those here to include them in my diary.

January 19, 2020: Forwarded message: In Order to Prevent the Spread of the Novel Coronavirus, Please Wear a Face Mask

---

Last month when I visited Chengdu, my classmate Xu Min gave me an N95 mask to wear because the air pollution there was so bad. But the air quality in Wuhan isn't any better than Chengdu; I've long grown accustomed to breathing shitty air. So I just put the mask in my pocket and never wore it. Over the course of the past two days there are more and more rumors about an outbreak in Wuhan and I don't normally keep any face masks at home. Yesterday when I went to the hospital to visit a friend I thought I had better be careful, which is when I remembered the mask that Xu Min gave me. I quickly found it but at first I couldn't even figure out how to put it on. I checked online and I think I got it right, although I wasn't that careful about following all the details.

I haven't worn a face mask in probably 50 years; putting it on makes me feel like I have returned to my childhood.

January 20, 2020: Forwarded message: Jiang Yanyong: Everything I Am Saying Is a True Record of What Happened in 2003

Jiang Yanyong said: "When you must be thinking that Zhang Wenkang's remarks are wrong, whereas Zhang Liping, Minister Wang, and others are able to freely speak the truth because they are already retired. In the past our country has suffered far too many consequences as a result of telling too many untruths; I hope that moving forward we will try harder to speak the truth."

Today there are a lot more speaking untruths than there were back in 2003. And there are no media outlets that dare to speak the truth. I just hope that all the official news we are now seeing about the new virus is all accurate.

January 20, 2020: Forwarded message: 40,000 Families Enjoy Banquet at Baibuting

I think that the community deciding to move forward with this large-scale gathering while this "new virus" is still spreading is basically a form of criminal action. No matter how much you love showing off for the leaders or how much you love displaying the power of this great era of peace and prosperity, for the time being the municipal government should ban all large-scale public gatherings like this; even if the participants are willing to take the risk, the government should still step in and prevent them from doing so.

January 21, 2020: Forwarded message: Paying My Respects! 432 Hours of Caregiving, They Say This Is My Responsibility

The doctors in Wuhan have it the worst. I'm afraid that this year the doctors won't have a break during the Lunar New Year. I salute them.

Don't gather in groups, don't go outside, don't try to be cool. If you do have to go out be sure to wear a face mask, keep washing your hands, and keep gargling with salt water. Taking care of yourself is the best way to help.

January 23, 2020: Forwarded message: In the Face of the Outbreak, The Bold Actions Taken by the International Alumni of Wuhan University Are a Shot of Adrenaline

---

I'm forwarding a message from one of my fellow alumni from Wuhan University.

I usually go down to Hainan every winter to escape from the cold weather. This year was a bit warmer than usual and the Lunar New Year came a bit earlier than normal so I planned to go down after the New Year. But in the end I ended up stuck here because of the quarantine, forced to share the same fate as the rest of the Wuhan people.

I'm sure that the government had no choice but to implement this quarantine, even if they did miss the boat early on by delaying their response. (There were two large-scale provincial meetings scheduled for early to mid-January. Everyone knows that in order not to disrupt those meetings, there is a moratorium on reporting any negative news. Moreover, all the government offices basically shut down to prepare for these meetings and nobody does any real work. All the reporters understand how this works and they are in a very difficult situation; what can they do? Although human lives are important, those officials believe that their meetings are even more important. The political is the first killer here. Once this outbreak has passed, those officials who failed to take action had better think about how they are going to beg the people for forgiveness!) But right now as citizens we need to follow the government's orders and follow their plans. We need to remain calm; we can't afford to let fear win; we have got to keep it together. It is best if we can restrict going out to a minimum. When we have to go out we should all wear face masks (even though it is very hard to find N95 masks for sale now and when they are available they are being sold for many times the normal price!). Keep washing your hands and make sure you are eating well. I suggest you try not to forward messages that might incite panic. Just lock yourselves up at home and try to live as normal a life as possible. Not causing additional trouble is one way to help out.

Thanks to all my friends for reaching out to show your support.

And for those of you with means to help out Wuhan, please do what you can!

January 23, 2020: Forwarded message: Latest Bulletin on the Availability of Daily Necessities in Wuhan!

Right now the entire world is watching Wuhan; everyone in China is sending aid to Wuhan. These days our transport networks are quite well developed; there is no way that people will starve here during the lockdown like they did in Wuchang during the war. So there is absolutely no reason for people to hoard supplies. I think we can completely trust the government on this.

The government should implement a policy prohibiting pharmacies from raising prices on necessities during this period. Yesterday afternoon I went to the pharmacy on Dongting Road (I won't print the name of the store) to buy N95 masks. They wanted nearly 900 yuan for a bag of 25 masks. These are disposable items; an average person uses three a day (I've been told that after wearing them for four hours they become ineffective), which adds up to 100 yuan. I was going to just buy a few but they didn't have individual packaging. The saleswoman handed me a few masks with her bare hands, which immediately made me decide not to buy them. I asked her: "How can you sell them at such a markup during a time like this?" The saleswoman replied: "Our suppliers raised their price, so we have to, too."

Every family is going through a huge quantity of these disposable masks. They can't be sold for such a high price. The government should really clamp down hard on all these people trying to make a buck through price gouging during a time like this.

January 23, 2020: Forwarded message: Saluting the First Group of Shanghai Pulmonologists Who Have Already Departed for Wuhan

I saw a video of some Wuhan patients begging for treatment; seeing that line of sick people crying and screaming was enough to make you break down. Those patients are in such desperate straits. And there is a shortage of doctors and hospital beds. For a long time now, the government hasn't taken effective measures (I heard that only today did they finally decide to build a quarantine hospital like the Xiaotangshan Hospital in Beijing). Besides staying at home and not adding to the mess, there's really nothing I can do to help. It is very rare for me to feel this helpless.

Right now I just want to express my deep thanks to the Shanghai doctors who have come here to help!

January 24, 2020: Forwarded message: All Hands on Deck in Wuhan to Test Patients with a Fever, Each District Is Arranging Transportation to Take Patients to the Hospitals

Forwarding this for a friend. They may have gotten off to a slow start, but at least the government is now taking action. The Hubei and Wuhan local officials' lack of skills and inability to take the initiative has been instantly revealed by what happened this week. What is the point if all they can do is give speeches, conduct political study sessions, and clamp down on people who speak the truth? I won't say too much for now, but let's see how they apologize to the people once all of this is over.

I went out this afternoon looking for a place to buy face masks. I finally found a small supermarket that had a few N95s in stock. All the other stores on the street were closed, including the pharmacies. Only a few mom-and-pop stores were still open. They were pretty well stocked and had a good stock of vegetables available for purchase. They were just a bit pricy, but not too bad. I talked to the storeowner and he said that they were even open during the Lunar New Year; they didn't close for a single day. I got some degree of comfort hearing that.

But what really moved me was seeing the sanitation workers still out there sweeping the streets. They were all out there, as always, on each and every street, even though Wuhan is now cold and rainy with a gusty wind.

Thanks to all these hardworking people! Their ability to stay calm while working hard gives me so much comfort.

January 25, 2020: Forwarded message: On the Eve of the Lockdown, 299,000 People Leave Wuhan

---

Let's be tolerant and understanding of the people who have escaped from Wuhan. They are all just everyday people who are scared and want to stay alive.

I'm thankful that this year I didn't leave early for Hainan. Otherwise my daughter would have been left alone here in Wuhan and I would have been a nervous wreck. If I had left I would have made sure to come back to her, even if I had to walk to get here! But things are okay now; mother and daughter are each self-quarantined in our own apartments for the New Year. I feel much better this way.

I did see reports of some people from Wuhan who had been in other provinces who are now suddenly facing all kinds of prejudice and no hotels will take them. My god, what a world we live in!

The way of the world is in a state of constant flux; there are warm-hearted people and cold-hearted people. That's the way it's always been. We need to just accept that. The best thing we can do is take care of ourselves.

January 25, 2020: Forwarded message: Please Spread the News: Wuhan City Taxis Allocated Accounts Based on Districts

---

Forwarding for a friend. A few days ago my colleague went in for surgery and she needs to go back to the hospital tomorrow to change her bandages. We already reached out to the community workers for assistance, and they said that they should be able to help arrange transportation.

Everyone feels helpless right now, but at least things are starting to get a bit more organized. It is good to know that the country is stepping up and there are people now taking the reins, so hopefully things wouldn't be as chaotic as before. After all the rumors and gossip that had been exploding over the internet, it seems that, starting today, people are beginning to calm down.

The first day of the Lunar New Year has come and gone in an instant. But I would still like to wish everyone a happy Chinese New Year. I hope that all the bad demons will disappear with last year; and here is hoping that things start to get better each day.

January 26, 2020: Forwarded message: Seeking Emergency Help: Appealing to All Hotels Nationwide to Accept Guests from Hubei and Wuhan

---

Forwarding to help get the word out. Everyone in China, please take in the people of Hubei, including those from Wuhan. No matter how they got out of Hubei, they all need food and a place to stay. Your enemy is the coronavirus and not these people from Hubei or those from Wuhan who are truly suffering.

I preserve these early posts on the coronavirus for the record.

MARCH 7, 2020

Who could have imagined that a second catastrophe
would befall the Chinese language itself?

It is a clear day and even a bit hot for this time of year. Nature seems to be quite pleased with itself; as soon as the sun emerged, it seemingly completely forgot how gloomy and cold it was just yesterday, which didn't feel at all like early spring weather. I had a headache yesterday and took a sleeping pill, which allowed me to get an extra hour of sleep. I didn't get up until noon and when I awoke I was feeling much better. The express delivery company delivered a package; someone sent me a fitness smartwatch. Even after racking my brains, I still couldn't figure out who the kind soul was who had sent it; looking at the return address didn't help. Friends, next time you send me something, please leave a note, okay? I won't mention you in public, but I would at least like to be able to privately express my thanks. After taking some time to figure out how the watch works, I'm now using it. Not bad.

This morning one of my doctor friends sent me a message that was brimming with positive news. The new cases of coronavirus in Wuhan on March 6 finally fell below 100. "After four days of seeing new coronavirus cases linger at just over 100, we have finally entered a new phase which will allow us to start getting things back to a basic operating level. The coronavirus outbreak in Wuhan is now seeing a tangible breakthrough. Our health management resources are now replenished and now even presumptive cases are able to receive in-patient treatment at the hospital. Specialized clinics and departments at various hospitals have begun to reopen; there is a very good chance that we will be able to get numbers down close to zero by the end of the month. We can now see the light at the end of the tunnel! Let's keep going!" Those are his exact words. Just yesterday we were still worried about the dead-lock we were in with the number of new patients, but now things seem to have suddenly turned around. In some ways, it is just like the way yesterday's gloomy weather unexpectedly cleared up.

Such a bright beautiful day. Everyone has played a role in turning the tide against the coronavirus. More and more people online are call-ing for the quarantine to be lifted. There are many hospitals in Wu-han that are beginning to resume normal operations, and their various departments are opening back up. But a lot of people unable to get treatment for other ailments have also passed away during this out-break. This is a secondary catastrophe brought on by the coronavirus. Two elderly people in my complex died from non-coronavirus illnesses during this lockdown period. If they had access to normal medical care, they both may have made it. Besides this, there are a lot of people facing economic hardships; they have no income coming in and are unable to support their families. This is another monumental problem we need to address. Today I heard that the Nanjing poet Han Dong[9] has been stuck somewhere in Hubei and was forced to stay in a hotel for more than 40 days. It's hard to imagine how he got through this period; I hope I will one day get to read Han Dong's record of his time under lockdown.

Yesterday I was chatting with a few of my old schoolmates. They were telling me about what happened to Shen Huaqiang, the Secretary-General of the Wuhan-Ningbo Business Association. Two of my class-mates were very close to him: H was his former supervisor and X was his classmate in college. Speaking of classmates, H and X were my classmates from elementary school all the way up through high school. I once wrote about the Ningbo businessman Shen Zhusan; Shen Huaqiang must have read that book because when he visited Wuhan with the Secretary-General of the Ningbo government, he told H that he was a big fan of mine. Shen Huaqiang wanted to meet me, so he asked H to introduce us. Shen Huaqiang was also the editor of the book *Natives of Ningbo in Wuhan* and he took care of a lot of the general affairs in his office. Who could have imagined that Shen Huaqiang would catch the novel coronavirus and all five members of his family would also be infected? He fell ill on the second day of the Lunar New Year and died on February 7—the same day his mother also died from the novel coronavirus. The other three people in his household were all under hospital quarantine. It is truly a tragic story. Neither Shen Huaqiang nor his mother was ever officially diagnosed with the coronavirus, so I'm afraid their deaths are not even counted in the official government tally. We kept saying we should meet so we could talk about Shen Zhusan, but we never got a chance. But I wanted to say something about this friend whom I had corresponded with numerous times but never got the chance to ever meet face-to-face.

I was talking with a classmate about all the cremations taking place and we were wondering how they are going to manage all these funerals; right after that I followed up with a professional psychologist I know about this issue. I asked her: "I'm afraid that there is still one more big obstacle ahead for the people of Wuhan. Once the outbreak is over, there will be thousands of families that will need to hold funerals. How are we going to get through this? This will be another large-scale collective trauma that people will have to face." My psychologist friend responded: "Since all these people died at the hands of an infectious disease, the funeral homes immediately cremated all the bodies; but all the ashes will be preserved until after the outbreak. At that time, they will inform family members by telephone that they can come and pick up their relative's remains. At that time families can make arrangements for various memorial ceremonies. But because arrangements will need to be made for thousands of deceased individuals, I suspect that the government will have to get involved to help with some of the logistics. Because part of what went wrong was due to human error, if we want people to get over their pain, they will need some kind of explanation. If there is no accountability, it will be very difficult for people to truly get past this. There are so many families that have suffered losses; but how they get through it will be up to each individual family's network of support and their level of functionality. Disadvantaged families will need more hands-on support from the government; psychologists will not be able to provide for all the practical needs that many of these families will have."

Another friend of mine who is well-versed in the field of psychological trauma told me: "Currently, most of the public is still in a state of psychological stress, but more serious psychological problems will start to emerge after this period of initial stress has passed. Once the outbreak has passed, we will start to see large numbers of people with post-traumatic stress disorder (PTSD). Many families suddenly lost loved ones and they were not only unable to perform their filial duty of taking care of their relatives before they died, but they were even prohibited from paying their final respects; no matter what people do, this type of trauma will always leave behind a deep scar. I suspect that there will be a very high ratio of people suffering from post-traumatic stress disorder among these surviving family members. And then there is a group of people who will suffer from traumatic reoccurrence disorder, which will cause them to replay the events that happened over and over like a nightmare they cannot wake up from. Still others will respond by going numb and shutting themselves off, and finally there will be others who will respond by becoming neurotic and overly sensitive."

While I am hoping this outbreak will end quickly, I am at the same time terrified about the day that all those thousands of Wuhan families will have to hold funerals for their lost loved ones. I'm not sure if there are other psychologists out there who can provide other useful and practical measures that can make things even a little bit easier for these grieving families.

Today the word appearing most frequently in group chats online is "gratitude." The political leaders here in Wuhan have requested that the citizens provide a public expression of gratitude toward the Chinese Communist Party and the nation. Their thought process is really strange. The government is the people's government; it exists to serve the people. Government employees are servants of the people, not the other way around. These government leaders spend all their time studying political doctrines; how could they end up getting this so backward? Professor Feng Tianyu[10] from Wuhan University said: "As for this question of gratitude, let's not mix up the relationship between the people and those who hold power. If you are going to take those in power as gracious benefactors who require that their people get on their knees and thank them for their benevolence, I think you had better go back and listen to what Marx said during a speech in 1875. Marx despised Ferdinand Lassalle's notion of state supremacy and argued that: 'the state has need, on the contrary, of a very stern education by the people' (*Critique of the Gotha Program*)." I'm sure that all the political leaders in Hubei and Wuhan very much respect the views of Professor Feng; if this current group of new leaders are educated, I wonder if they will really hear what Professor Feng is trying to say.

That's right, the outbreak is now basically under control and we should indeed express our gratitude for that. But it should be the government standing up to express *their* gratitude. The government should start off by expressing their gratitude to the families of those thousands of victims; their loved ones were the wrongful victims of a terrible scourge. They weren't even able to say goodbye to their family members or have a proper funeral; all they could do was keep the pain inside and bottle everything up and, meanwhile, virtually no one uttered a word of complaint. The government should express their gratitude to the more than 5,000 people still lying in hospitals beds as they struggle for their lives against the god of death; it is their stubborn will to live that has slowed down the number of deaths. The government should express their gratitude to all the healthcare professionals and 40,000 angels in white who came to Wuhan from around China to save people's lives; they worked in the face of great peril, pulling people from the grip of death, one soul at a time. The government should express their gratitude toward all those workers and laborers who hustled all over the city during the course of this outbreak; they are the ones who kept this city functioning amid the crisis. And the government should save their biggest thanks for the nine million residents of Wuhan who locked themselves in their homes, even though it meant facing all kinds of difficulties; without their cooperation this virus would never have been brought under control. No compliments or beautiful words would be considered excessive in describing the contributions that all these people made. My dear government, please suck in your pride and humbly extend your gratitude to your masters—the millions of citizens of Wuhan.

Next the government should make haste and beg for the people's forgiveness. This is the time for reflection and assuming responsibility. A rational government with a conscience that listens to the needs of its people and understands how to console them should, at this very moment, quickly establish an independent investigative team to piece together the full details surrounding the outbreak, who was responsible for delaying the response, who decided to withhold information about the outbreak from the public, who were the leaders that in order to save face decided to twist the truth when reporting to their superiors and hide the truth from the public, who was it who put political correctness above the lives of our people, how many people contributed to this disaster? Whoever had a hand in this should take responsibility; the people need someone to assume accountability. At the same time, the government should urge officials from various departments whose actions misguided the public, leading to casualties, to resign. Individuals to be investigated should include high-level government administrators, top officials from the Ministry of Propaganda, those in the media who helped cover things up, and top officials from the Department of Health. If any of them are criminally liable, let the courts decide their punishment. However, based on my observations, most Chinese government officials are lacking when it comes to self-reflection, not to mention those willing to take the blame and resign. In a situation like this, citizens should, at the very least, draft a public call for all those officials who took politics as the center of their world while treating people like trash to resign. How can we let these people with blood on their hands continue strutting around in front of the people of Wuhan, gesticulating as if they are heroes? Supposing that 10 or 20 officials stand up and resign as a result of this, at least we will know that there are at least a few officials left who still have a conscience.

Tonight around dusk a famous writer sent me a text. He wrote something that I found to be quite profound: "Who could ever have imagined that a second catastrophe would befall the Chinese language itself?" Gratitude is a beautiful word, but I'm afraid it has been forever sullied. I wonder if, moving forward, it will now become a "sensitive term" that we aren't allowed to use.

MARCH 8, 2020

When clues appear, shouldn't we follow through with them?

It's raining again, quite a downpour, actually. It is also quite chilly and all day the sky has been as dark as it normally is at dusk. A certain

Mr. Liu all the way out in Chengdu had his friend in Wuhan deliver some fresh fish to me; I tried to politely refuse, but in the end I wasn't successful. The fish had already been prepared for cooking; in fact, he even sent over sliced scallions, ginger, and radishes so I could conveniently make fish soup. And because they figured out from my diary that I have diabetes, they also delivered some dried fruits. They left the package with a letter at the main entrance to my compound. I felt quite embarrassed to accept their kind gift, but I was also quite moved. Thank you, my friends, for caring.

Today is March 8, Women's Day in China. Everyone is sending flowers to women online today. Every March 8 when I was a kid, my girlfriends and I would always sing: "March 8 Women's Day, the boys will work, the girls will play, the boys will stay inside, doing their homework all day." We would sing it in the Wuhan dialect, which created a certain melody and rhyme scheme that you could never get tired of. Thinking about it now, if feels like such a distant memory.

In Wuhan dialect we called children *ya*. Boys are referred to as *nanya* and girls are referred to as *nüya*. When kids grow up, we replace *ya* with *jiang*, so men become *nanjiang* and women become *nüjiang*. These forms of address function irrespective of a person's status, class, or title; everyone is either a *nanjiang* or a *nüjiang*. The word *jiang* often refers to a "general" in the military, but here there is no association with anything military. It is really an interesting way to refer to people; I'm not sure if other regions in China also use it.

While it seems that in Wuhan the *nüjiang* always look like they are in charge, inside the home it is usually the *nanjiang* who calls all the shots. But what is interesting is that if a family runs into trouble, it is mostly the *nüjiang* who step up to deal with it. It's not that the *nanjiang* is incapable of dealing with these things, it is just that the *nüjiang* seem to have an innate instinct to protect the *nanjiang* of the family.

Sometimes, she takes the lead on things because the *nanjiang* has a profession of some social standing that doesn't allow him to behave in certain ways in public; however, *nüjiang* never care about those things. Most women are relegated to a lower social status than men, which means that when trouble comes, the *nüjiang* are the ones who step in to put things back in order. Wuhan's *nüjiang* speak quickly in high-pitched voices, and it is rare to see them lose an argument. And when you get two *nüjiang* arguing with each other, now, that is a quite a sight. During the Cultural Revolution, my former father-in-law was a professor at Huazhong Normal University when the Red Guards stormed his house to struggle against him. That's when my former mother-in-law told him to sit tight and she brazenly strutted outside and started arguing with those Red Guards! Those Red Guards had nothing on my former mother-in-law—she was a real *nüjiang*—so, in the end, those Red Guards had no recourse but to scurry away. I've told this story before in other essays. But now in this age of the coronavirus, a lot of *nüjiangs* feel like it's their duty to deal with things like all the complications of online shopping and dealings with the community. Since that is the case, you usually see more *nüjiang* taking care of these issues. Wuhan *nüjiang* are brimming with energy and tend to talk loudly; there have been a few videos of them circulating on the internet that have really shocked a lot of people. So at this time, I'd like to take a moment to wish all the *nüjiang* a happy Women's Day!

It's day 46 of the quarantine. At this stage in the outbreak there is an increasing amount of positive news coming out. Some districts are beginning to start incrementally easing the quarantine orders; I've also been hearing some occasional rumors that people might be getting back to work soon. One friend told me that the airport was already preparing to resume flights. This news is both encouraging and frightening at the same time. If this is all true, then the city should be opening back up soon. My fellow Wuhanese, I think the light of day is almost here?

The messages I'm getting from my doctor friends are also positive. It has now been two days since we entered this new low-infection-rate stage, and the numbers of patients are clearly dropping. The temporary hospitals have begun to successively shut down, and the largest one that was set up at the Wuhan Keting Expo area just announced today that they are shutting down, too. New patients can now all be directly admitted to regular hospitals for treatment. Some hospitals have gotten their outpatient clinics back up and running again. In this fight to control the spread of the coronavirus, we are currently clearing the battlefield; the day we can start over again is now in sight. But right now we still have over 5,000 patients with serious symptoms, and more than 17,000 people are still hospitalized. Thanks to the coordination of a team of leading medical specialists, doctors are now able to share their experiences treating the coronavirus and improve on standard treatment methods, which has helped to ensure that all patients receive the best care possible. My friend's optimism makes me believe that it won't be too long before these final 17,000 patients will be discharged.

Actually, we can now see that the last stages of this battle against the coronavirus and our own lives are all gradually becoming more and more orderly. Most community service workers have been quite meticulous, and everyone has a very good attitude. One of my colleagues is always showing us pictures of community workers helping local residents with all kinds of tasks; he said that they are amazing, even helping residents with shopping. To win the people's approval like that, they must be doing a really good job. You should know that those Wuhan *nüjiang* can be really hard to please, and sometimes really fierce! To be fair, those community workers who volunteer to go out to these smaller communities really have a tough job; they basically end up doing all kinds of odd jobs; they have to do a little bit of everything. This is especially the case in those traditional old neighborhoods where the buildings have no elevators; they end up lugging groceries up many flights of stairs, teaching elderly residents how to use cellphones, and in some cases helping residents who don't even have cellphones make phone calls. There are all kinds of people living together in this city. There is no shortage of people who love to bicker; they are very stubborn and won't think twice about getting in a real fight. Dealing with these types of people makes community service particularly challenging. The fact that most Wuhan people have been able to make it this far and are able to still hold on is, in large part, due to the hard work of those community workers.

Some of my colleagues at the Hubei Writers Association are starting to get back to work. *Changjiang Literature and Art Magazine* plans to get its next issue out on time, which is something that cannot be done if everyone just stays home. Originally I was supposed to submit a novella to them after the Lunar New Year, but I ended up eating my words. Reporters keep asking me the same question about what I'm most looking forward to doing once the city reopens. My response: I want to take a good rest; and then I want to finish that novella. If I don't take care of those lingering debts, I'll probably end up ostracized from all my friends!

The outbreak is already easing up here, yet the tragedies continue. The Xinjia Express Hotel in Quanzhou where people were being housed under quarantine just collapsed. My classmate just sent a message to our group chat; the collapse occurred this evening just after 6:00 p.m. and 71 people were trapped inside. As of 4:00 p.m. firefighters on scene had already rescued 48 people, 10 of whom have already died and the other 38 were taken to the hospital for treatment. There should be another 23 people still trapped inside. I'm so anxious! A lot of these people who were quarantined were from Hubei. Somehow they escaped from the grip of the coronavirus, yet couldn't escape from this unsafe building. Perhaps this qualifies as yet another secondary disaster?

Today I saw an interview in *Caixin* with the Hong Kong microbiologist Yuen Kwok-Yung.[11] Dr. Yuen was a member of the third team of specialists that came to Wuhan. During this outbreak he was appointed as a specialist to the World Health Organization's COVID-19 task force, and he is also a member of the Advisory Council for the Hong Kong Special Administrative Region. Some of the information he revealed to the reporter in this interview was quite shocking.

Dr. Yuen stated: "I want to tell you the truth; the places we visited in Wuhan were likely all 'model hospitals.' They answered all the questions we asked, but it felt like their answers were all prerehearsed. But Zhong Nanshan was particularly sharp; he kept repeatedly asking them questions like: 'Are you sure there weren't any?' 'Are you positive there aren't any more cases of infection?' 'Is the number of cases you reported really accurate?' But their answer was always: 'We are still testing. That's because the Hubei Center for Disease Control didn't receive test kits from the central government until January 16.' After repeated questioning, they finally told us that: 'It seems that one patient being treated in the department of neurosurgery infected 14 medical practitioners.' Then they added: 'But none of those medical workers have been officially diagnosed yet.' The reporter from *Caixin* was really good; he followed up by asking: 'So just who does "they" refer to? When you conducted your investigations at Wuhan Hospital, who were the primary people you met with?' Yuen Kwok-Yung responded: 'We met with people from the Wuhan Health Organization, the Wuhan Center for Disease Control, representatives from local Wuhan hospitals, and the Hubei Health Organization.' The reporter pressed him further: 'At

the time did you suspect that any of them were concealing the facts?'
Dr. Yuen responded, 'During lunch I saw the Vice Mayor sitting next
to Zhong Nanshan and he looked terrible. Judging from the stern look
on his face, I'm sure that they already knew at that time that something
really bad was happening. After all, we were already the third team of
specialists to visit Wuhan. I believe that even if there had been things
they were concealing, by that point there was already nothing left to
hide. Yet they kept emphasizing the fact that a shipment of test kits
had only just arrived in Wuhan so they hadn't yet had enough time to
conduct tests and confirm cases.'"

Now that we have some leads, we need to keep investigating! If we
keep asking the right questions, we will eventually get to the cause. All
of us want to know why there was a need to conceal such an important
thing from the public.

It was only thanks to Zhong Nanshan's sharp and stern questions
that we were able to learn that human-to-human contact was, in fact,
possible with this virus. It was only then that the people of Wuhan
quickly awakened from their ignorance. Otherwise, had they continued to conceal the facts for much longer, it is hard to imagine just how
much worse things would have gotten. Of the more than ten million
Wuhan residents, how many would have survived?

Right now the questions we want to ask are: (1) Do we want to
investigate all the people that Dr. Yuen Kwok-Yung mentioned? How
far do we want to take this investigation? And (2) The two earlier
groups of specialists who visited must have clearly seen how serious
this was, so why didn't they pursue their questioning with the same
rigor and aggressiveness as Dr. Zhong Nanshan? During the course
of his interview Dr. Yuen, at one point, uttered the following words:
"Our scientists should know better than to ever overlook the value of
soft intelligence."

MARCH 9, 2020

If someone has to take the blame and resign,
let's start with the secretary and director of Central Hospital.

The downpour was quite heavy last night and this morning it continues. In my mind, I always think of spring rain as being gentle and silent, perhaps even a little romantic, but today it is just flooding down from the sky; I suppose I'll have to keep the lights on inside all day today.

From the tone of my doctor friend's texts today, I can tell he is in a good mood. It is now the third straight day that we have had fewer than 100 new cases, and that number continues to drop. After they put in a new set of leaders at the municipal and provincial levels and started implementing a set of new stricter policies, the virus has quickly been brought under control. When the number of patient infections was at its peak, there was a plan to build an additional 19 temporary hospitals, but now those will clearly not be needed. According to my doctor friend, 11 of the temporary hospitals have already been shut down, and the remaining three will be closing down operations within the next two or three days. Wuhan's fight against the coronavirus is finally nearing its end; it feels like they are now cleaning up the battlefield. The number of cases of serious infections continues to decline. This decline is due to two primary factors: Some of them have recovered and others have passed away. But right now there are still 4,700 patients who are considered to be in serious condition. This is still a fairly large number. Medical workers are providing them with the best care possible, and we hope those patients will be able to hang in there and recover quickly.

Central Hospital, which has faced multiple calamities over the course of this outbreak, today lost yet another physician, ophthalmologist Dr. Zhu Heping. Before this, Central Hospital had already lost ophthalmologist Dr. Li Wenliang on the evening of February 6; Director of the Department of Thyroid and Breast Cancer, Dr. Jiang Xueqing, on March 1; Director of the Department of Ophthalmology, Mei Zhongming, on March 3. That is four specialists that they have lost, three of whom are from one department. I've been told that on the list of patients currently in critical condition, several of them are also doctors from Central Hospital. In the face of such horrific losses, you can't help but ask, *what exactly went wrong at Central Hospital*? Why were so many doctors and medical personnel infected? How are the top hospital administrators, including the hospital secretary and director, going to explain this? Was it a simple case of not understanding how this novel coronavirus spreads? Or, using the perspective of "positive energy," were the doctors at Central Hospital trying to use herd immunity to build a protective wall around the people of Wuhan? Does that make any sense? But these are all questions we should be asking. Today alone I saw several articles that took issue with the actions of the Central Hospital administrators, including an appeal from an insider at the hospital who berated the people in charge. I have no way of knowing if the content of that appeal is accurate, but I know without question that four doctors from Central Hospital have died and 200 other medical workers are currently admitted as patients at hospitals all around the city. Based on those figures alone, I wonder if the secretary and director of Central Hospital even deserve to still be in charge. I'm quite confident that even without them, the rest of the hospital staff would still be able to carry on with their fight against the coronavirus. And so at this point I would like to say: if someone has to take the blame and resign, let's start with the secretary and director of Central Hospital.

Actually, stepping down to resign is also a matter of common sense. Wouldn't any reasonable person with a conscience resign if their negligence resulted in the deaths of numerous colleagues? Wouldn't they want to make up for their mistakes by trying to take actions to repair the damage they caused? But in reality, it is very difficult to find people in China willing to step up and do this. We have a lot of people who understand all kinds of big, abstract theories, but none of them have basic common sense. Sometimes when it comes to these most fundamental concepts, they are a blank, completely lost. It is similar to us listening to those officials give speeches or reading those government directives in the newspaper; it is often torturous enough just to get through it, but in the end we still have no idea what the main point was. Even when there is a clear theme, most of it is usually bullshit anyway. But there are so many commonsense issues that get buried under the dense language of those big concepts; it is hard for even a sliver of common sense to dig itself out from all of that. But these kernels of common sense remain absolutely essential for us.

Yesterday when I was writing about Dr. Yuen Kwok-Yung's interview, the term "soft intelligence" came up. I think scientists should place more emphasis on soft intelligence. Actually, it's not just scientists who could benefit from this; people like hospital and government administrators should also start paying more attention to "soft intelligence." I started wearing a face mask when I went outside way back on January 18; I even told our housekeeper to wear one when she goes shopping. Why is that, you ask? It's because I had gotten a lot of "soft intelligence" from the people around me, telling me to be extra careful. A shame, then, that our government officials, who are responsible for the lives of millions of people, didn't exert an ounce of caution. They continued on with their concerts and other mass events all the way up until January 21. Even after Dr. Zhong Nanshan made the announcement on the 20th saying that the virus could indeed spread via human-to-human contact, they *still* carried on with their big concert! My colleague YL told me what happened to a group of her cinematographer friends; four of them were assigned to shoot the performance at the Tian Han Theater; three members of that team later died from the coronavirus. If the government had informed the public earlier, if they had canceled performances like this one, perhaps we could have saved a lot of lives? So how come everyday people were already taking precautions, while our leaders just ignorantly carried on with business as usual? It is due to a lack of common sense. Their idea of common sense is rooted in a political notion of the term, while our idea of common sense is rooted in life experience.

Today there is an essay being forwarded like crazy on the internet. The title of the article is "The Fourth Round of the Shirking Responsibility Summit Meeting Opens in Wuhan." Part of the essay mentioned a telephone meeting that was held by the National Health Commission's Division of Disease Prevention on January 14. I asked my friend to check if this really happened and, indeed, there is a record. There is an article from that date entitled "In Deploying Preventive Measures Against the Infectious Novel Coronavirus, the National Health Commission Holds a Nationwide Tele-Conference." Here are two paragraphs from that story:

> During the meeting it was pointed out that there is currently a high level of uncertainty regarding methods to control this outbreak. Although the outbreak is currently limited to the city of Wuhan, we have still yet to discover the source of this novel coronavirus, nor have we fully grasped its method of transmission. We still need to keep strict watch in order to ascertain its potential for human-to-human spread. Since the Thailand Ministry of Health[12] has confirmed a case from Wuhan, efforts to control the outbreak have undergone considerable change; the spread of the virus may rapidly increase, especially with the onset of spring, and we cannot rule out the pos-

sibility of its spreading to other regions. We also cannot rule out the possibility that it could spread outside China into other countries. There is a need to prepare for worst-case scenario possibilities and increase our risk awareness; in terms of risk management, even if a given outcome is highly improbable we need to proceed as if it is the most likely outcome; we need to research the protective measures being used against the outbreak in the areas being affected by the outbreak; we must promptly figure out the most effective means of dealing with what might possibly be a new disease outbreak.

The meeting requests that the direction we take on a national level to control the outbreak follow the lead taken in Wuhan in terms of preventive measures. Hubei Province and the city of Wuhan need to adopt strict control measures with an emphasis on regulating produce markets and close monitoring for individuals with a fever; temperature monitoring stations and hospital clinics admitting patients with flu-like symptoms will be two important lines of defense. We need to increase supervision at various events, decrease large-scale public events where people gather, remind patients with fever-like symptoms not to leave Wuhan, bolster treatment plans for patients, and monitor those people who have had close contact with patients. We must implement the strictest measures and take a resolute stance to limit the outbreak to one location and do everything in our power to prevent the further spread of the virus within Wuhan.[13]

That is from a meeting held on January 14! *January 14!* That is a full six days before Zhong Nanshan publicly stated that the virus was indeed possible to spread between people! That was a full nine days before the quarantine was imposed! The author of the article "The Fourth Round of the Shirking Responsibility Summit Meeting" is a man who works in engineering, and he really is quite the detective. He was quickly able to figure out exactly when that memo was first posted; in his essay he writes: "This article was posted online in February; sometime before February 21 since it was last edited on February 21 at 8:39 a.m. But the date listed for initial posting was revised to read January 14." I find that very interesting.

It has now been verified that this document does indeed exist. This means that that meeting did indeed take place. This essay led to a lot of discussion in my classmates group chat. K commented by saying: "First of all, there must be a very large number of people who participated in this nationwide teleconference, so it would be very hard to fabricate details about it after the fact. If there had been any question as to the authenticity of the content, I'm sure that policymakers from the Hubei and Wuhan Health Commission offices would have taken issue with this report. Secondly, I wonder just who it was that 'refreshed' the content on the National Health Commission website? Who ordered them to do this? What was the actual process involved? Did someone just temporarily make a mistake and later corrected it? Or were some officials trying to 'mend the fence after the sheep had escaped'? In actuality, the National Health Commission could leak an unofficial report of this meeting in any way they might choose in order to ensure that a correct record of the details got out. But it is a bit unimaginable that they would instead choose to use this rather secretive method. That's because no one would ever claim that the National Health Commission's forgetting to upload a meeting summary to their website was somehow responsible for the tragedy we are facing today in Wuhan. Should a summary of that meeting have been made public? Who decided that that meeting should be an internal session? And who decided that the content of that meeting should be withheld from the public?"

There are simply too many suspicious things about what happened. I figure that if it was a nationwide meeting, then there must have been officials from Hubei who also participated. Who from Hubei was on the line during this teleconference? And why didn't they enact any of the suggested safety measures after that meeting? And why didn't they share the content of that meeting with the media so that things could be made public? Instead, they did not take any of the recommended actions, like monitoring people with fevers, shutting down large-scale public events, reminding people with fever and flu-like symptoms not to leave Wuhan, limiting public gatherings, and taking other similar precautions. If they had made all that information public on January 14 and urged the public to take precautions, would Wuhan have had to endure such a terrible loss of human life? Would such a horrific catastrophe have still befallen us? Would the nation have suffered such heavy losses? If they already knew that the virus was spreading and that the consequences would be severe, then why didn't they take action? Was it an intentional dereliction of duty, or were they simply being careless? Or were they simply ignorant? Did they think that everything would somehow straighten itself out after a few days? Whatever the case, I truly don't understand what happened.

Reflection and responsibility are intricately interconnected. If we do not staunchly pursue those responsible for what happened, we will never be able to seriously reflect. At this stage in the outbreak, this is the single most pressing issue for us. We need to push forward with this now while we still remember everything that happened and all the details of the complete timeline are still fresh in our minds. And so I again call on our government to quickly establish an investigative committee to thoroughly examine the core reasons that allowed the coronavirus to spread and expand to the point that it could turn into the calamity that we are now all facing. At the same time, I recommend that all people in Wuhan who have writing skills start recording everything they have seen, heard, experienced, and felt since January. I also hope that amateur writers also establish working groups to seek out families who lost loved ones to the coronavirus in order to help them document what their family members went through in search of treatment and what they experienced before their death. They should set up a website where all these testimonials can be uploaded and categorized for convenient searching. If possible, print versions of these testimonials published in multiple volumes would also be an important contribution. Let all of us in Wuhan leave behind a collective memory of what happened. I promise to do my part in contributing whatever help I can muster to support this cause.

Today among the texts my doctor friend sent me, there was the following passage: "Nine million Wuhan residents along with one million people originally from outside the city have all been trapped here in Wuhan, there is still no accurate count of how many people originally from Wuhan are now stuck outside the city where they have been subjected to untold prejudice and discrimination while being unable to return home, more than 42,000 heroic warriors have traveled to Wuhan to support the efforts here, and there are 1.4 billion Chinese who have still been unable to get back to their normal lives; we are all utterly exhausted and at the point where we simply cannot take any more."

Another doctor friend told me: "Based on what people who have been calling into our hotlines are saying, people's biggest concern is now starting to shift from getting infected with the coronavirus to the question of when they will be able to get back to work and what protective steps will be put in place once they are back to work. As of now, most people are still unable to return to work, and many are currently unemployed. The massive economic pressure people are facing is causing a lot of anxiety. For some this will result in depression and even cases of mental breakdown."

I pray that all these disasters may soon come to an end.

MARCH 10, 2020

Remember, there is no such thing as victory here,
there is only the end.

The weather is truly amazing today and the sun is shining brightly. All my colleagues are showing off photos of the flowers blooming in their courtyards; they are all glowing with beautiful colors. I'm reminded of the fact that I had originally bought an airplane ticket to Hainan island for February 6, and today was the day I was originally scheduled to return home. Because of the quarantine, I got stuck here and never made the trip. From the beginning of the outbreak until now, this is the first time that I truly feel like the difficult days are now behind us. All the temporary hospitals have now been completely decommissioned, and there are very few new reported cases of patients testing positive for the coronavirus; I think that we might be down to zero new cases in another one or two days. The horror is finally about to come to a close. But friend, please don't you dare talk about this as being some kind of victory. Remember, there is no such thing as victory here, there is only the end.

I truly never imagined that the quarantine would last this long. I remember the last time I went to the pharmacy to pick up my medicine, thinking that a month's supply would be more than enough; the reality couldn't be further from the truth. In the end, I had to go to the hospital to get my prescription refilled. I also had to deal with some hand issues during this lockdown. Several years back the palm of my hand split open; it took nearly a full year of treatment before it was back to normal. However, over the course of the past few days it started to open up again from the finger. Today my finger was in so much pain that it is affecting my ability to type, so I don't think I'll be able to write too much today.

It is a good thing, then, that a few days ago a magazine called *Soulker: Art & Literature Review* (apologies for my ignorance, but I never read this magazine before) emailed me with a few questions. Since they are an arts magazine and not a news organization, the questions they sent over were pretty open-ended. Since we are all in the same field, I decided to answer their questions somewhat freely. Today I'll share the interview with you below:

Your diary is so true to life; you record all kinds of little details about the everyday, even those emotional things that make you sigh. Did you ever consider revising it with a more polished literary language?

FANG FANG: It is only if you have a different view of what literature is that you would think that. This is a diary; so there is no need for further revision. When I first started writing this diary, I would post each entry on Weibo, which is an informal platform where you can basically speak your mind. Moreover, I'm not just some idealistic artistic youth, I'm a professional writer. I write from the heart and try to truthfully capture what is in my heart; for me, that is enough.

There are a lot of people saying they would rather read Fang Fang's diary than read reports from official media outlets like *Yangtze Daily*. What do you make of that? Did you ever imagine that your *Wuhan Diary* would elicit such a huge response?

FANG FANG: I think those who say they don't trust the media are being a bit overly biased. In order to understand the general trajectory of how the coronavirus is spreading, you still should be reading what the mainstream media has to say. All I present in my diary are my own personal thoughts and feelings. You can't get a complete perspective from just reading my diary; that should be obvious. When I first started writing I never imagined that so many people would be reading it, which was very strange to me. I even asked my colleagues and classmates why they think that so many people have been following my online diary posts; but they didn't have a good answer, either.

There is a line from your diary that reads: "When an era sheds a speck of dust it might not seem like much, but when it falls upon the shoulders of an individual it feels like a mountain." Those words have become the single most widely circulated sentence of this entire coronavirus outbreak; somehow that sentence has been seen as emblematic of everything we have experienced. Looking back, do you feel that those words have transformed into a kind of prophecy?

FANG FANG: That sentence isn't prophetic, it is reality—a reality that is with us during every era.

Every day you seem to spend a lot of time following news stories about individual people. Besides your *Wuhan Diary*, do you have any plans to record the fate of some of these individuals during this outbreak, perhaps as a novel? Or are there any individual stories that have had a particularly powerful impact on you?

FANG FANG: There are a lot of people whose stories have moved me, but I don't have any plans to write a novel about what has happened here. I already have too many writing projects that I'm doing right now.

Some people have accused the majority of Chinese writers of being mute throughout this coronavirus outbreak; what drove you to speak out? Especially considering how frequently your diary places blame on government officials and raises criticisms . . .

FANG FANG: I don't really agree with that. There are actually quite a few local writers who have all been documenting what has been happening. What's more, the method with which people record things is very different; some people are writing novels, others are recording things privately, and there are actually quite a few people publishing accounts on public platforms like I am. As for Chinese writers outside of Wuhan, since they don't understand the local dynamics it is hard for them to know how to even approach this subject. When the Ebola outbreak took place in Africa, I never published anything about it because I didn't have any firsthand knowledge and wasn't that clear about many of the details. This is perfectly natural. I think it is unreasonable to expect every writer to speak out on this issue. For the outbreak in Wuhan to spread like it has is the result of multiple forces. Government officials and specialists from Hubei and Wuhan, including members of the Wuhan Health Commission, all have a responsibility for what happened here; a very large responsibility at that. Since they are among the responsible parties, why shouldn't I speak out?

"If you are just going to fawn all over the officials, please restrain yourselves. I might be old, but I will never tire when it comes to speaking out." This line reminds me of a lot of things that have happened to you, such as those open letters you published criticizing some things that happened with the Lu Xun Literary Award or a certain poet's assessment for promotion. These criticisms were all directed at people in your field whom I'm sure you will encounter in the future; yet you still insisted on speaking out. What is the meaning of criticism for you?

FANG FANG: When I was serving as the chair of the Hubei Writers Association, there would sometimes be things I saw that were against our regulations. Whenever I encountered these situations, I would discuss them with the Chinese Communist Party representatives in the Writers Association and ask them to step in. In situations where they failed to take action, I felt it incumbent on me to speak out online about what was happening. I feel like I was just doing my job. Now that I'm retired, even if they were to all turn completely rotten, it would still be none of my business anymore.

Do you agree with the idea that writers should shoulder more social responsibility besides just writing?

FANG FANG: That depends on the individual. Not everyone's personality is suited to take up that additional social responsibility. It is easy to "shoulder it" but if you don't have the courage, insight, and ability it can be a tall task, especially if you have a weak personality, tend to be timid, or get anxious easily. If you fall into that latter category, then there is no reason to take on that responsibility. In this world there are people who just bear it and others who enjoy taking up that responsibility; that's how it has always been. But you can't force people to do these things; it comes down to a matter of individual choice. There is no such thing as what people "should" or "shouldn't" do.

Back when *Soft Burial* was published, it elicited attacks from all sides; how did you look at those attacks? And were you ever scared when there were so many agitated voices of criticism attacking you?

FANG FANG: I never let it get to me. What's there to be scared of? I suppose they are the ones who are scared of me? As for written polemics, as a professional writer, I live by the pen. So what is there to fear? Of course if they showed up at my front door with clubs in their hands, that would be another matter. But all they do is write essays, and that is what I do for a living. Some of those critics you are referring to must be those ultra-leftists? They operate at a very low level; their writing skills, ability to make logical judgments, and critical thinking skills are all quite pathetic. It would be an utter waste of time for me to even respond to their essays. It would be a waste to use the beautiful Chinese language on them. So I prefer not to get into arguments with them. But government officials are a different story, especially high-ranking officials. They wield a lot of power; even after they have retired they can still have a profound influence on a lot of people. So when they attack me I think it is important to fight back. But I'm too lazy to pay much attention to most of those ultra-leftist hooligans; but when they are wearing an official government hat, why shouldn't I push back? When I fight back I'm not the one who ends up losing, it's them. They have now learned their lesson and know not to go after writers like me. Let's see if any more of those retired high-ranking officials dare to come after any more writers. If they do, they will only be making themselves look bad.

Many years from now when critics look back on your work, do you hope they regard Fang Fang as "an admirable woman writer with a strong social mission and a good conscience" or "as an outstanding writer with incredible literary skill and talent"?

FANG FANG: I really don't care. I really have no interest in how other people perceive me. As long as I can face myself, I am happy. How critics view me is their business, not mine.

Back when you wrote the novel *The City of Wuchang* how did you balance the actual history with your fictional imagination? What is the meaning of recording history for contemporary people's lives?

FANG FANG: Novels are, after all, works of fiction; they rely on the imagination. But when you write a historical novel about actual events that happened, you need to also respect the history. I just place my characters into that history. There are always fissures that exist within historical narratives. When I write historical fiction, I always have the broad historical map in my mind and then I search for those fissures where I can set my characters free to roam. The meaning of recording history for me comes down to "using history as a mirror."

There are actually a lot of voices out there online that have been criticizing you or raising suspicions about you. Do those voices ever make you uncomfortable or depressed? Amid all this fear and chaos, how do you manage to maintain a normal healthy outlook?

FANG FANG: I don't get depressed, but sometimes I do feel a bit uncomfortable, but, even more than that, I get angry because I find what they are doing to be utterly incomprehensible. You get angry about why these ultra-leftists are doing what they do, and I find it difficult to understand how these people could have so much hatred inside themselves. I don't personally know a single one of them, nor have I even had contact with them; yet their hatred for me runs so deep it is as if I killed their fathers in a past life or something! I really can't understand it.

And I don't always maintain a normal healthy outlook; sometimes I get anxious. And then there are times when I am really at a loss as to what to do. When there are so many unknown factors that you face, you can sometimes be left very confused inside.

Does the fact that you are the former chair of the Hubei Writers Association serve as a kind of protection? Or does it come with a negative impact?

FANG FANG: I don't think either one. I didn't let this title affect me when I was the chair, so I certainly don't let it affect me now that I have retired.

This title has never provided me with any sort of protection, nor do I feel that it has brought any negative consequences. I had a good life before serving as chair, and things didn't change much after I took over. Now that I'm retired, things are still like before. Those people who think serving as chair is a big deal really don't understand the Chinese system, or me.

A large number of your stories all depict the people of Wuhan's lives. What traits of the Wuhan people are you fondest of? Has the corona-virus outbreak revealed any new characteristics about the people of Wuhan that you never saw before?

FANG FANG: The people of Wuhan have always been straightforward and they place a lot of emphasis on what is right and wrong. They are generous when it comes to helping people out and have a sense of honor. Perhaps a lot of this is connected to the geography and climate here. But Wuhan has always been a city of commerce; most people are careless and casual, yet they aren't the bravest. They tend to follow whatever the government tells them. They like to enjoy life but aren't particularly interested in politics; they are very practical. Whether or not there is an outbreak, the people of Wuhan always behave the same, at least that is my impression. They are the same as they ever were.

How do you view the relationship between a writer and their city?

FANG FANG: It's like the relationship between a fish and water; or a tree and the soil.

Once this outbreak has passed, what are you most looking forward to doing?

FANG FANG: Completing the novel that I have been working on.

MARCH 11, 2020

> *Once things get to this point,*
> *do you really think you can delete it all?*

Another day of nice weather. It feels good to have the early spring sun shining down. I'm thinking about how East Lake must be completely desolate and empty right now. I'm sure the plum blossoms all shed their flowers during that rainy night a few days ago. Tens of thousands of plum blossom trees and they all bloomed and withered for them alone to see and enjoy. If you had to put that in a poem, how would you convey that? "The flowers whirl and scatter as the water flows." My old dog has been locked up at home for so long now that he doesn't even want to go out to the courtyard anymore. He just likes to stay curled up in his dog bed. In some way, I feel the same; I don't even want to go out anymore, I just want to stay here in my apartment. A few friends have sent me invitations; they are all telling me to come over to visit and rest for a while once the outbreak is over. They are all telling me how gorgeous the spring scenery is, trying to entice me with the images of beautiful mountains and rushing water. The old me would have been there in a minute. But right now I don't even want to leave the house; I wonder if this is some kind of post-traumatic stress syndrome I'm going through.

My doctor friends have continued to forward me news about how much the coronavirus situation has improved. The number of new cases is now down to under 20; it should be down to zero soon. And thanks to the hard work of all the doctors, the number of deaths has also dramatically decreased. But I really can't wait until the number of deaths gets down to zero. Today the Hubei Province Outbreak Control Center released a statement: All work units in Hubei Province will begin to gradually resume work and production according to each district, level, and type of industry. That means that we should be able to get back to our normal lives soon?

One of my friends (all these friends are real people, but I do not always reveal their names here in order to protect them from potential attacks) sent me a photo this morning—it was a group photo of Central Hospital's Department of Thyroid and Breast Cancer, which was Dr. Jiang Xueqing's department. The day that Dr. Jiang passed away, someone replaced the heads of all the people in the photo with candles, only leaving one person's image untouched—and that was Dr. Jiang Xueqing. I was quite touched by that photo and by his colleagues' sense of friendship and loyalty. If Dr. Jiang can somehow see this, I hope it gives him a sense of comfort.

For the past two days now, the name Ai Fen,[14] a physician at Central Hospital, has been circulating all over the internet. All the internet censorship has begun to elicit the wrath of the people. It is as if everyone is in a relay race; as soon as the censors delete a post, netizens repost it again online. They just keep passing the baton forward. They just keep forwarding those posts, using all kinds of different methods to the point that the internet censors can no longer keep up; there is no way for them to delete everything anymore. Over the course of this process of resistance, posts get deleted, then reposted, over and over again. Preserving these deleted posts gradually becomes a sacred duty of those netizens. This sacred duty comes from an almost subconscious realization that keeps telling them: Protect those posts, for protecting them is the only way to protect yourself. Once things get to this point, I have to ask my dear internet censors, do you think you can really delete it all?

It is really hard for me to understand how those internet censors work. They delete my posts over and over; I suspect that it is the ultra-leftists who bombard the internet companies with complaints that my posts threaten social stability, so they try to solve everything by just deleting everything in one fell swoop. I understand the psychology behind this because I do the same thing; whenever someone posts things out of line on my social media accounts, I just blacklist them. But why would someone censor an article about Ai Fen published in the magazine *People*?[15] Unless, of course, someone was scared that she might reveal the inside story that someone doesn't want told? I wonder what that inside story really is. The essay was about what happened at Central Hospital and addressed exactly the kind of things that we have all been eager to find out: It was about the who, what, and where behind the 20-day delay in reporting the outbreak. Don't the internet censors also want to know these things? If we don't unravel the details behind what actually happened between the initial outbreak and its spread, how will the people of Wuhan, and the people of China for that matter, ever get over this? I don't believe that the internet censors would just haphazardly delete that article for no reason; the order certainly had to be coming at the request of someone. So who was it who made the call to delete that article? Officials from Wuhan? Or was it an order coming from Hubei? Or was it . . . anyway, the whole thing is very difficult for me to understand, even hard to imagine.

Ever since the novel coronavirus first appeared in December of last year, everything that has happened since has seemingly gone against normal rules and conventions; and there are so many questions that will never be answered. We are now starting to see some of these things gradually emerge in reports being published by various journalists. Some of the details in these reports have left us utterly dumbfounded and at a complete loss for words. Whether these officials and specialists failed to perform their assigned duties, careless and inattentive, flippant and perfunctory, or just plain stupid, they need to be held accountable and punished, which should also serve as a warning to others. I don't believe that the government will let those responsible off easy after what they have done; I don't think anyone is going to get a pass on this. After all, if you don't pursue this and hold people accountable, at the end of the day, the biggest victim will be the nation itself. It will result in the government's loss of credibility with the public, not to mention the pain that citizens will feel. And that would lead to all kinds of other continued catastrophes. But right now, for a lot of people, it doesn't seem to matter if these people don't do their jobs or completely screw up their jobs; they just don't care. If they don't take responsibility, the nation will still be able to absorb the damage. But we can't go on like that anymore. To quote a famous line: If we continue on as we have in the past, the country will cease to be the country it once was.

Today I took the time to look up some official documents relating to the resignation of government officials in China. One item I found was entitled *Provisional Resignation Rules for Party and Government Officials and Cadres*. I'm not sure what year this version was published or whether or not it was later revised, but I will nevertheless quote it here. Chapter four of the document is entitled "Resignation After Assuming Blame," and the fourteenth article states: "Party and government officials who commit professional mistakes that result in large-scale losses, catastrophic impacts, or bear the responsibility for major accidents should no longer serve in any official capacity and they should resign their position and accept blame for their mistakes."

Article 15 is even more specific: "(1) In cases in which a dereliction of duty results in a serious incident affecting the public, or when a group incident or sudden incident is handled improperly, resulting in serious consequences or adverse effects, those leaders primarily responsible shall accept blame and resign; (2) For serious mistakes in decision-making that result in large-scale economic losses or other negative impacts, the leaders primarily responsible should accept blame and resign; (3) In cases of serious negligence as relating to disaster prevention and relief operations, prevention of epidemics and infectious outbreaks, etc., which lead to major losses or adverse effects, leaders bearing the primary responsibility should accept blame and tender resignation; (4) In instances of serious negligence in terms of work safety, continuous or multiple major liability accidents, or if a major accident occurs, the leader in charge should accept responsibility and resign; (5) For cases of serious negligence in the management and supervision of economic markets, environmental protection, social management, etc., continuous or multiple major accidents resulting in large-scale losses that are the result of bad leadership decisions, the individual in charge shall accept blame and tender resignation; (6) In cases where poor implementation of the articles contained in *Regulations on the Selection and Appointment of CCP and Government Leaders and Cadres* results in serious oversights, mistakes, and negative impact, leaders bearing responsibility should accept blame and resign; (7) In cases where negligent management or supervision results in team members or subordinates repeatedly committing serious legal violations or actions that breach the discipline code resulting in a negative impact, those leaders responsible shall accept blame and tender resignation; (8) If the spouse, children, or staff of government officials commit actions that seriously breach the code of discipline or commit illegal acts resulting in negative consequences, those leaders who were aware yet took no actions are to be held responsible and shall tender resignation; (9) In addition, there are other additional actions that can also result in leaders' being forced to accept blame and resign."

It is quite clear from the regulations recorded above that assuming responsibility and offering one's resignation is something required for a society to function properly. Upon review of the nine items listed above, who from Hubei Province and Wuhan city should accept responsibility and tender their resignation? I recommend that all officials involved in what has transpired consult the above articles and decide if any of the items are applicable to their own actions. If they do not feel any of the articles apply to their own actions, then the public will probably still submit a formal list of officials that they feel need to bear responsibility; but it would be terrible if it had to come to that. Instead I feel that, from now on, government officials need to understand the importance of being able to step up and accept blame for their mistakes *before* they even take office; and then they need to learn how to resign. In short, we have so many ignorant, arrogant, and thick-skinned officials who refuse to admit their own mistakes that the people can no longer stand by and take this anymore.

As I get to this point, my friend just sent me an investigative report from the magazine *Southern Weekly* entitled "Four People Dead in the Line of Duty, Four People Critically Ill: Wuhan Central Hospital's Darkest Moment." The essay begins with: "There are still four doctors from Central Hospital who are critically ill. Dr. Yang Fan, who has been on the front lines with these patients, stressed the fact that all four of them are experiencing multiple organ failure, including respiratory failure, and other severe complications. 'Some of them are currently completely reliant on respirators and life support to stay alive.' They include Assistant Director Wang Ping, Medical Ethics Committee Member Liu Li, Assistant Director of the Thoracic Surgery Department Yi Fan, and Assistant Director of the Department of Urology Hu Weifeng." My god, it really breaks your heart. How can the secretary and director of Central Hospital bear to sit comfortably without taking responsibility for this? Someone needs to cry out: "If you have a conscience, stand up and resign!"

MARCH 12, 2020

Someone has probably been trying to use this
incident with the police to harass me?

The sky is bright but you can't see the sun. But there is still a strong feeling of spring in the air.

Today is an unusual day. Ever since I got out of bed, there has been a constant stream of bad news. It started with a post that a few of my friends sent to me. The title of the article was: "What Do You Think of Netizens' Denouncement of Fang Fang?" and it included a compendium of more than 200 vicious online attacks against me. What can I say? These people are rotten to the core; it seems they don't have even an ounce of goodness left. At the very least, shouldn't they have balanced the article out by including voices from some of my supporters? Half and half would be nice. The publisher of this post was a website called "Hubei Today Online," which is run by the Hubei Province Journalists Association. Is this even an official site? Don't tell me that someone put this site up after I starting calling for some officials to take responsibility and resign? Is that what they are resorting to?

But the other thing that happened today was even more unusual. Moreover, once it happened, the news was everywhere. The basic gist of the accusation is that I abused my special authority to get the traffic police to escort my niece out of Wuhan, so she could escape to Singapore. There were quite a few verified users on Weibo who have been trying to put on a good show by earnestly publishing essays about this. It really seems like those ill-intentioned people intent on attacking me really have nothing better to do with their time.

My niece has lived in Singapore for more than a decade and is considered a Singaporean-Chinese. She took a flight home that was arranged by the Singapore government to evacuate Singapore citizens who had been living or working in Wuhan. The whole thing was arranged jointly by the governments of Singapore and China. This happened back around the time of the Lunar New Year, and I believe that the flight departed sometime around 1:00 a.m. (I don't recall all the details, but I think the flight was later pushed back to 3:00 a.m.? In any case, the flight departed very late.) My brother and his wife are both in their seventies and neither of them drives. And that day the order had just come down banning private automobiles from the roads. I always follow the rules, so I decided to inquire about what we should do to get her to the airport. Frankly speaking, I have lived in Wuhan for more than 60 years and know quite a few police officers. Some of my colleagues also have relatives who serve on the force. The Wuhan Police Department even has a writing class that I once visited, on their invitation. I also used to get invited to a lot of conferences organized by the police department. I have even written several stories with police officer protagonists, and some of the material for those works actually came from hearing their stories. So, based on this experience, isn't it only natural that I would have some police officer friends? Since I know these officers and I had an emergency situation, I reached out to them for help; which all makes perfect sense to me. Officer Xiao and a few of his fellow officers even came to my apartment about two years ago. When I reached out to them for help, I was told that Officer Xiao was actually off duty, so he would be free to help me out. I sent him a text and he immediately agreed to help. Although he is technically a member of the auxiliary police, I still refer to him as Officer Xiao. There are quite a few auxiliary police on the force and I always treat them with respect, as I feel one should. I think that was around Day Five of the Lunar New Year (although I'm not exactly sure of the date, but I'm sure I still have his texts saved on my phone). So if anyone wants to

investigate, please go ahead. If this is what is called "abusing my special authority," then I'm not sure what "special authority" means. To be
truthful, I think what is really going on is that someone has probably
been trying to use this incident with the police to harass me?

I already responded to these accusations earlier today on Weibo
because I was very concerned that Officer Xiao might face repercus-
sions if his superiors didn't understand what actually happened, which
is why I have taken the time to provide a full explanation. Otherwise, I
never look at Weibo as a platform for dealing out judgment; I normally
don't feel obliged to respond to accusations just because someone posts
them on Weibo. Writers are allowed to have friends who are police officers and police officers are allowed to help their friends out on their
day off; this is all a common part of human relationships. Don't you see
plots like that on television shows every day? The fact that this issue has
become so overblown is really a sad joke.

While I'm at it, why don't I share a few things about myself for those
people lacking common sense (including those who have been reporting on me) in order to prevent mistakes with their future posts:

1. This year I am 65 years old and recently retired. I have quite a few
   health conditions. I was actually admitted to the hospital just before
   the Chinese New Year last year for a herniated disc, which didn't end
   up resolving itself until the end of the year. All my colleagues at work
   can attest to the health problems I have faced. For the first half of last
   year I could barely walk, I was in so much pain. So those people online who have suggested that I should get out and volunteer need to
   know that it is simply not a practical option for me. Moreover, at my
   age, I don't think I could handle the physical strain involved in most
   volunteer work. If I were to slip and reinjure my back, then I really
   would become more of a burden than anything else.

2. I am not a Department-level cadre! I am not a Department-level cadre! I am not a Department-level cadre! Since this is important, I need to repeat it three times! I'm not even a public servant anymore! So there is no rank-level at all attached to my name. I'm sorry to disappoint all of you who keep referring to me as a "department-level cadre!" After retirement I became just an ordinary citizen. And, of course, I never joined the Communist Party of China. I have always been one of the people. Sure, I previously served as Chair of the Hubei Writers Association, but those who understand how the system works know that this title doesn't involve active administrative duties. Almost all the tasks taken on by the various provincial Writers Associations are decided by party organizations. That being the case, there have been several literary events in which I helped the Writers Association out when it came to planning and organizing.

3. I received a special appointment with the Writers Association back in 1992, so I suppose I now qualify as a senior figure in the organization; that means that my salary, while not terribly high, is not that bad, certainly enough to live on. And now I am receiving social security and money from my retirement fund. The Writers Association has always taken good care of retired writers. That has always been the case, even going back to veteran writers like Xu Chi and Bi Ye, and the tradition continues on to this day. That means that even after retirement, the Writers Association has continued to take good care of me, just as it has for many other writers. My colleagues here are also very good to me; I have watched many of them grow up, so we have always been quite close. My lifestyle is indeed a bit different from your average person's because I'm a professional writer who has published nearly 100 books. There are a lot of people out there who have read my work and they seem to respect me, especially people here in Wuhan. The fact that I have won a small amount of notoriety for my writings cer-

tainly has led some people to go out of their way to help me out; I have to admit that. Sometimes when I go out to eat, the restaurant owner will bring out a special dish, and I even once had a cab driver who refused to accept the cab fare after he recognized me. I am very thankful and moved by all these people's generosity.

4. Those ultra-leftists have been continually looking for any excuse to attack me; they must have gone through my Weibo posts with a toothpick in search of the slightest flaw. And God knows how many times they have officially reported me to Weibo, even though I can't figure out what they would report me for. I've actually never been afraid of people reporting me; I'm more scared when they *don't* report me! It's when they don't report you that people start believing all the rumors. But when they report you, they really expose all your good traits! To be honest, even people from the Central Commission for Discipline and Inspection have told me that I should serve on their commission, since I'm honest, I'm always abiding by the rules, and I dare to speak the truth.

5. The attacks that they launched today were particularly fierce and came quite by surprise. It was a collective attack and they all followed the same talking points, used the same language, the same images, and even posted their attacks at the same time. They also all reported me to Weibo for infringement of online rules at the same time, in order to make their case more powerful. It is almost like the meeting was held last night where they picked a specific time and decided to take collective action. Isn't that an interesting coincidence? So who was chairing this meeting? (Even an idiot would know that such a meeting must have been orchestrated by a government office.) And who was it that fanned the flames? When you really think about it, the whole thing is actually quite terrifying. If the group one day decides that instead of just coming after my

diary they want to start an insurrection or do something really destructive, I'm sure the consequences would be exponentially worse.
This organization and their members have incredible resources to
recruit and mobilize large numbers of people; they attack whom-
ever the organization tells them to. They collectively attack any individual with views that oppose their own. (I even heard that two
professors who spoke up for me on Weibo were also targeted; those
hacks went through their accounts and even reported them to the
government. All it takes is one wrong word for them to send down
an order and they immediately let their dogs loose, who unleash a
flurry of insults and curses against you. I'm really not sure what the
difference is between them and any other terrorist organization.)
Doesn't the government feel they should be concerned about these
organizations? They must have also threatened the government on
more than one occasion?

6. Here I am, a writer quarantined in the epicenter of an outbreak,
locked up in her home, recording all the things she thinks, feels,
and experiences. If you want to support me, support me; if you want
to criticize me, criticize me; all that is perfectly natural. I really still
don't understand why so many people are interested in reading my
diary. But a few days ago I saw one reader comment, "Fang Fang's
Wuhan Diary is like a breathing valve to save us from our boredom."
That felt good to read; it's really hard to describe in words. As I myself struggle to breathe, I have also been helping others to breathe. It
is only because I have had so many readers leaving me encouraging
comments that I decided to push forward and carry on. It is those
readers who have brought me the most warmth throughout this
period of life under quarantine.

7. But what I really don't understand is why a rather unassuming diary
like this would elicit such malicious denunciations and attacks from

so many people? When did this all begin? Who incited all these people to attack me? Who exactly are these people who are coming after me? What kind of intentions lurk behind their attacks? What kind of system of values drives people to do this? What kind of education and upbringing did these people have? What kind of work do they normally do? There is always a record left online; perhaps some people who care can look into this and do a little research to uncover the truth behind these attacks and the people launching them. It's something worth looking into and I am quite curious.

8. I really feel sorry for all those young people who are part of this. Once they start to take those ultra-leftists as their teachers and mentors, I'm afraid that many of them will be spending the rest of their lives in a dark abyss.

The outbreak situation continues to improve. The number of new confirmed coronavirus patients today dropped to below 10, and most districts in the city are now down to zero. That's a number that makes a lot of people happy. I started today in a lousy mood, but thanks to the good news about the coronavirus numbers dropping, I suppose things evened out a bit.

MARCH 13, 2020

Open up a space so we can all have a good cry.

It was still quite sunny at noon, but later in the afternoon it started to turn cloudy and the wind picked up. The old man in heaven can be unpredictable, changing on the turn of a dime; sometimes we would prefer a transition period, but often we can't even get that. The cherry blossoms on the campus of Wuhan University must be in full bloom now. Looking down at them from the rostrum of the Laozhaishe, the belt of flowers would always resemble a trail of white clouds. Back when I was in college there, we would always go there to take pictures when the cherry blossoms were in bloom. At that time there were no tourists, just us students. Years later that place became a major tourist destination, and during this season each year the campus is swarming with so many people that you can barely walk without bumping into people. There are more faces in the crowd then petals on the flowers, and the scenery is more dominated by the throngs of people than by the cherry blossoms.

The coronavirus situation continues to improve. More and more people are being discharged from the hospitals, and there are now only a handful of new patients. But one strange thing today was that the daily coronavirus press conference was held a bit later than usual. In the afternoon I looked at several of my group chats and discovered that a lot of people were all discussing this; no one knew why there was this delay. My doctor friend also wondered why just a short delay would suddenly send everyone's imagination to run wild. I wonder what everyone is thinking?

It has now been more than 50 days since the quarantine was implemented. If they had told us in the beginning that this would last 50 days I wonder how we would have taken that news. But no matter what, I certainly never imagined it would last this long. Last month when I picked up my prescription at the hospital, I got a one-month supply, which I thought would be plenty—I never thought the quarantine would still be going on. Looking back, I clearly underestimated this virus. I underestimated its ferocity and endurance. While the number of new patients continues to decrease, there is some strange news that has been coming in that reminds us that we can't take any half-measures, otherwise this virus could rear its ugly head again. Therefore, we continue to stand at the ready. One thing on our side now is the fact that we now have more experience about how to fight this virus; if you get sick, it usually isn't too bad if you immediately go to the hospital and get treatment. As long as you don't let it progress to the later stages, treatment isn't that difficult.

We are almost halfway through March and the Qingming Festival is almost here. Honoring and remembering our past relatives, burning incense for them, and sweeping their tombs are all traditions that have persisted a long time in our culture. This is also a rite that most families partake in every year. For the people of Wuhan, who are usually stubbornly traditional, this year's festival will be a big challenge for people. In just over two months' time, we have lost several thousand people, impacting tens of thousands of their friends and relatives. Their loved ones are gone, yet they are not only unable to prepare their tombs in remembrance; they cannot even pick up the ashes of their deceased relatives. This is especially the case for those families who lost relatives during early to mid-February; the first seven days after someone's death are supposed to be reserved for various rites, but they were instead thrown into a state of chaos and pain; for many people the official 49-day mourning period wouldn't end until after the Qingming Festival. Everyone realizes that this coronavirus period is an era unlike any other time, however, when the moment comes that you must face a personal loss, how can you be expected not to feel sadness and longing for your loved ones? That's simply not a possibility. I'm quite concerned for families that have lost someone. I'm worried that when the reality really sets in, they won't be able to handle this extended period of repression and it could lead to a lot of people having a nervous breakdown. Just thinking about it now, even I have trouble holding in my tears.

You need to talk to people and cry in order to get over the death of a loved one. This is an effective method to help one psychologically heal. A few days ago I read an essay about all the people who have been posting messages on Li Wenliang's Weibo page; their messages have transformed Dr. Li's Weibo page into a wailing wall. These messages are not simply in commemoration of Li Wenliang; their more important function is providing an outlet for people online to release those things that have been pent up inside them. I figure that now that we are at the tail end of the outbreak and it is still a few days before the Qingming Festival, we should really establish a website that can function as a "wailing wall"; perhaps we can call it the "wailing web." That would provide a place for mourning families to go where they could post photos, light candles, and have a good cry. Actually, it isn't just family members of the deceased who are crying. Everyone in the entire city of Wuhan needs a good cry; this "wailing web" could serve as a portal for people to mourn and cry for their family members, friends, and themselves. We need to release the sadness in our hearts and we need to express our grief over all the loss we have witnessed. Perhaps the website could also feature some comforting music, which might make it even better. Perhaps after we have all let out our tears and cries of mourning, we will all feel a bit better. We still don't know the exact date that this epidemic will be over, but during this uncertain period the sadness of countless people has already become pent-up to the point that it is forming a wall; moving forward, this could become a big challenge for people. That is why we need to open up a space so we can all have a good cry.

Besides this, there is another group of people that we should not be overlooking. During the early phase of the outbreak, there were large numbers of people getting infected, and it was very difficult to secure a hospital bed for patients; sick people were not getting the treatment they needed; and many have been unable to even get a nucleic acid test, let alone a coronavirus test. Some of these people died at the hospital, but most passed away at home. One of my high school classmates told me that her husband has a colleague who lost two family members during that early stage. Their grandmother died at home but the funeral home was so busy that they weren't able to come pick up the body until late that night. There were a lot of deaths like that in Wuhan early on; that is by no means an outlier example. And since they were never officially diagnosed with the novel coronavirus, they are not even counted as part of the official coronavirus death toll. How many people fall into this category? I have no idea. I discussed this issue on the phone today with a psychologist friend of mine; we both felt that if each district in the city is able to officially register all these deaths as coronavirus fatalities, it would allow those surviving family members to also take advantage of any future national policies the government sets up for victims. At the same time, it would also be helpful if each district is able to calculate how many non-coronavirus patients died of other ailments during this lockdown period because they were unable to receive proper medical care. All these different categories of patients should be accounted for, so that the government can take things into consideration when they decide how to placate victims' families in the future.

For the past few days the coronavirus outbreak has improved greatly, yet the public outcries have been deafening. The strongest voices have all been speaking out against the practice of using garbage trucks to deliver food to Wuhan residents. There was a video circulating online yesterday that left a lot of people utterly shocked. Who could even possibly conceive of using a garbage truck to deliver food!? The level of ignorance and audacity is simply outrageous. Are these officials completely lacking in basic common sense, or do they look at citizens as somehow less than human? I'm not sure if there were some special circumstances that led them to make this decision, but no matter how desperate they may have been, that is still no excuse for them to do something this unbecoming.

Sometimes I think that if a particular government regime doesn't place their citizens on top, the next time there is some other virus, we will again face another catastrophe like this one. When you have a group of government officials who don't care about the people and the only thing they seem to really care about is what their superiors think, then you can expect more garbage trucks delivering food in the future. One major problem facing a lot of government officials today is that none of them ever look at the people as the fundamental core of society; and none of them ever consider things from the perspective of everyday people. If they just continue looking at things from their bureaucratic perspective, I'm afraid it will never be enough. This is not entirely an issue of character; it also has a lot to do with the system they find themselves in. This fast-moving machine trains their eyes to only look at their superiors, while making it impossible for them to clearly see all the lives below. It's what is often referred to as: "When you are in the game, you don't always have full control of the circumstances around you."

Allow me to digress for a moment: Today I read an article in *Southern People Weekly*, which featured an interview with Dr. Du Bin, a member of the Senior Advisor Team to the National Health Council. The title of the article was "This Has Nothing to Do with Heroism." It was a great article, but there was one sentence that made me laugh. Dr. Du Bin said: "I don't believe that when you are in a treatment facility the virus can fly into your eyes and infect you." I distinctly remember Dr. Wang Guangfa, who is also a specialist in this field, saying that he was personally infected when droplets went into his eye. Dr. Wang's comments are what led to protective goggles selling out everywhere overnight. One of my friends even insisted on sending me a set of goggles. I really didn't want to give her any trouble, so I just told her to send me the website address and I would order one directly. I still haven't even opened the package.

One final item I want to mention: Today I saw an official user group on Weibo called "Fang Fang's *Wuhan Diary*" Editorial Group, which was forwarding essays written by other people. I just want to publicly state that this group has absolutely no connection to me. I hope the manager of this group changes the name in order to prevent various misunderstandings.

MARCH 14, 2020

Whose turn will it be to step up and
become the next whistleblower?

A bright clear day. I wonder if the cherry blossoms are still in bloom? Normally when they bloom the weather tends to be rainy and windy, so after just two or three days the trees are already bare. That's why seeing the brief duration between the cherry blossoms' blooming and withering always seems to leave us with all kinds of reflections about the fragility and precariousness of life.

The coronavirus situation continues to improve as new patient cases are still on the decline. For the past few days, the number of new cases has been fluctuating in the single digits. Yesterday a concerned friend asked me if I thought the numbers might be fake. After officials hid the details of the outbreak early on, a lot of people are still harboring doubts about the accuracy of official statistics. "What if they are lying to make the numbers look better? What if those officials are lying to make themselves look better? What are we going to do if they lie to us again?" I completely understand my friend's concerns; as the saying goes, "once bitten, twice shy." What happened could lead people to be suspicious about a lot of different things. And so I decided to put in a call to one of my doctor friends to get their opinion on whether or not there was a possibility that people may be fudging the numbers. My doctor friend was quite confident as he responded, "They wouldn't hide anything; there is no reason to hide anything!" That's the answer I was hoping to hear.

This afternoon my old classmate who goes by the nickname "Old Fox" sent me a message. Old Fox's father, Mr. Hu Guorui, was once my poetry teacher. Mr. Hu was an excellent lecturer; a lot of students from other departments also enrolled in his classes, which were always packed. Eventually they had to move his class to a larger classroom in the Laozhaishe building. Back when I was in his class, there was a poem he taught us that wasn't in our textbook. He recited it to us:

> Coming and going amid the misty water,
> for ten years I claimed to be Lord of the West Lake.
> On my light rowboat,
> I float past the bay overgrown with reed-catkins.
> In my pleasure I break out in song,
> on this silent night my voice rings clear.
> But there is no one present to appreciate it,
> instead I clap for myself,
> as my song reverberates through the endless mountains.[16]

I can still remember the way Mr. Hu kept the rhythm and exclaimed his appreciation for this poem as he recited it. The image is as fresh in my mind as yesterday. Old Fox was a member of the class of 1977; he loved to travel, he even went to America to hike the entire Appalachian Trail. The whole trip took several months and he kept a complete record of his journey as he went. It was really an incredible trip. At first I thought he was the first Chinese to complete the entire Appalachian Trail, but he later told me he wasn't, but he was quite confident that he was the first person from Wuhan to do it.

The news that Old Fox forwarded to me today was really quite shocking. I'll copy the two items he sent below:

1. I wanted to report some good news; Yi Fan has been taken off the ventilator machine and is awake. He even recorded a short video to say hello to some of his old classmates. Yi Fan's nine-year-old daughter also made her dad a whole bunch of get-well cards. Hu Zha also came out of his coma; this is really a miracle for the Sino-Japanese Friendship Hospital in Beijing.

2. Yesterday you mentioned two doctors from the front lines who were now struggling for their lives, Dr. Yi Fan and Dr. Hu Weifeng (Hu Zha is Hu Weifeng's nickname); they both happen to be classmates of my jogging partner. She sends me updates every day on how they are doing, and today she told me that they have both woken up.

There is no better news to get than that as we are struggling through these depressing days. Dr. Yi Fan is the assistant director of the Thoracic Surgery Department at Central Hospital, and Dr. Hu Weifeng is the assistant director of the Department of Urology at the same hospital. Two days ago the newspapers were reporting that both of them were still in critical condition; I also mentioned that in my diary. The fact that both of them have now woken up is simply marvelous news. I hope these two doctors can hold on; I'm confident that their physicians will be able to find a way to help them both recover.

The heavy number of casualties suffered by medical caregivers at Central Hospital remains a widely discussed and controversial topic. But up until now, I still haven't heard any news about any of the hospital administrators facing any kind of disciplinary actions. Even as endless appeals for the hospital leaders to take responsibility continue to appear online, the people running Central Hospital have remained unusually silent on this issue; it is as if they can make the criticism disappear by ignoring it. This is very different from the situation with the district head of Wuchang and the assistant district head of Qingshan, who were both removed from office before there was even a public call for them to step down. It's hard for me to understand what standards top leaders go by when making decisions about how to discipline officials in situations like this. All I know is that the number of people killed or injured in an incident never guarantees that a leader will step up to take responsibility for what happened. But I had better stop talking about this particular topic here; it won't be good if I keep going.

There has also been all kinds of online chatter on the topic of journalists today; some of the discussions have been quite detailed and interesting. I would also like to chime in a bit: Dr. Ai Fen from the Central Hospital is now calling herself the "whistle-giver"; the public has been referring to Dr. Li Wenliang as a whistleblower. That means that the whistle has been passed from Ai Fen to Li Wenliang, which makes me wonder who the torch will be passed to next. Although Dr. Li Wenliang was reprimanded, they never confiscated his "whistle." It was actually the police's action that amplified the sound of his whistle. The appearance of the novel coronavirus was already made public on December 31, 2019. At the very least, that is the day that I received the news. The following day, reports that local police had reprimanded "eight netizens" appeared all over the media, including CCTV. But that doesn't necessarily mean that the "whistle" had been confiscated. So who should now take up the whistle? Whose turn will it be to step up and become the next whistleblower?

There are two large media groups here in Wuhan; the largest is, of course, the Hubei Daily News and Media Group, and the second largest is without a doubt the Yangtze Daily Newspaper Group. How many reporters are employed between these two companies? I'm not sure, but according to the search engine Baidu, the Hubei Daily News and Media Group "controls 7 newspapers, 8 magazines, 12 websites, 5 mobile platforms, 1 publishing company, 56 companies (in which they are the sole investor or controlling stockholder), and they have 17 station offices located throughout Hubei Province, making them the largest news and information platform for the outside world to understand important news coming out of Hubei." Looking at this structure, I'm sure that the Yangtze Daily Newspaper Group also has its fair share of subsidiary publications, magazines, websites, and companies, but I'm too lazy to look all of that up. But I think it is safe to assume that these two massive companies employ quite a large number of reporters and journalists.

This brings us to ask what the professional responsibility and mission of journalists really is. There may be multiple ways to answer this question, but according to my understanding, the single most important mission for them should be to pay close attention to our society and the people's livelihood. If that is indeed the case, then I have to ask, after the explosive news of the discovery of the novel coronavirus and then the news of the "eight netizens" who were admonished by the police, which was also a pretty big story, how come they didn't follow up on these major stories that were directly connected to our society and the people's livelihood? How come they didn't investigate *how* the coronavirus was discovered? How come they didn't investigate whether or not is was contagious? Why didn't they look into who these "eight netizens" were, and why they were "spreading rumors"?

When it comes to incidents like these, professional journalists should have a high degree of professional sensitivity; they should have been the ones to carry Li Wenliang's torch as whistleblowers. But where were they? Don't people often say that "If a reporter isn't at the scene already, they are on their way to the scene"? If at the time there had been reporters who took a deep, hard look at the origins of the novel coronavirus, if they had understood that doctors working at Central Hospital were collapsing at record numbers, or if they had uncovered the fact that the "eight netizens spreading rumors" were in fact all doctors, then perhaps, just perhaps, things may have turned out differently. But that would have required them to have a higher level of professionalism; they would have had to have worked hard to build ties and negotiate with various platforms to ensure that their voices were heard. If all that had happened, I wonder if Wuhan would be facing such a horrific scene as it now faces. Would we have this phenomenon of everyone in Hubei Province being quarantined and abandoned? And nationwide would we still be facing all kinds of different losses?

Of course, I'm more than willing to believe that there are a lot of outstanding journalists not just in Wuhan, but throughout Hubei Province. It is very possible that you indeed investigated these issues, you may have even written up some articles, but then they were not approved for publication. It is also possible that journalists requested permission to pursue some of these stories, but they were not even approved. If that is indeed the case, it would actually give me some sense of consolation. It's just a shame that up until today, I have not heard a single case of anything like that having happened. Dr. Ai Fen already sounded the alarm; Dr. Li Wenliang also made some noise; but who is there to carry on their mission? The sound of the whistleblowers has disappeared under the triumphant songs and laughter blaring from those two big media companies. The coronavirus mercilessly spreads and expands; one after another, doctors fall in the line of duty; and yet each issue of our newspapers continues to be filled with vibrant colors, smiling faces, red flags, beautiful flowers, cries of joy. Even a normal citizen like me knew about how deadly this virus was back on January 18, so I started wearing a face mask every time I went out. But what about our media organizations? On January 19th they covered the government's big 40,000-person banquet, and on January 21st they reported on how all the major provincial leaders had attended the big Chinese New Year concert. Every day, they were blindly leading the public to believe that we were still riding high on this great and prosperous era; and there was not a single word warning the public that a new viral monster had its jaws open and was already on its way to our front door. Looking back on the period from the Chinese New Year all the way up through the time that construction of the temporary hospitals was completed—there were thousands of people who suffered and died during that time—I wonder if there is anyone out there with a conscience who feels bad that they abandoned the single most important professional responsibility they had during that time. For those two major news organizations that misguided the public instead of informing them, I wonder if either of them plans on taking responsibility and resigning?

One reporter from the *Yangtze Daily* named W claimed in a report that all Fang Fang knows how to do is make "wild accusations." Well, there, I might be a slow learner, but it looks like I picked up this term pretty quickly. So I decided: Why not go ahead and make some more "wild accusations" today?

MARCH 15, 2020

> *These days fewer and fewer people are discussing*
> *the coronavirus while more and more people are*
> *discussing when we can get back to work.*

Another beautiful day and the sky is clear and bright, which tends to put you in a good mood. A few days ago, my maternal aunt's niece, who also lives in the same complex as me, dropped off some snacks, like steamed buns and dumplings. After eating them for the past two days, I now have a much better understanding of why northerners love eating that stuff so much. It is much more convenient if your staple diet is based around breads and noodles. There are a lot of semimanufactured goods you can make from wheat products; you just need to do a little preparation and they are quite filling. Having a wheat-based diet is much more convenient and less work than cooking rice and dishes for each meal. (By the way, in response to those people online raising questions about how I can pick up food from the front gate if we are supposed to be quarantined inside our homes, I want to clarify that I live within the Literary Federation compound and when I go out, I only go downstairs to the main gate of our compound to pick up groceries.) It is a good thing I like bread and noodles. These days everyone is talking about how much trouble cooking and cleaning up the kitchen has become. We used to be able to just call for takeout and throw everything away when we were done; it was so much easier.

Today my friend JW forwarded me an essay her little brother, Mr. Li, wrote. Mr. Li had two friends who are both members of the senior choir. It is very common for a lot of senior citizens in Wuhan to join various arts and culture groups like that. That is especially true for people of my generation who all grew up during the Cultural Revolution when every school had a cultural propaganda team. So a lot of us know how to sing and dance. Once they retire, people tend to have a lot of free time, and all those old artistic cells start to come back to life. During every weekend and holiday, these retirees really come to life. One after another, they participate in all kinds of performances and parties; they really know how to enjoy their golden years. This year was no different, except for the fact that the novel coronavirus came mercilessly sweeping down and ended up targeting many of them. Mr. Li's essay was a tribute to his two friends. The essay begins with: "How could I have ever imagined that the lives of my two close friends Bao Jie and Su Huajian would be suddenly taken from us this Chinese New Year?"

There is a moving story connected to this: A man fell ill with the coronavirus, and his 90-year-old mother was concerned that the rest of the family might get infected, so she took care of him at the hospital as they were waiting for a bed so her son could be admitted. This elderly mother stayed by her son's side for five days and five nights until the hospital finally had a room for him. However, because his condition had deteriorated during that time, he needed to be admitted to the ICU. His mother asked if she could borrow a pen from one of the nurses to write a letter to her son. The letter read: "My son, you need to hang in there and be strong to get over this terrible illness. Please listen to what the doctors say. I know the respirator might feel uncomfortable, but you need to put up with it in order to recover. Please tell the doctor as soon as your blood pressure returns to normal and you can breathe through your nose again. I forgot to bring any cash when I came to the hospital, so I asked your doctor to lend me 500 yuan so I could get someone to pick up some daily necessities for you." There's no one who read that letter without shedding a tear. But that's what a mother does; even though her son was in his sixties, he will always be her child. This son was Mr. Li's friend Bao Jie. Regrettably, Bao Jie never got to read that letter. He died the following day, leaving his family members behind, including a strong elderly mother who won everyone's respect and admiration.

According to Mr. Li, "The arts group of the Whampoa Military Academy alumni association was preparing a program for the big Chinese New Year concert; since Bao Jie has a connection with the academy through his parents, someone recommended that he join the arts group. As soon as he showed up, Bao Jie really shined. He had a great voice; he actually received professional vocal training and sang with real emotion. It only took two days for them to recommend that he be the lead singer for the choir. On the afternoon of January 17, Bao Jie successfully completed his task as lead singer during the Whampoa Military Academy Chinese New Year concert. He was standing right next to me at the time." But Bao Jie went on to also perform at another New Year event the following day on the 18th, and that is where he became infected. "Three people were infected at the same time, and two of them lost their battle with the coronavirus."

There is another local choir in Wuhan called the Xi-Wen Choir. It was first jointly established by students and teachers from the Xilida Girl's Middle School and the Wenhua Middle School in 1938. After the Reform Era began in the 1980s, some of the old alumni put the Xi-Wen Choir back together, but now its members were no longer limited to alumni of those two schools; anyone could now join. The Xi-Wen Choir held quite a few concerts throughout January. Mr. Li said that both he and Huajian were part of the tenor section and were quite close. "On January 9, some of the members of the Xi-Wen Choir had a concert luncheon at Fanhu; that was the last time I saw Huajian." He continued, "He was usually quite active in our group. But he suddenly stopped showing his face; my friends and I tried to call him, but he didn't pick up. He didn't even respond to WeChat messages we sent him. Everyone thought that it was very out of the ordinary for him, and we were starting to get worried." From that point on, no one was able to get back in touch with Su Huajian, all the way up until they received notice of his death. Su Huajian passed away on March 6. You can still find some videos of the Xi-Wen Choir performing online; there is one song in particular called "Holding Hands" that I find particularly moving. Perhaps it is because I have experienced so much in my life that I am so easily moved by these things. Part of the lyrics go: "I hold your hands and I want to walk with you again in my next life; I have you beside me on this road we walk together, there is never a time to look back." That is one song that could be the soundtrack for your life.

A neighbor had told me a while back that there were many members from those senior choirs who had been infected. That's because during the New Year and throughout the Lunar New Year they tend to have a large number of events and concerts they participate in; and they are all in an age group that makes them particularly vulnerable to infection. Mr. Li's essay included photos of both Bao Jie and Su Huajian; although they were both retired, they looked quite youthful and full of spirit. If they had been warned about the virus, would they have still participated in all those events? Would they have still attended that concert luncheon? Given their lifestyles and the fact that they both had active hobbies, I'm sure that these two men in their sixties could have easily lived another 20-plus years. "Not Contagious Between People; It's Controllable and Preventable." I wonder how many people were driven to their death by those words. When I think about that, I ask myself: *For those of us still alive, even if it means disturbing our comfortable lives, how can we not fight for justice for those wronged souls?* Holding people accountable is something we must do!

For the past few days, the coronavirus situation has continued to improve. The number of new confirmed cases in Wuhan has continued to stay down in the single digits for several days now. As the number of patients decreases, people's desire to go outside and return to work has been growing stronger. These days more people are discussing getting back to work than discussing the coronavirus. There are a lot of families and companies that can no longer take this quarantine anymore. It has been way too long and people are way too depressed; at this point the government should consider adopting a more flexible policy. The good news is that things are improving for some locations; today I saw that there are a few districts that have gotten down to zero new cases that are starting to bus people out so they can start working again. And starting tomorrow some of Wuhan's public transportation will officially begin service for the employees of certain industries that will be resuming operation. This is all excellent news. If we don't open up the city and get back to work soon, it won't be a question of economic collapse that we will have to worry about, it will be the more fundamental question of making sure that people are able to eat!

Let me say a little bit about some of the things I have been facing these past two days.

I have always liked Weibo as a platform, so ever since my account was unblocked, I have been posting my diary entries on Weibo each day. However, starting a few days ago there was suddenly a flood of thousands of users who started to attack me online. These trolls have been deployed in mass numbers, and their posts are ridiculous and offensive. I've gone from thinking the whole thing was just preposterous to a state of anger and, now, I'm just left numb by the whole thing. Part of the reason is that I have discovered from their posts that the vast majority of them have never even read my diary. All they have heard are a few quotes taken out of context and then framed with a particularly malicious analysis; and that is what they are attacking me on. They curse me just for the sake of it; for them it is like a game. Of course, there are a few who try to package their attacks with arguments that appear more logical; however, those arguments are all rooted in fabricated rumors that they have accepted as truth. They try to argue for truth based on the logic of rumors and lies; how can you reason with someone like that? At first I blacklisted a lot of the users who posted stupid, outrageous messages filled with profanities. But later this afternoon I suddenly had a second thought: Maybe it's not a bad idea to leave their ridiculous attacks and comments online for all to see.

It is pretty easy to figure out who these people attacking me are; you can view their profile photos, you can see what they have in common, which online clubs and groups they are members of, whom they follow, whose posts they typically forward, and which ones interact with each other. It is actually quite similar to investigating the origin of a virus; you start with where the outbreak began; when did they all begin to post their attacks, who has been instigating them, organizing them, and egging them on behind the scenes? You can also tell whom they have attacked in the past, whom they support, whose direction they seem to follow, where the language they use comes from and whose language it resembles; you can even see how the language they use when they attack people has changed over time, and other things like that. You can learn a lot about this group just by observing them online. You can even reach back as far as seven or eight years ago and find postings calling on students to upload messages advocating "positive energy." You can even discover the list of names of people recommended to be their advisors. I remember once asking the head of a certain government ministry, "How could you let people like that advise students? Some of these people are thugs!" A shame that they didn't listen to me back then. But now those people who were once called on to display their "positive energy" online have now been turned into these people who attack me today. A lot of these people would seem decent if you ran into them on the street, but once they log onto the internet their malicious dark side all comes out.

A good thing, then, that the internet has a memory, and that memory lasts a long time. And so I think I should preserve the message thread on my Weibo account as an observation point—a living record of this era to preserve for the future. Preserved in the memory of every era are beautiful and moving things right there alongside those painful and sad things. But what usually leaves the deepest impression is always shame. It is particularly important to preserve those shameful acts of this age, as well. This flood of collective curses and insults serves as a record of the most humiliating and shameful documents of this era. When people in the future one day look back and read these comments posted in 2020, they will see that, as a virus was spreading in Wuhan, another virus was infecting people's language online and spreading all over my Weibo message board. The spread of the coronavirus led to the unprecedented quarantine of millions of people within this city, while the virus infecting my Weibo account clearly unveiled the true shame of this era.

As a victim quarantined here in this virus zone, I record snapshots of my life and reflections. Most diaries are never preserved, but these thousands of collective curses and attacks will ensure that my diary will last forever.

MARCH 16, 2020

To borrow three words from the great Song poet Lu You:
Wrong, wrong, wrong.

Another overcast day, but the blooming spring displays itself in an array of color and forms. Those colors are able to cut through the gloom

and relieve some of our depression and sadness. My neighbor out in
Jiangxia, Tang Xiaohe, sent another photo from the front porch of my
apartment there; my winter jasmines are now in bloom, displaying a
glorious yellow, while the Chinese flowering crabapples, which had
bloomed earlier, are now starting to shed their petals, which are now
all over the ground. That blanket of petals on the ground creates a pic-
turesque scene against the green hanging leaves of the winter jasmine.
Tang Xiaohe's ruby orchids are always gorgeous this time of year; they
are so rich and vibrant that even when you pass by on the street the
tapestry of crimson flowers can brighten up even the most depressing
of days.

In terms of the coronavirus outbreak, there is no big change today
from the previous few days. It just feels a bit like we are stuck in this
period when everything is operating at a low level, but is not yet back
to normal. There are now only a small handful of new coronavirus patients, while there still remain 3,000 seriously ill patients who continue
to struggle for their lives. All the temporary hospitals have now been
shuttered. Although today some controversial discussions started popping up online, claiming that closing down those temporary hospitals
was actually a "political move," many of the patients hadn't yet really recovered. But if I remember correctly, even a few days ago I mentioned
that there were now more beds available at the regular hospitals, so patients from the temporary hospitals who have not fully recovered could
be transferred there for further treatment. Those who have recovered
can be transferred to hotels for an additional 14 days of quarantine
before returning home. But I'm still not sure if those accounts I read
online are merely unsubstantiated rumors, so I decided to ask one of
my doctor friends what he thought. He response was quite direct: "That
is certainly just a rumor! There would be no reason to shut them down
for political reasons, and it is utterly impossible that they would! Right

now, the only political angle here is to completely control the spread of the coronavirus; we want to completely eradicate this virus, and do our utmost to treat those infected patients. There would be no political pressure to close those hospitals earlier than needed. When you are dealing with an infectious disease, there is no hiding things! For issues like this, we need to have faith in our government! No matter how fearless you may be, no one can take on the world alone. For a strong and acute virus like this one, nothing short of complete containment will be able to stop the spread. And that is something that no one can conceal!" Those are my doctor friend's words, even the exclamation mark, and I believe him. This coronavirus has already overturned the notion that politics should be placed above all else; now that we find ourselves at this current juncture, who would dare attempt to conceal the truth? No one wants to relive the terror that the people of Wuhan went through a month ago.

A lot of people in my friends group have been forwarding an essay by the writer Yan Geling;[17] a few friends also sent it directly to me. The title of the essay is "To Borrow Three Words from the Great Southern Song Poet Tang Wan: Conceal, Conceal, Conceal." Yan Geling, who lives in Berlin, has been closely following the events in Wuhan from afar. Many years ago the Hubei Writers Association organized a conference of women Chinese writers from around the world. Yan Geling came to Wuhan to attend; we even invited her to deliver a lecture at Wuhan University. I wasn't there for her lecture, but I heard it was a full house. Yan Geling has a great sense of intuition; she was able to latch onto the most important keyword that has been in play from the very beginning of the outbreak up through the point it transformed into an unmitigated disaster. That word is: Concealment. While a lot of effort went into controlling the outbreak later on, if you pull apart and examine the key points in the development of the outbreak, you will discover that there is one concept that is ever-present: Conceal-ment. But why did so many things need to be concealed? Were they concealed on purpose or due to some kind of oversight? Or was there some other reason? But let's put that discussion off for the time being. Dear Geling, I read your essay and was quite moved; it also gave me a lot to think about; however, before I had time to forward it to my friends group online, it was deleted from the internet. You probably also already know that here in China concealment is the brother of censorship. We've already been tortured by this brother named "cen-sorship" to the point that we are wooden and numb. You never know when it might happen or why it happens or what rules you may have broken to be censored, because no one ever tells you. You have no choice but to just accept it.

Another piece of shocking news in the literary world today is that all of Mario Vargas Llosa's books have been ordered to be taken off the shelves of bookstores. Could this be true? It is really hard for me to be-lieve. I started reading Llosa back when I was still a teenager. Almost all writers from my generation back then were reading him. A lot of people really liked the tone of his writing and his experiments with structure and form. But actually, I don't think I have read more than three of his books, and those were all his most popular novels. When I heard this news, I went through the same emotional cycle as a lot of other writers: I started out shocked, then I was angry, and finally I just felt depressed. I just don't know what else to say anymore. Besides grumbling about it a bit, what else *can* you say? No matter what Llosa may have said, he's not a politician; he is still a writer. I remember reading an essay a few days ago that used the following words to describe what a writer is: "The greatest and most fundamental mission of a writer is to vanquish falsehoods, bear testimony to the truth of history, and restore dignity to mankind." I'm not sure who originally spoke those words. Llosa must be in his eighties now. Is this really necessary? Conceal, conceal, conceal—those three words are from the love story between Tang Wan and Lu You; it is a story that most Chinese know. But here I would like to borrow three words from the poet Lu You: Wrong, wrong, wrong.

Today I learned that the medical personnel who came to Hubei to help with the aid effort have already begun to leave in groups. Yet when it comes to when the city might reopen, there is still almost no news. There are all kinds of sensational things floating around the internet. There are a lot of rumors too. But no matter how fierce this virus may be, there is something even more terrifying that is now rushing out in front—there are a lot of people who simply can't go on anymore. Today a reporter in Beijing sent me an appeal written by someone here in Hubei. It reminded me of that telephone recording I heard a few days ago. Rereading this appeal now, I feel it is actually quite objective and sensible. Part of the appeal mentioned some issues that the author hopes the government might consider. I would like to cite a portion of that appeal here:

I take legal responsibility for everything I am saying here. As you fought the coronavirus, average people like us were extremely supportive and gave you our full cooperation. But after having been locked down for so many days, more than 50 days, even those who may have been sick to begin with should have recovered by now. You should arrange some chartered buses for us, but how come you government people haven't taken any action?

We keep staying at home wasting time every day and you won't even give us a clear answer as to when it will end so we can at least have a target in mind. The end of March? The end of April? Whatever the case, you need to give us a time frame! Right now, without any time frame for when the quarantine will end, we have nothing to hope for; instead we just sit at home waiting. Day after day, we all have living expenses and we have families to raise; how is a breadwinner supposed to make money to support a family?

Each and every day we need to eat, drink, we need oil and salt for cooking, and all this costs money. Of course, everything ends up in our stomachs, but it still adds up as part of our expenses. Every morning we get up and the first thing we look at are the headlines from all the major newspapers; we check whether the number of infections has gone up or down. We look at the statistics all over, but it only seems to be here in Wuhan that the number of sick people is higher. But that doesn't mean that all the other cities in Hubei Province also need to go through the same torture as Wuhan; it really doesn't.

I returned home on January 21; you can calculate just how many days that it has been now. Every day since then I have been sitting at home eating and sleeping, eating and sleeping. The main thing is that I just don't know when this will all end. At first they said the quarantine might be lifted on March 1, then they pushed it back to March 10, then March 11; later they said March 15; now Zhong Nanshan is saying it might last until late June.

If you continue on like this, where is the end?

You can quarantine the sick; however you want to quarantine sick people, we will cooperate. But you need to quarantine the virus, not the people of Hubei Province! What's more, since you have us all quarantined at home, and if we leave Hubei we would also be quarantined, then why not just let us leave and be quarantined somewhere else? We could leave Hubei, self-quarantine for 14 days, let local officials confirm we are healthy, and then let us get back to work! We need to create income; things need to get back to normal! Instead you have us quarantined at home, you want us locked down until late May or late June, then after that we'll have to be quarantined for another two weeks; are we going to get any work done at all this entire year? What kind of people waste their time like this?

You people in charge need to hear what the people are saying; you need to pay attention to what we are requesting. I'm not speaking just for myself; most members of the public all feel the same way, and I am speaking for all of us. We are not trying to cause trouble; we are just trying to make a living. We need to put food on the table. You need to try to think about the situation from our perspective, the perspective of ordinary citizens.

What family isn't facing this burden? All day from morning until night we put up with the loudspeakers blaring: "Do not go outside! Do not go outside! Do not go outside!" How long is this going to last? How far are they going to take this? What are the conditions that aren't allowing us to go outside? What are the reasons? All day long they are trying to attend to big and small affairs at once with a one-size-fits-all strategy. "Do not go outside, no matter what happens, do not go outside!" You have to realize that we should be quarantining the coronavirus, not the entire population of Hubei Province! Only after you really understand this and let it sink in will you be able to truly carry out the spirit of all those documents you send down.

One more thing: Everything costs money. Let me tell you, if pumpkin seeds are 15 yuan for every half kilo, are you going to buy any? When meat is 32 yuan for every half kilo, would you pay that price? What about cucumbers for 7 yuan a half kilo, any takers? Potatoes are also 7 yuan, cabbage is 8 yuan . . . so how about it? Are you buying? If you don't, you still have to eat . . . so in the end, everyone buys. But then you have to pay. Without a job, where is that money going to come from? Who is thinking about us here?

My god . . .

That last frustrated exclamation at the end really makes your heart break. The people have already done everything they can to cooperate and be reasonable, but the question of taking care of their basic living needs is dangling right there before us. We have been relying on the government's great resolution to bring the coronavirus outbreak to a screeching halt. My impression is that many places throughout Hubei Province are already down to zero new infections, yet they still have not yet lifted the quarantine order. Back when I was in college, one of my professors taught a course on Modernism and I remember us reading *Waiting for Godot*. Two men sitting there waiting for Godot, but he never arrives. As we now sit here waiting for the quarantine to be lifted, I am suddenly reminded of that play. Stand in the shoes of the people and think about the issue of the people's livelihood; it is all right there on the table before you. There are a lot of things that can be handled simultaneously; you don't need to necessarily line them up and take care of them one after another.

It is now day 54 of the lockdown; this hand of poker is over.

MARCH 17, 2020

It is clear that life will gradually start getting back to normal.

Day 55 of the Wuhan quarantine.

The weather is nice and clear. I stepped outside to empty the trash and through the branches caught a glimpse of the peach blossoms in full bloom on the slope across the way. I'm reminded of a line of poetry: "The shrubbery conceals not the colors of spring, as a branch of crimson peonies hangs over the wall." Besides the fact that there is not a single person outside, the rest of the Literary Federation courtyard looks the same as always.

According to the daily coronavirus report, there was only one new case of infection today. We are getting close to the point where everything can start over. An increasingly large number of patients who had been suffering from severe symptoms have been saved, but there is still a long road ahead for them before they will be able to fully recover. I know it is hard, but I hope they are able to hold on and get through this; they can always take their time recovering, once this critical stage is behind them. Currently, the government is officially reporting that the death toll from novel coronavirus in Hubei Province has reached 3,000; this is indeed a depressing number to have to face. Now that the outbreak is over, I'm afraid that the job of consoling family members of the deceased should now be our most important task. Looking broadly now at the trajectory of the entire outbreak, ever since the moment the nation committed all their efforts to saving Hubei and began to enact a variety of measures to control the virus, it is clear that their methods have been very powerful and effective. It hasn't been easy for us to get to this stage.

Even more good news is starting to flood out; I see people in my friends group posting the latest news everywhere. The most important news is that, with the exception of Wuhan, all other cities in Hubei Province have lifted their lockdown orders and people are now returning to work; a lot of workers who have been trapped outside the city are also now starting to return to Wuhan. This is great news, and it is exactly the kind of news that a lot of people have been waiting to hear. Wuhan has always been a city bustling with life, and I really can't wait to see it get back to its energetic and chaotic old self.

Actually, besides those industries, there is another group of people even more eager for the city to get back on track again: They represent a massive number of people, I am talking about those elderly people who are living alone. They normally rely on maids or hourly help to take care of them. But every year during the Lunar New Year holiday, these caregivers and part-time workers all go home to the countryside to celebrate the holidays with their own families. But due to the quarantine this year, most of these caregivers were unable to return to Wuhan, which created a lot of difficulties for the elderly whom they normally care for. A few days ago, my friend Mr. Zeng was chatting with me about his mother's situation.

There is a very famous restaurant in Wuhan called Lao Tong City; it is located in the Hankou district and there is basically no one in the city who hasn't heard of this restaurant. The tofu skin they make at Lao Tong City is considered one of Wuhan's most popular delicacies. The founder of Lao Tong City was a man named Zeng Guangcheng. Many years ago, the Hubei Writers Association organized a literary program to invite local residents to write about local topics. A certain Mr. Zeng registered for the event; he was working on a book called *The Story of Lao Tong City and the Zeng Family of Hankou*—he was the eldest grandson of the restaurant's founder, Zeng Guangcheng. Over the years, the Zeng family's history has given him a lot of forward motion, but it had also brought him a lot of pain; Mr. Zeng decided to get that entire history on paper. We ended up selecting his project for inclusion in our program. Mr. Zeng went to great lengths to get his story on paper and ended up publishing it as a trilogy. A few days ago Mr. Zeng told me that his mother, who is 97 years old, was living in the faculty dorm of Hubei University. Meanwhile he and the rest of the family were all working outside the city; he only had one little brother still in Wuhan, but he was quarantined in another district and unable to get to his mother. Mr. Wang's mother enjoyed living alone; she was still sharp and in good health; she just has a helper she pays by the hour to come and take care of household chores. But after the outbreak, her helper also ended up quarantined elsewhere, so she was left alone. All her children were worried sick about their elderly mother being left alone at home. She didn't know her way around the kitchen and there is no way for her to buy daily necessities; she certainly didn't know how to sign up for those group delivery services, and even if they delivered a bag of fresh vegetables right to her doorstep, she still wouldn't know how to cook them. How was she supposed to eat? On top of that, she was almost out of medicine. And without a cellphone or access to WeChat, how was she going to get in contact with anyone if she needed something? Everyone in the family was so anxious about her that they "almost broke the phone by calling her so much."

They were lucky that the community workers in the district near Hubei University quickly stepped up. Mr. Zeng said that the community volunteers delivered a bag of vegetables, but that wasn't much help since she didn't know how to cook. All she wanted was some pickled vegetables and a steamed bun you can quickly heat up. She got in touch with those community volunteers for help, and people from the neighborhood committee arranged for hot meals to be delivered right to her door. They even got in touch with the doctor on call at the university hospital to check on her. Her old colleagues and students from the university all reached out to help; they delivered all kinds of food to her door, and even after she brought the food inside, they would wait for a few minutes outside the door to make sure there wasn't anything else that she needed. Only after they heard her say she was having trouble opening a jar of honey or a bottle of soy sauce would they ask for her permission to come in and help her open them. Mr. Zeng said he called her every day to check in and "every time I talked to her I could tell how happy she was from the sound of her voice. She even got passionate about learning and would endlessly tell me stories about [historical figures like] Qu Yuan and Li Si over the phone. She told me that she was writing 1,000 words a day and would recite what she wrote to me." His mother said: "They delivered another three dishes to me; no one has ever taken care of me like this before in my entire life! The university really has their act together this time."

Can you believe it? She is 97 years old, living alone, and still manages to do creative writing every day, calmly passing the time during this extended quarantine period. How can you not respect and admire such a strong woman! That said, long term, this is still not the best option for someone like her. In Wuhan there must be thousands and thousands of elderly people like her who rely on caregivers and helpers for their daily needs. They can barely wait for the day that their caretakers are able to return to help them; even I count myself as one of them. Yesterday someone left a message on my Weibo page, stating: "I live in Qichun County in Huanggang; this is the sixth day since the quarantine was lifted and for the past couple of days they have been arranging for buses to take workers back to the cities. A lot of cities in Hubei are doing the same thing right now. There are also some counties in Hubei that are gradually starting to allow private cars to leave Hubei for work. . . . In short, after all of Hubei was locked down for so long, things are slowly starting to improve." This is great news! My housekeeper is from Shanchun; I should get in touch with her today. Although I have heard that not all the roads are open yet, it is probably still a few more days before she can return to Wuhan.

Something else happened today that I need to record: Starting today, Hubei's medical aid teams have all started to clear out of the city. They all braved terrible dangers during the most critical period of the outbreak in order to help save people's lives; there is a special place of gratitude in our hearts for what they have done. All told, there were more than 40,000 medical workers who came in to help, and not a single one of them was infected; it's truly a miracle! Thanks to them, all of us can now breathe a collective sigh of relief. It's always difficult to say goodbye. Today I saw a video posted in my friends group chat; the video was shot just as the medical aid teams were departing; as they left, all the Wuhan residents who still cannot leave their own homes stood on their balconies calling out "Thank you! We know it's been hard! Farewell!" Seeing that was enough to leave you in tears. Wuhan people from all walks of life stood together to give these angels in white their most heartfelt salute; after all, these were the people who saved our city—these were the people who saved *us*. It's been said that the city of Xiangyang has recorded the names of everyone in their medical aid teams, and they decided to grant lifetime free admission and accommodations to visit the top scenic destinations in the area. I'm not sure if this is fake news or not, but I figure "why not!" In fact, I think we should open up every scenic and tourist location in all of Hubei Province to them for free! Of course, as I am so moved, something funny also happened: As the medical team from Sichuan Province was leaving for Hubei, one medical worker's husband yelled out to the bus: "Zhao Yingming, once you're safely back home, I'll do all the household chores for the next year!" Now his dear Zhao Yingming has finally come home. Almost immediately someone put up a video online calling for netizens everywhere to monitor this husband and make sure he keeps his word for the next year. Everyone got a good laugh from that video. I wonder if they will set up a 24-hour livestream from their apartment to make sure he does his chores.

The hottest topic being debated online these days is all those Chinese who have spent time overseas who are now returning to China. One meme put it this way: *China fought half the battle, countries outside of China fought the other half of the battle, but Chinese studying abroad have fought the entire battle.* This refers to the fact that a lot of Chinese international students left China just before the Lunar New Year, but now that China has largely controlled the outbreak—even Hubei is now safe—while the coronavirus situation abroad is starting to heat up, all those students are now flooding back into China. Actually, this meme is not entirely accurate, because when the outbreak began most of those international students were already abroad. During the initial outbreak, many of these international Chinese students went all over the place trying to help secure donations and supplies for Wuhan; they really worked hard. And while it is true that many of them have now indeed returned to China, we should still keep the facts straight. What is interesting is how many people have asked me what I think of this.

I feel like these kids are like our own children; we need to be empathetic. If my daughter were abroad right now, I would probably also tell her to return home. Not everyone can be a hero. So I can completely understand why they would make those choices. The fact that they are all coming back home shows that deep in their hearts they know they can always rely on their own country. Doesn't this say a lot about their sense of trust and patriotism? Actually, back during the War of Resistance against Japan, there was the term "seek refuge." When the Japanese invaded, large numbers of people all went south to seek refuge. No one blamed them for that; no one asked, "How come you don't stay behind to fight those Japanese devils?" That's because the urge to seek refuge is a basic human instinct. Those who stayed behind to fight the Japanese were the ones considered heroes. Those who escaped to seek refuge may not be heroes—none of them would certainly claim to be heroes—but that doesn't mean they did something deserving of blame. They are now saying that more than 100,000 Chinese currently abroad are all about to come back. China is a large country and all the provinces are now calling their children home. Those who are ill will be admitted to hospitals for treatment, those who are healthy will just go home for quarantine; that's how it will work. But whether you are seeking refuge or just flying home to China from abroad, it is essential that everyone follows the rules. We need to protect ourselves, but that should never come at the expense of hurting other people; this is, after all, common sense.

One of my old high school classmates just sent me a timeline for the lifting of the quarantine: "On March 22 all personnel outside of Hubei and Wuhan can return. Personnel in Hubei and Wuhan can also leave those regions on the same date. On March 24 all public buses and subways will be disinfected and undergo technical tests to ensure that all public transit is ready to resume service. On March 26 residential doors will be opened back up and residents will be able to move about freely within their own residential communities. On March 29 the quarantine will be lifted for small residential districts, and residents with a work permit and health certificate QR code will be able to return to work by car, bicycle, or on foot. On March 31 businesses and production enterprises will gradually return to normal operating levels. On April 2 major shopping plazas and malls will resume normal business operations. On April 3 buses and subways will resume operations. On April 4 all airports, high-speed trains, light rail, and highways will return to normal operating status." My classmate forwarded this and when I passed it on, I made sure to write: "I'm forwarding this, but not sure if it is real or not." But whether or not it is true, it still gives us a lot of encouragement. It is clear that life is going to start getting back to normal.

I would like to express my sincere thanks to my readers. Yesterday I was unable to send out my daily entry on WeChat; Er Xiang also tried to send it more than a dozen times, but it wouldn't go through. Later I just put it up as a message without the comments section attached, but that was also deleted. I really don't understand why. Finally, Er Xiang just logged onto her official account, "Er Xiang's Eleven Dimensions of Space," and just posted a short, four-word message: "I did my best."

Just those four words. But a reader saw that and copied my entire post from yesterday in the comments section, one paragraph at a time. That was something I completely didn't expect, but also something I found quite moving.

MARCH 18, 2020

Where we were back then is where you are now.

Day 56 of the quarantine.

It is clear and the sun is bright, so bright, as if it is racing straight into summer. Although it is sunny, it's not too humid. This is the best kind of weather in Wuhan. Actually, one of the major reasons I like Wuhan so much is the weather. The seasonal changes in Wuhan are quite pronounced; each season has its own character. As people in Wuhan say, the summers are hotter than hell and the winters freeze you to death. There is a humid period every spring, while every day in autumn is usually filled with clear skies and crisp air; that's the most comfortable time of year. When I was younger I used to get annoyed by the weather in Wuhan; I always hated the heat and I hated the cold. Later as technology became more advanced, our quality of life began to improve; we had AC during the summer, heat during the winter, dehumidifiers during the spring, and then, come fall, we could just enjoy the beautiful weather. Just like that, all the flaws the climate here had were suddenly fixed, thanks to the wisdom of man; and that allowed the good things about the city to really shine through. These days I really like experiencing the four seasons here in Wuhan. A long time ago when I was making a documentary film, there was one summer when it got up to 40 degrees Celsius. One old-timer I talked to commented on the heat by saying: "It has to be that hot! That's what makes you sweat out all the poisons in your skin. People never feel really good until they get all hot and sweat it all out." At the time his words really surprised me. If one summer the temperature didn't make it up to 40, a lot of people in Wuhan would be deeply disappointed; how can you call *that* a Wuhan summer!

But let's get back to the coronavirus. After getting through the early stage of suffering and chaos, the coronavirus situation has been improving each and every day up until now, when it has clearly been contained. Today there was just one confirmed new case in Wuhan. There were 10 deaths today and there are currently no new suspected cases. The people of Wuhan are eagerly waiting for all the numbers to come down to zero, and then this will all be truly over. I suppose that day should be here soon.

This afternoon I had a long phone call with a doctor friend who has been working on the front lines of the outbreak. Some of our perspectives on things were not quite in line with one another; for instance, on the issue of assigning blame, my doctor friend feels that if we start trying to hold people accountable now, he is afraid that no one will do anything if the leadership suddenly disappears. I feel that whether we are talking about the government or hospitals, I just can't believe that people would be that weak. There are a lot of capable people working in these hospitals and in the government; there are plenty of people who could step in for officials who might resign. Now that we are finally at the tail end of this outbreak, this is the time to settle up, while everything that happened is still fresh in everyone's minds. But as far as holding people accountable goes, this is an absolute necessity; how else can we face those thousands of dead souls and the countless number of Wuhan residents who have suffered through this? As I have said numerous times before, this outbreak was the result of numerous forces coming together. These forces came from many different levels, and there were many reasons behind what happened. Each of those reasons was different, but they all ended together in the same big pot. Now nobody wants to take responsibility for what's in that pot. But it is our job to monitor what has happened and make sure no one shirks their responsibility. Those who had a hand in this should carry their own burden.

But my doctor friend mentioned two things that I found especially interesting. I will share them with you here for reference: (1) He feels that there is a problem with the hospitals' construction. Many hospitals are poorly ventilated, which easily increases infection rates in confined spaces. Apparently, many hospitals have constructed new buildings these past few years in order to respond to the call to save energy and reduce emissions, but those measures are not always suitable for hospital safety measures. My doctor friend said that if you remember what happened back during the SARS epidemic, the climate in Shenzhen was quite warm, so his friend who was working in a hospital there opened up all the hospital windows, which diluted the density of the virus spores in the air and helped reduce the number of infections. I didn't look up the number of infections in Shenzhen during SARS, but what he said seemed fairly reasonable to me. But right now in Wuhan it is winter and we can't really open up the windows, which left me a bit dismayed. But I do think that the ventilation issue with hospitals, especially in the ER and the Infectious Disease Department, is a big problem. (2) My doctor friend also feels that the interval between winter and spring each year is always a period when a lot of infectious diseases spread. This is when SARS first broke out; it is also when the novel coronavirus appeared. Therefore, he wondered why the government insisted on holding their big meetings during this time every year; they should move them all to a season much less likely to be affected by infectious diseases.

My friend's suggestion opened up a slew of ideas in my head. I'll be honest with you, ever since 1993 I have been attending the Provincial People's Congress Meeting and the Provincial Political Consultative Conference each year for a full 25 years now. I know all too well what all the various government offices are like every year when these meetings approach. In order to ensure that everything runs smoothly with these meetings, all the various media outlets are prohibited from covering any negative news reports. And during this time every year, employees from all government offices put aside their normal tasks because the leader of every government office has to attend these meetings. This year was no different. You can clearly see that the day the Municipal Health Committee stopped reporting the number of people infected corresponded almost perfectly with the date of those two government meetings. That is no coincidence. At the same time, I wouldn't say it was really intentional, either; it is simply how government offices have grown accustomed to functioning. And these practices are not some-thing recent; they have been developed over the course of many years. For years now, every government department has gotten into the habit of putting various tasks off until after the meetings are over; while, at the same time, in order to ensure the success of these meetings, the me-dia has for years been following the practice of reporting the good news but not the bad. All the cadres are used to this; so is the media, so are the leaders, and so are the people. And so they put off their work and suppress negative news reports; usually nothing unexpected comes of any of this. After all, there are a lot of small matters in life and most of it can always wait a few days. It turns out good for everyone; people seem to like the arrangement and everyone saves face. But infectious diseases don't care about etiquette, and they certainly don't care about saving your face; in fact, they'll rip it right off. That's what SARS did, and that is what the novel coronavirus did; will there be a third one? I'm a bit worried. And so in following my doctor friend's thoughts, I would like to make a suggestion: If we don't change the timing for these meetings, then we should change the ugly habits we have fostered around them. Or if we can't change the disgusting way we run these meetings, then we should alter the timing to hold them during a time of year when the weather is unlikely to spawn an infectious disease outbreak. Actually, it shouldn't be very difficult to change both these things.

Something else occurred today that I cannot ignore; I suspect that many of my readers are actually awaiting my response. Someone who claimed to be a 16-year-old "high school student" published an open letter to me online. There were a lot of details about the letter that didn't feel right, and numerous friends thought it was obvious that the letter could not have been written by a 16-year-old; it felt more like something one of those men in their fifties who impersonate teenage girls online would write! However, whether that's the case or not, I decided to go ahead and respond to the letter as if I were writing to a 16-year-old high school student.

What I want to say is: My child, it's a good letter that you have sent me, filled with the uncertainties of someone your age. The ideas you expressed are quite what one would expect, and I'm sure that those things that are bothering you came directly from those people who have been educating you. But I need to tell you that I'm not the one who can dispel the doubts you have. Reading your letter actually reminded me of a poem I read many years ago. It is a poem by Bai Hua;[18] I'm not sure if you've ever heard of him, but he was a talented poet and playwright. I first read this poem when I was 12 years old; that was in 1967 in the middle of the Cultural Revolution. All summer long that year, Wuhan was filled with Red Guards fighting in the streets. I was in the fifth grade, and that was the year I received a copy of Bai Hua's collection of poetry called *Distributing Flyers in the Face of the Iron Spear.* One poem in that volume was entitled "I Too Was Once Young Like You." There is one line in the poem that goes: "I too was once young like you, and back then we were as you are today." I was so excited when I first encountered that poem, so much so that I remember that line even today.

My child, you say you are 16 years old. I was 16 years old back in 1971. If someone had tried to tell me back then that "the Cultural Revolution was a terrible calamity," I would have thrown down my gauntlet and gone at them until we were both bruised and bloody; and I know that even if this person had spent three straight days and three straight nights trying to talk sense into me, there was absolutely nothing they could have said to change my mind. That's because ever since the age of 11 I had received an education that repeatedly reinforced the fact that "the Cultural Revolution was good." By the time I was 16, I had been exposed to those views for a full five years. Three days of trying to change my mind wouldn't come even close to doing the trick. So it is based on that same principle that I know it will be impossible for me to clear up those things you have misgivings about. I'm afraid that even if I took three *years* trying to convince you and wrote eight books explaining why, you probably still wouldn't believe me. That's because, just like me when I was young, you have received at least five years of that sort of education.

That said, I still need to tell you, my child, that you will one day find an answer to dispel all your uncertainties. But only you can provide that answer for yourself. Perhaps in 10 or 20 years there will come a day when you will remember this and realize how childish you were back then. That's because by then, you will be a brand-new you. Of course, if you end up following the path of those gangs of ultra-leftists, you may never find that answer you are looking for; instead, you might into fall into an abyss of lifelong struggle.

My child, I also want to tell you that when I was 16 years old, I was much worse off than you are. At that time, I had never even heard of words like "independent thought." I never knew that people needed to learn how to think for themselves; we just did whatever our teachers told us to do, we followed whatever the schools told us to do, we followed whatever the newspapers told us to do, and whatever the radio broadcasts instructed us to do. The Cultural Revolution broke out when I was 11 and it wasn't over until I was 21; that's the world I grew up in during those 10 years. I never thought of myself, because I never thought of myself as an individual person; I was just one screw in a much larger machine. I functioned in step with that machine; when it stopped I stopped, when it moved I moved. This is probably quite similar to where you are today. (When I say "you," I am not referring to everyone from your generation, because there are actually a lot of 16-year-olds today who have very strong independent thinking skills.) But I got lucky because I had a father whose greatest dream in life was to send all his children to college. I still remember when he told me that. So even when I was working as a porter, I knew that I had to do whatever it took to make sure my dad's final wish was realized. I ended up getting accepted into Wuhan University, which has the most beautiful college campus in China.

My child, I often feel that I have been quite fortunate. Although the only education I received during my childhood was filled with nothing but stupidity, I was still able to somehow get into college. While I was there I read and studied like someone who had been starved for knowledge for her entire life. I discussed all kinds of fascinating topics with my classmates, I started writing fiction, and finally one day I came to understand the importance of independent thought. I am also fortunate to have witnessed the early days of the Reform Era and then go on to experience the entire series of reforms that would unfold from there. Emerging from the catastrophic toll of the Cultural Revolution, I watched as, one step at a time, China turned itself around from a backward country to a powerful one. You could say that if it were not for the Reform Era, we wouldn't have any of the things we have today, including the right for me to publish my diary online and the right for you to publish your open letter to me. We should both be thankful for that.

My child, do you realize that for the first 10 years of the Reform Era I was basically struggling against myself for that entire decade? I needed to clear all that accumulated garbage and poison out of my brain. I had to fill my mind with new things, I needed to try to view the world through my own eyes, I needed to use my own mind to think through problems. Of course, all this is built on the foundation of my own childhood experience growing up, what I have read, what I have observed, and what I have worked so hard for.

My child, I always thought that this process of struggling against myself that I went through in order to clear out all the garbage and poison inside me was something that only people from my generation had gone through. I never imagined that you and some of your peers will also go through something similar in the future. You too will one day need to struggle against yourself in order to purge all that garbage and poison that infected your brain as a child. It is a painful process; but with each purge comes a kind of liberation. And with each liberation you gradually transform from a dead, fossilized, rusty screw into a real person.

My child, do you understand what I have been trying to say? Now I'd like to leave you with a line of poetry: "I too was once young like you, and back then we were as you are today."

MARCH 19, 2020

I may be retired, but I still have
enough energy to take you to court.

Day 57 of the quarantine.

That news we have been waiting day after day to hear has finally arrived: Today there are no new cases of novel coronavirus in Wuhan and
no new suspected cases! My doctor friend also seems to be extremely
excited: "We are finally at zero! Zeros across the board! The outbreak
has been contained and we can now control all traffic from the outside
coming in; now the main task is treating the patients we already have."

At the same time, today we also saw the Hubei government's goodbye ceremony for the army of service workers who are leaving; they
also appealed to everyone in China to treat the people of Hubei with
kindness! That's right, please treat us with kindness. Not everyone in
Hubei was infected with this virus. Millions of people here in Hubei
spent nearly two months quarantined in their homes in order to help
control the spread of the disease; it is hard for outsiders to understand
the stress and difficulties that they had to deal with. But the Hubei people's strength and forbearance in the face of this calamity ended up being the biggest contribution to China's efforts to contain this virus. And
so it is important for me to say it out loud: Please, my friends from all
over China, treat the people of Hubei well, be kind to these people who
sacrificed so much for all of you.

The next step should be for people outside Wuhan to start returning.
If you ask me personally, I'm already desperate to get my helper back;
I really hope she can come back soon. After two months, my house is
in need of a deep cleaning. My old dog is now dirty and smelly; and his
old skin problem is starting to come back. My hand is also still badly

injured; I've been trying not to wash it or get it wet. I wonder when the vet's office will reopen. Every day when I let him out into the courtyard I tell him that he just has to wait a few more days and then he'll be all clean again. All the businesses are waiting to reopen, and we wait too.

Just like always, I got out of bed today and ate breakfast as I looked at my cellphone. One thing I didn't expect was after receiving that letter from a "high school student" yesterday was that today a bunch of her "relatives" suddenly came out of the woodwork to publish a series of open letters supporting her. (Wow, she sure has a lot of "relatives"!) Naturally, a bunch of other people also wrote letters, including some university students, middle school students, and even elementary school students. I have to be honest; some of them made me laugh harder than I have in a long time. Now that we are down to zero, I guess it is finally an appropriate time to have a good laugh. My old classmate Yi Zhongxue jokingly referred to today as National Letter Writing Day; I really lost it when I heard that one!

The result of the investigation into what happened to Li Wenliang was also released today. I have no idea if people are pleased or not with the results, but I feel that I have said enough on this issue. Li Wenliang is gone; his Weibo page has become a wailing wall where countless people can go to forever remember him. Everyone knows that he was not a hero; he lived a normal life like everyone else, and the actions he took are the kind of actions you would expect any ordinary person to take if put in his position. All we can do is make sure he is remembered and do everything we can to support his family. As for the results of that investigation, I really don't care anymore. To be honest, our commemorations are in some sense a way for us to commemorate ourselves, to commemorate this experience we went through, and there was one important man who was part of that experience—his name was Li Wenliang. That said, it appears that the younger generation are much angrier than I am. This afternoon one young man left me a message: *When an era sheds a speck of dust it might not seem like much, but when it falls upon the shoulders of the Zhongnan Police Station it becomes a buck to be passed on to the next player.* Just like the second letter I got from that "high school student," this message also made me burst out laughing. But I still want to say that things might be a bit more complicated than we all think. They are complicated in a way that common people like us have no means to truly understand. Some things just take time, even though I'm not sure if time will help in this case.

Although we are still prohibited from going outside, virtually everyone knows that for the past several days now the city of Wuhan has been fairly safe. Even though everyone continues to reinforce that we should continue to stay on guard, psychologically we are all now much more relaxed. Whether it be the reality of what is going on inside the city or everyday people's state of mind, we are now in a completely different place than where we were a month ago. I have faith that lives will soon get back to their old rhythm. When they imposed the quarantine it was as if they suddenly slammed on the brakes, but I'm afraid the process of opening the city back up will be slow and gradual. I figure I don't have to necessarily stop my diary when some government leader proclaims that "the city will reopen tomorrow." Perhaps such a day will never come; that's because they have already gradually begun to reopen some parts of the city, so it will likely be a slow process of transition until the city is completely open again. That's why a few days ago I told Er Xiang that I planned to stop writing once I completed my 54th diary entry. It's like a perfect deck of poker cards, and now my hand will soon be finished. What I didn't realize was that yesterday was actually my 54th entry. It would be impossible for me not to reply to the open letter from the "high school student" who somehow already has more than 100,000 Weibo followers. Anyway, it now seems that I missed my chance to say some concluding words to close out this diary. But today I'm wondering when should I close up shop and bring this diary to a close?

I should, by the way, mention that all my diary entries have been uploaded to WeChat from the official account of the writer Er Xiang. The reason for that is quite simple: The day my Weibo account was frozen happened to be the same day that Li Wenliang passed away. I suddenly lost my one public platform. I'm not very adept with public posts on WeChat, but I often follow Er Xiang's official account there, so I reached out to her to see if she might mind helping me forward my posts. As a fellow writer, Er Xiang immediately agreed to help out. At the time, besides the fact that I knew she was a novelist, I really didn't know anything about her, and we have never met in person (of course, that isn't even possible now). It was only later when I read an essay about her that I learned something about her background. In short, it just comes down to an author with a verified official public account on WeChat helping out an old writer who doesn't know how to create an official account and share essays on that platform. Who would have thought that such a simple arrangement would lead to all kinds of conspiracy theories online?! I'm extremely thankful for Er Xiang's help and I hope she is able to one day visit Wuhan where I look forward to treating her to the seafood here! Seafood is one of Wuhan's specialties and there are a lot of talented seafood chefs in town.

I would like to digress again with a story from my youth. I was thinking back to many years ago when I was a member of the literature society in college; we would often discuss all kinds of literary topics. But after discussing things over and over, we could never seem to come to a mutual understanding. Later I grew a bit impatient with them and came up with a nickname I used behind their back; I called them the "Three Old Essays"[19] group. The three topics the group kept going back to were the tensions between praise and expose, comedy and tragedy, and darkness and light. More specifically, we found ourselves continually discussing whether or not literature should only be about works that express praise, are comedies, or shine light on the positive side of society. We also discussed whether or not those writers who expose social ills, portray human tragedy, and reveal the dark side of society were all reactionaries. This was back in 1978 into 1979. Since we never seemed to come to a conclusion about these questions, we for some reason just eventually stopped discussing them. Later we even organized a big discussion around the topic "Is Literature a Tool for Class Struggle?" but I don't think we came to a conclusion on that, either. Eventually, time passed by, I graduated, I started working, and I became a professional writer; then one day I discovered that somehow not only my old classmates but also the entire literary world had already reached a common understanding about how to approach this question: Can you write about anything you want? The main issue came down to the *quality* of your writing. So sometimes when I deliver lectures I say that there are a lot of questions that really don't need to be discussed, as time will eventually answer all those questions.

But this time I suddenly realized that I was wrong. Even though 42 years have passed, time hasn't completely answered those questions. Our views of literature seem to have somehow returned back to those same old questions. Those people who endlessly attack me—aren't they doing that just because I refuse to approach this catastrophe with praises, make it into a comedy, and shine a light on the positive things being done? When I think about how things have come back full circle like this, it is quite a strange feeling.

As I get to this point, a friend just forwarded me an essay from the website "Investigative Web" entitled "A *Wuhan Diary* Brimming with Malicious Intentions" by Qi Jianhua. I would like to begin by sending out a warning: "Mr. Qi: You can curse me if you like, but your essay is spreading false information and lies, in an attempt to portray me in a way that does not reflect the truth. I suggest you delete your post and publicly apologize. If your post is not deleted and an apology is not issued, I will use legal means to resolve this issue. This notice also pertains to the website 'Investigative Web'; you have the freedom to criticize me every day in your posts, but by posting essays like the one authored by Qi Jianhua that attempt to publicly slander me and spread rumors and untruths, you will force me to take legal action. I don't care about your background, or which government officials you have backing you, or how much support you have behind the scenes; I will pursue legal action against you, as well. China is a society based on the rule of law. I can tolerate your vicious curses and attacks—after all, all they do is speak to your lack of character. However, once you slander me, invent rumors, and try to frame me with lies, you are breaking the law. Here I make a special announcement to 'Investigative Web' and Mr. Qi Jianhua: Please get yourselves in order, or I will see you in court!"

Can't you see? Wuhan is on the verge of reopening. I may be retired, but I still have enough energy to take you to court.

MARCH 20, 2020

Let's see if I'm scared of you!

Another clear day. By the afternoon the temperature was already up to 26 degrees Celsius. I still haven't turned the heat off, and I suddenly realized that it was the same temperature inside and outside. When I opened the window to get some fresh air, I was surprised to discover a few magpies that had flown into my courtyard. They were hopping back and forth between the branches of the camphor tree and the magnolia tree; one of them even came into my doorway to drink from a puddle on the stone mortar. Just watching them was enough to really fill me with joy, and I wonder if this might be a sign of some good news coming.

There isn't much more to say about the coronavirus. The numbers are still holding at zero. We hope that continues; if it can continue for another 14 days, we will all be able to go outside again. Yet there is some other news online that is quite concerning; it has also been spreading very quickly. One news item is claiming that there are 20 new patients at Tongji Hospital who are sick with the virus, but the hospital is afraid to officially report these cases. I sent this information to two of my doctor friends to get their opinion. One doctor said that it was simply a misunderstanding. Now that there are a lot of patients being discharged from the hospitals, some of the remaining patients are being transferred to other, larger hospitals designated for coronavirus treatment. But those are not new patients, they are just newly transferred patients. My other doctor friend was more direct: "In a strict system you either speak the truth or get out of class."

There is a post that everyone has been forwarding like mad. A patient recently tested positive for coronavirus after being released from the hospital and is now having difficulty getting readmitted. This incident has also triggered a lot of fear. So I again reached out to two doctor friends to get their input. One doctor friend confirmed that there was indeed a case of reinfection, but that is extremely rare. The other doctor started out by saying almost the same thing as the first doctor, but he actually had a more concrete understanding of this particular case. He explained that because they had already changed which hospitals were designated as coronavirus treatment centers, the patient ended up going to the wrong hospital, which was not one of the designated treatment centers. Later he got in touch with an administrator he knew and convinced them to admit him anyway. My doctor friend wanted to confirm two points: There are very few patients who test positive again after recovery, as some of them have no symptoms and are not contagious; besides that, hospitals are keeping track of all patients, so if any of them start to feel sick again, they just need to return to one of the designated hospitals (there is no such thing as patients not being able to get admitted anymore). I'm not going to check if the doctor's interpretation matches up with the patient's account; I am just providing an accurate report on what the physicians told me.

For most Wuhan residents right now, no matter whether they have been infected or not, they are all in a relatively fragile state of mind and prone to anxiety. Since they have changed which hospitals are now designated as coronavirus treatment centers, I suggest that this information be made clear to the public so everyone knows. If there are any changes like this, information should be immediately updated. As for patients who are feeling sick, they should double check which hospitals are currently accepting coronavirus patients in order to avoid showing up at the wrong hospital. There is no way around it: Spending several hours in the middle of the night trying to get treatment at an ER is always a torturous experience.

More bad news just came in from Central Hospital; Medical Ethics Committee Member Liu Li died this morning from the novel coronavirus. She is the fifth doctor from Central Hospital to pass away from this illness; I still don't know how the hospital's administrators are able to continue on in their current posts.

Yesterday there were a lot of people writing letters in response to a certain "high school student," and that seems to have continued all the way up until today. And today there was even a letter that appeared online entitled "A Letter from a Group of High School Students to Another High School Student." At first I didn't pay much attention to it; I just thought it was some kind of prank. So I was quite surprised when a friend told me it was written by a group of real high school students. This piqued my curiosity and I decided to read it. The first thing I noticed was that these high school students were indeed quite different from *that other* "high school student." Not just in terms of their writing level, but they were on a different level entirely. There was one sentence that was so good that I can't help but quote it here: "What we really want to say is that in many cases the problem does not lie with someone paying too much attention to the dark side of things, it is actually due to our overemphasis on bright and positive things—sometimes that brightness can be so blinding that it damages our ability to see things clearly." I suppose these kids are not all as vulnerable as I imagined them to be. They really do have strong, independent thinking skills; and they reveal very strong powers of observation. From that letter I can see that, on many issues, they actually have a deeper understanding of things than many adults.

Yesterday I started off intending to write about literary debates from back in the day; I got some of that down on paper, but then I saw that article published in "Investigative Web" that derailed me for a while. I even contacted a lawyer to provide evidence in case I need to file a defamation lawsuit. This afternoon I received several messages telling me that the essay published on "Investigative Web" by Qi Jianhua has already been taken down. He surely knew what he had published was illegal and the fact that he deleted it in some ways indicates that he knows he was wrong; I will consider whether or not I want to forgive him. Then in the afternoon someone said that an ultra-leftist from Shanghai seemed to have trouble accepting this outcome; they started screaming and hollering that Fang Fang wouldn't dare to sue— she wouldn't dare! That is quite funny; okay then, don't delete the essay, and let's see what happens!

Originally I really wanted to continue the discussion about literature from yesterday; I wanted to pick up from where I left off and cover the period up to the present day. But then I received another essay forwarded from a friend, which interrupted me again. It's a good thing that the discussion about literature is an old topic that I can come back to anytime.

It seems that Peking University Professor Zhang Yiwu[20] has now personally come out to address what has been happening. Zhang Yiwu is a really big name in the field. Is he the one who has been supporting the group attacking me? Or is he the one who has been directing their attacks? This is something that I cannot ignore. I heard that Professor Zhang uploaded an essay on Weibo, but I haven't yet had time to read it. Instead I will just post an excerpt that one of my friends just forwarded to serve as a record. Professor Zhang writes:

There is an author who has been focusing specifically on a diary about the outbreak. She has been raising all kinds of criticisms and suspicions about these [letter] writers, saying how dark they are and hinting that they may all be following orders from somewhere; there was also a letter from an anonymous high school student that she criticized for being so stupid, etc., etc. To be perfectly frank, if you want to know why people don't trust her diary, it's because when the outbreak was at its peak, she employed a reportage literary style to describe a photo of a pile of cellphones on the floor of a crematorium; it is said that the photo was sent to her by one of her doctor friends. This brought widespread attention to her diary and became the incident that garnered her a lot of followers.

But a lot of people have suspicions about this incident; some are asking if this photograph even exists. The author has consistently been unwilling to address this question; instead she repeatedly brushes it under the rug while telling everyone that there are people out there trying to incriminate her. But the crucial issue here is that every writer should abide by a basic fundamental standard when it comes to the pursuit of truth. You cannot sacrifice the basic principles of human dignity; you cannot fabricate information to deceive naive readers who trust you; moreover, during a crucial time like this, fabricating facts will certainly not be tolerated; such acts are only committed by those without a conscience and shall become a mark of eternal shame on a writer.

Reading Professor Zhang's comments makes it clear to me that he has not even read my diary; perhaps he just read a summary that someone prepared for him? A summary tailor-written for his specific tastes at that. Take, for instance, the sentence "there was also a letter from an anonymous high school student that she criticized for being so stupid." I clearly never said anything like that. He also wrote, "if you want to know why people don't trust her diary." I wonder about these "people" he is referring to; how many people are we talking about here? Is he referring specifically to the people in his circle? How would Professor Zhang know anything about how many people trust me? If we follow Professor Zhang's methods to make judgments and inferences, then I could say that I have basically never met anyone in the field of literature or academia for that matter who trusts Professor Zhang. Moreover, there is that line about fabricating "information to deceive naive readers who trust you." I wonder if in using such categorical language Professor Zhang might be going a bit too far with his own fabrications? But that's okay, he has always been quite fierce in the way he pushes his viewpoint. When he was complimenting Zhou Xiaoping on what a wonderful example of a model youth he was, Professor Zhang's language was also quite over the top; he used language that was so exaggerated and laudatory that one would think Zhou Xiaoping was even *more* qualified to teach at Peking University than Professor Zhang himself.[21] Actually, Professor Zhang likes to use his own petty mind to speculate about other people, and in the past he has also paid a price for that. Didn't Professor Zhang once accuse a famous novelist of "plagiarism" but only ended up losing the case and embarrassing himself so badly that he could barely show his face?

As for that photograph, I have already explained that in great detail in an earlier post. So it is a real shame that Professor Zhang seems to have never taken the time to read what I wrote. Actually, Professor Zhang should really come out to Wuhan to understand the true situation firsthand: Then he would understand things like just how many people died each day, how the dead bodies were transported from the hospitals to the crematoriums, what happened to the personal articles of the deceased after they died, what kind of situation the hospitals and crematoriums were in, why lithium batteries cannot be burned, what kind of sterilization methods are being used, and why so many crematoriums all over the country have been supporting Wuhan. But I will have to stop here. For Professor Zhang and others who are willing to understand what is happening, all the information is here; if you don't want to see the truth, that is your choice. I'm sure that one day everyone will see that photograph; but it won't be from me, it needs to come from the person who took that photo. I really recommend that Professor Zhang visit Wuhan so that he can conduct his own firsthand investigation; of course, I should add that all these things occurred during the early stages of the outbreak, not later and not now. I think it would be more in keeping with Peking University's standards if Professor Zhang first took some time to understand the true situation before rushing to make categorical conclusions. I'm sure that will also make the parents of the students he teaches feel much more at ease.

I'll stop here for today, but I want to emphasize one thing: The presence of those ultra-leftists represents an existential threat to China and her people. If the entire Reform Era is destroyed at their hands, it would be the ultimate slap in the face to my entire generation. So come at me with all you've got, bring out all your dirty tricks, and tell all your big-name supporters to show their faces too! Let's see if I'm scared of you!

MARCH 21, 2020

The coronavirus outbreak seems to have stabilized,
but people's hearts have not.

We are now 59 days into the quarantine. It has been such a long time.

The sun was so bright yesterday but today it suddenly turned cloudy. There were even some light afternoon showers; but this time of year, my plants and trees in the courtyard all desperately need that rain. Two or three days ago the cherry blossoms on the Wuhan University campus blossomed; and although the campus is empty, I suspect there must have been some reporters there taking pictures, because everyone in my classmates group was forwarding photos of cherry blossoms in bloom. There is something so perfectly beautiful about seeing cherry blossoms in full bloom, devoid of any humans in sight.

The sky was extremely dark and when I went down to the main gate at dusk to pick up a parcel, there was a light spring drizzle; I didn't bring an umbrella, but it felt great to let the rain fall on me. Just as I got back to my front door the rain suddenly turned into a downpour; if I had arrived home just a moment later I would have been soaked. I guess I got lucky.

The coronavirus outbreak seems to have stabilized, but people's hearts have not. People are scared that patients who have recovered from the coronavirus might get reinfected; they are scared that hospitals will not report new cases because they don't want to spoil the perfect new record of "zero" new infections. Since people are talking about these issues, I decided to ask my doctor friend and he gave me a clear answer. However, online I see that a lot of people are still very worried about this. This virus works in strange ways; it is crafty, it is elusive, and there are still a lot of unknowns concerning how it works. People are extremely scared, especially those of us here in Wuhan. We have all witnessed the tragedy firsthand during the early stages of the outbreak, and I think the fear we felt is still lurking deep inside us. But no matter what happens, we need to stay calm and collected. It is no use to get panicky; I think that the terrible situation early on was, to some extent, related to the state of panic we were thrown into. Anyone who had even the slightest fever rushed straight to the hospital; that led to a situation where a lot of people who didn't have the novel coronavirus ended up getting infected by going to the hospital. That, in turn, put even more stress on a medical system that was already on the verge of collapse and led to even more deaths.

Now that the outbreak has gotten to its current point, things have more or less stabilized and there is no need for us to be in panic mode. The hospitals now have enough experience treating patients of novel coronavirus so patients who are newly infected or recurring cases don't need to be as anxious as before; you just need to go in for treatment. We are, after all, not made of steel; people often get sick and, just like always, we need to seek out treatment when we fall ill; it just takes time to go through the treatment. During the period between winter and spring, it was already flu season, which is also contagious; but didn't we all get through that? According to a doctor in Shanghai named Dr. Zhang

Wenhong,[22] the death rate from novel coronavirus is less than 1 percent. If that's the case, there isn't that much to be scared of. Except for those few lethal cases, we shouldn't be so terrified of infection; weren't those patients in the temporary hospitals singing and dancing? Once they got discharged, they all seemed happy as can be, as if this illness is no different than any other.

But, on the other hand, I am having trouble understanding this desire to keep all the numbers at zero. Just how big is the difference between one and zero, anyhow? I feel that neither the government nor the people need to be so fixated on this issue. During normal times, there are always various infectious diseases out there; we just need to be cautious and if we get sick, we seek out medical help. Don't tell me that if we are at zero we can all go back to work, but that even one confirmed case will affect our ability to return to normal? Can't we just solve the problem by sending that one patient to the hospital for quarantine? We can't necessarily always get a perfect zero; sometimes perfection simply isn't practical.

When it comes to precautionary measures against the novel coronavirus, I trust the judgment of Dr. Zhang Wenhong in Shanghai. According to Dr. Zhang, there are protective measures you can take. You need to adopt effective personal protection measures such as practicing social distancing, frequent hand washing, and wearing a face mask; all three of these are essential. Dr. Zhang said: "Up until this point, we have still not seen a single example of someone who carefully and consistently implemented all three of these measures and still got infected. If you follow these guidelines, it is highly unlikely that you will be infected." I very much agree with his view on this. There is a meme that says, "You can send anything you want to Hubei, except for Dr. Zhang Wenhong!" So why *do* the people of Shanghai hold Dr. Zhang Wenhong in such high regard? It's because most of what he has said has already been proven to be true. It is said that the reason Japan has been so successful in controlling the coronavirus has a lot to do with the high hygiene standards of the Japanese people. There is some truth there; if you travel around the world, it is indeed hard to find a country cleaner than Japan. That is also why Japanese people tend to have long life spans; implementing strict hygiene standards can prevent a lot of illnesses.

Since the outbreak, concepts like "love" and "goodness" no longer seem as empty as before. People are now able to clearly see what true love and true goodness really are. It is just a shame that there are some people who insist on shouting these phrases, yet when it comes time for them to take real action, you can't find them anywhere. They are used to passionately expressing love and goodness as empty, politicized concepts, but once you bring them down to the real world and put these concepts in real concrete terms, you won't see an ounce of passion; in fact, you won't even feel the slightest warmth. During the past few days I have seen a few videos of people cursing and insulting Chinese who have just returned from abroad; I also saw footage of people from other provinces getting into heated conflicts with Hubei workers who have just arrived to get back to work. These videos have left me utterly flabbergasted. Why can't they love these people with the same passion they put into loving their country?

I remember that when the coronavirus first broke out in Wuhan and our local cache of medical equipment and supplies was facing a severe shortage, a lot of overseas Chinese really stepped up to the plate; they basically cleaned out the shelves from stores in whatever country they were in and sent it all to Wuhan to help us get through this difficult period. But who would have expected that, once they started facing difficulties themselves and decided to come home, so many people would come out against them. How quickly people change; it just goes to show you how evil human nature can be. And then there are the residents of

Hubei who, in order to stop the spread of the virus, faced a myriad of difficulties staying at home for more than 50 days, yet once they tried returning to work, they still had to face all kinds of resistance. Our country has so many grand slogans that we shout, so many official government documents, yet when it comes down to it, they all amount to nothing. In both of these cases, the government provided amazing support to both those compatriots abroad who decided to return to China as well as those Hubei residents who wanted to resume work outside their home province, yet in both cases there were many citizens who simply seemed intent on making it hard for these people; the whole thing is very strange indeed.

There are a few more things I would like to record: Several countries are now giving out cash payments to their citizens to help them get through this difficult period! This news is going viral online; and the way they are distributing the cash is quite admirable. This has led some people to ask if China will also be making payments like that to its citizens. Will they do it in Hubei? Today I saw that someone suggested that the government should distribute cash vouchers so that citizens would be able to purchase goods once the epidemic is over; this could also help get sales going again and maintain the vitality of the market; that would help us get back on track more quickly. From the message board it looked like a lot of people support this suggestion. I heard that in Wuhan there would be some special policies in place to help underprivileged groups and others who might need additional help. I just saw this news from the Office of Poverty Alleviation and Development: "In order to do our best to alleviate the economic burden that low-income families are facing due to the coronavirus, we have approved a one-time relief payment to benefit urban low-income families and urban and rural flexible workers whose employment has been impacted by the epidemic. One-time payments will be made at four times the average monthly salary rate

(780 yuan/month in urban districts and 635 yuan/month in rural areas)." Compared with the payments being provided by other countries, this rate seems quite low; however, I suppose something is better than nothing. Moreover, perhaps there will be more to come?

At this point, hospitals are now gradually starting to reopen their normal departments. But I'm not sure if they are now already back to how they were before the outbreak began. But this is actually an extremely urgent task. In normal times, these hospitals are always brimming with patients. Yet for the past two months all those patients with urgent medical needs and chronic conditions have been putting off their care and waiting until the coronavirus situation is cleared up. But all this waiting comes at the price of damaging their own health. For instance, those cancer patients who interrupted their chemotherapy treatments due to the coronavirus—how are *they* doing? Those patients with scheduled surgery that needed to be delayed—will they still be able to get their surgery in time?

One of my friends forwarded me a letter written by someone recounting his sister's experience. It said that his sister used to practice Tai Chi every day, but after more than 50 days stuck at home she ended up having a sudden stroke. They called 110, but no hospitals were initially able to take her; by the time they finally got her to a hospital, they were required to first test her for the novel coronavirus. By the time the test results came back to rule out coronavirus, that most critical window to save her life had already passed, and she died a week later. The letter writer said: "I need to get this out soon; on the one hand I need an outlet for all the sadness and anger inside me, but even more importantly, I need to warn those people in charge here in Wuhan how important it is to immediately resume normal hospital operations. Public transportation in Wuhan is all returning to order, but what about the hospitals; we need to take precautions against the virus but at the same time we also must get back to the normal order of things; if the hospitals don't get back to normal there will be a lot of wrongful and unnecessary deaths in this city! My sister-in-law's mother had cancer in her biliary duct, she was unable to eat, and couldn't get any medical care; we called 110, and 120 numerous times, but no one picked up. She died of the pain on the second day of the Lunar New Year." He continued, "I truly hate the fact that this coronavirus has been spreading throughout the city. And I hate the fact that the Wuhan Health Commission was not transparent early on and didn't warn the public; think of how many innocent people died because of that. Before the quarantine, those useless leaders really had no idea how to deal with this crisis; now nearly two months into the quarantine and they still have absolutely no policy for how to help the large number of elderly residents suffering from chronic health conditions, cancer patients, and those dealing with the sudden onset of acute illnesses. The whole situation is really terrible!!!!" This is a direct quote and I have even preserved his punctuation marks.

Seeing people around you dying one after another is indeed a horrific experience. Right now the lack of treatment options for patients with chronic and acute illnesses has become a very real and pressing problem. I passed this issue off to my doctor friend to get his comments. I started off by asking him: "Is it true that all ordinary patients who go in to see a doctor need to have a blood test to first check whether or not they are positive for the novel coronavirus, and they can only register after that step?" My doctor friend responded: "We have implemented security measures for all non-coronavirus patients who come in for treatment; we have implemented security measures which include setting up special safeguard zones in every hospital. If there is a patient who is suspected of possibly carrying the coronavirus, we then admit them to a quarantine room; once we have ruled out coronavirus, they are then transferred to a room in the safeguard zone.

Every patient has their nucleic acid level and antibodies checked and they undergo a chest CT scan. If a patient is accompanied by a family member, they will also need to have a chest CT and an antibody test to rule out coronavirus before being allowed to stay with them at the hospital. For patients suffering from myocardial infarction or strokes, our neurologists and cardiologists take them directly into the ER to administer lifesaving procedures and they do not wait for the results of those coronavirus screening tests." A shame that the sister of the person who wrote that letter couldn't hang on long enough.

Medical practitioners also have their own concerns; right now, as the coronavirus situation has not yet completely stabilized, there is still some uncertainty when it comes to which patients may or may not be coronavirus carriers; after all, after so many medical workers have been struck down by this virus, it is only natural for them to be traumatized and fearful. But there seems to be a deadlock here. My doctor friend explained it: "If we don't rule out novel coronavirus in patients and admit them into the hospital, it could lead to other patients getting infected; so we have a huge responsibility here. If we aren't careful, all that we have achieved with our 50-day lockdown could be wasted in a single day." Now you see how serious this issue is.

My doctor friend is also worried that doctor–patient relationships are about to start getting tense due to increased cost burden on patients for all the extra tests. My friend says: "Why do you think the public is so happy with the treatment they have been receiving for the novel coronavirus? It's because the government has been footing the bill. For a low-income family, 1,000 yuan is a huge expense. The cost for just those initial screening tests is close to 1,000 yuan and that doesn't even mean that you will be admitted right away; this has resulted in a lot of anger toward those ER doctors working on the front lines. Right now all patients go through the ER for normal visits; the ER is basically functioning as an outpatient clinic; currently in the entire city of Wuhan you can only go through the normal medical insurance reimbursement plan if you are admitted to the hospital. When patients register at the ER, they are expected to pay up front and be reimbursed later. If the government were covering these costs up front, we wouldn't have so many angry patients yelling at us. But when the patients are forced to foot the bill, the doctors are the ones who take the heat." And then there is the problem of hospitals being understaffed, which is clearly an issue. "During the early stage of the coronavirus outbreak there were large numbers of medical caregivers who were infected and most of them are still recovering at home."

The hardships that the people are facing and the difficult position that doctors have been put in are all laid out right there before our eyes. And this situation is no less serious than when the novel coronavirus was at its height. To solve these problems that have revealed themselves, we need to act quickly and resolutely. I hope that professionals are able to offer suggestions about what strategies might work, in order to find a method to resolve these issues. For instance, perhaps it might be possible to waive all fees associated with coronavirus screening, regardless of the patient's illness?

MARCH 22, 2020

The wildfires cannot eliminate the grass,
which shall be reborn when the spring winds blow.

Day 60 of the lockdown; these days have been hard to imagine.

The rain last night was quite heavy but today the sky has cleared up. Those communities with no coronavirus cases are now gradually opening up; today I even heard the sound of a child outside laughing—such a long time since I have heard that sound. As long as residents limit their amount of time out, they are also permitted to venture outside local developments for shopping, although people are still recommended to avoid peak times. There are special shopping hours for seniors in the morning, while younger shoppers are encouraged to go in the afternoon. There are also other recommendations, like all people maintaining a 1.5-meter distance between themselves and other shoppers when in line. The area in which people are allowed to freely move about is also gradually being expanded. After two months of silence, Wuhan is now beginning to loosen up and breathe again; the noise of bustling traffic will soon return to our streets and lanes. It will still be some time before Wuhan returns to its old lively self, but right now just getting out is good.

Although official word of the city's opening up has not yet come down, the door is gradually starting to open. Instructions for returning to Wuhan have been issued for both personnel from Wuhan as well as personnel from other provinces. Those instructions being: "According to the principle of 'ask and apply,' that is, all you have to do is apply and it will be approved. All provincial personnel with a 'green health QR code' can pass without having to go through any additional procedures. Those from outside of Wuhan who have a health QR code from other provinces will just need to scan their health QR code and have their temperature taken and then they will be able to enter Wuhan; they will no longer be required to provide a certificate of health (unless they have been unable to attain a health QR code), a travel pass, an approved entrance application, certificate of acceptance, vehicle pass, or other certifications." This is really wonderful news. My days of hardship are almost over. Since my dog's skin disease has been acting up, I made an appointment to take him to the vet tomorrow. It really feels like the sky has suddenly brightened up. Since I also need to periodically go to the doctor, I started looking into what the current situation was to make appointments at places like Zhongnan Hospital, where I usually go. Although their outpatient clinic is still closed, their ER is now back to normal. There were also quite a few doctors and nurses from Zhongnan Hospital infected by the coronavirus, but most of them are now doing much better.

In the afternoon I was sweeping my courtyard when my colleague's son Y, who lives next door, asked me if I would mind chatting with some of his fellow volunteers for a while. I had to politely refuse; I simply had too many chores to tend to; I really just didn't have the time. But they quickly told me a little bit about their volunteer group. I added Y as a friend on my WeChat account so I could look up his group and learned that Wuhan has a volunteer group called "Shadow Dream Team." They have been volunteering around the city ever since the first day of the lockdown. The members of the team are all ordinary people from all different walks of life; right now their primary mission is to deliver donated food to some of the smaller districts in the city. I was quite surprised to learn that today they had just sent a shipment of medical supplies to Canada. Back when we were in dire straits, a lot of overseas Chinese bought up all the local medical supplies and sent them here to China. Now that things have turned around and we have an ample supply of personal protective equipment and other items, young people here have begun to donate them back to countries overseas. The only problem is that the process of sending them back is sometimes a bit more complicated than it was when we first received them.

Now that the threat of the virus has waned, the main task at hand for the hospitals is the treatment of those patients still struggling with serious illnesses; meanwhile, there remain no new cases of novel coronavirus. Even though this remains quite controversial, I still can't claim to know the truth. But at this moment there are now a lot of countries outside China that have fallen into the abyss of this coronavirus. Today one of my doctor friends shared some news with me: "500 Chinese-American physicians have established a large group which includes all kinds of different doctors." All of them are front-line doctors. They plan to collect and organize some of the main issues deserving of attention. Once the results are ready, they will also organize discussions to understand the typical case histories of novel coronavirus patients in order to deepen our understanding of this illness for their colleagues worldwide! My doctor friend said: "China has found a set of effective methods that the whole world can learn from. If we are able to provide some help on this front, perhaps there won't be so much hatred toward the Chinese people; we are trying to transform something negative into a positive." He added: "This project is being led by Massachusetts General Hospital, which is affiliated with Harvard University. I saw this news on a WeChat group; the US is really quite impressive with what they are doing."

That bit of news was the happiest thing I heard today. This virus is humankind's common enemy; we have no choice but to stand side-by-side to get through this difficult time together. This is what is most important right now. Doctors around the world can now use the internet to collectively discuss which medicines are most effective and share which treatment methods have been best suited to coronavirus patients; these should be the most important things to work out during this coronavirus era. This would be a great contribution to humanity. Doctors from Wuhan should be able to provide even more insights, since they have already gone through the entire process, from the initial lax period up until the point the entire system was brought to the brink of collapse. Since they have lived through this, they would be the ones with the most reliable information to share. I truly feel that this group of doctors is really just too amazing for words; what they did was truly an act of kindness and love for this city. Normally, this doctor friend of mine gives the impression that he might have a slightly anti-American tendency; so I was happy to discover that once he and his colleagues in the medical field started working together against this virus, that sentiment seemed to completely disappear.

So what are ordinary people's lives like these days? Yesterday I was chatting with my middle brother and he sent me another one of my sister-in-law's sketches of daily life under the quarantine. Her previous preoccupation with online shopping has now been displaced by other things; one of these posts is about what happens when you need medical help; there are two entries that I will share with you:

March 18: Last night Z had a toothache so in the middle of the night he got up and rubbed some oral pain relief cream on his tooth, but it only seemed to help a little. The next morning, besides rubbing on some more cream, he also tried gargling with saltwater, but he was still in a lot of discomfort. It was a good thing he was able to calm down and carefully examine his mouth; he discovered that it wasn't actually a tooth problem, he had a mouth ulcer in the gum area. I remembered that there was a spray that can treat mouth ulcers, so I quickly had him contact the pharmacy over WeChat and we were able to easily purchase the spray as well as a traditional Chinese medicine that was supposed to relieve internal heat. After I paid via WeChat I quickly went down to the west gate of our complex and picked up the medicine, which the storeowner next door passed to me through the iron gates of the fence. It was so convenient. I felt much more relieved once I picked up the medicine. You have to know how very difficult it is to go to the hospital during this current situation; first of all, just getting out of our complex is difficult and then getting into a hospital is also very hard. Since Z suffers from a serious chronic health condition, what worries me most right now is his illness's suddenly acting up and requiring him to go to the hospital.

But going down to the west gate to pick up the medicine was actually quite enjoyable because I got to enjoy a full five minutes of sunlight on the way there and back; what a treat! Both of our main meals today are soups or soft dishes that won't irritate his mouth; but waxed-duck and Chinese radish soup with some century eggs on the side was enough to fill us up while being quite tasty and nutritious. The medicine I bought is fairly easy to use; you just spray it in your mouth once every two hours. The Chinese medicine needs to be taken as a hot drink three times a day; I'll start that one tomorrow. The good thing is that with Chinese medicine it doesn't really matter if you use a bit extra in the beginning. By the evening, Z's mouth was already much better; I don't think it will keep him up again tonight.

March 19: Today is our 59th day at home. Z's mouth ulcer is much better. I guess we bought the right medicine. This afternoon for lunch I reheated the waxed-duck and Chinese radish soup from yesterday, but threw in a bunch of other ingredients like cabbage; that way, with a bowl of rice, it will be a full nutritious meal: another delicious soup dish. Hopefully, tomorrow his mouth will be good enough for us to start eating normal solid foods again.

L's old partner had a stroke last year; at first it didn't seem that serious and he had made a decent recovery, but the whole process was very stressful for him and he ended up with a long-lasting depression. Over the course of this extended lockdown, the two of them started to really get on each other's nerves. I remember last time she texted me on WeChat she told me how terrible it was. Everyone is ecstatic today since the number of new cases just went down to zero so I thought I'd reach out to see how she and her husband were doing. I never imagined that the first thing she would say would be that she broke down crying as soon as she saw the number get down to zero. I never imagined her to respond so strongly; compared to her, I wonder if I've turned into a zombie after being locked up at home for so long. Of course I'm happy, but I also quickly realized that today only marks the first day at zero, we still have a long way to go.

Before I even had a chance to share what I've been going through, she just unloaded all kinds of complaints on me: "Oh my, we can't go on like this! We're just stuck at home every day. All day all he thinks about is his illness, he's a real hypochondriac, oh my goodness, I'm so frustrated! Every day at home all he talks about is his illness coming back! He keeps babbling about wanting to go to the hospital yet at the same time he's scared to go; so he ends up just sitting at home fixating on his illness. He gets so wrapped up in it that he can't even sleep. I'll tell you, this old man is going to make me have a nervous breakdown!"

I tried to talk some sense into her by explaining that once you enter old age there are a lot of times where you simply need to calm down and let things go. I told her what was most important was having someone there beside her to keep from feeling too lonely. I even suggested that she try looking at herself as a carefree big sister who has to take care of a naughty child; if that doesn't work try to just laugh it off or pretend you are brain dead. I feel like people with psychological problems all have a common trait; when they say something crazy, you just nod your head in agreement, and then once that is out of the way you can do whatever the hell you want to. When you run into situations where you simply can't agree with them, never try to talk sense into them, that will just make things worse. Instead you had better just shut your mouth and say nothing. There's nothing else you can do because the person you are dealing with is not entirely normal.

When I read this entry written by my sister-in-law I thought it was really interesting, especially the part about "the person you are dealing with is not entirely normal," which was particularly funny to read.

Today is a day worth commemorating: Day 60 of the quarantine. Today there were quite a few people who got in touch with me, asking me to stop writing. They are probably afraid about the number of people now attacking me online. Actually, I only intended on writing 54 chapters—a perfect deck of poker cards—I joked with my friend about playing out my entire hand. But I didn't end up stopping on Day 54; instead I have decided to go up to 60. Today all my friends suddenly seem to think that the danger level has risen. I'm also starting to sense that. This afternoon the number of people attacking me on Weibo seemed to clearly double. My friends probably all know who these people attacking me are.

A few years ago there was a popular slogan online: "When the Emperor's Bar sets out on an expedition, not even a single blade of grass grows."[23] At the time I also thought this whole controversy was quite something and even forwarded a few posts about it. Someone in my friends group also forwarded me a "command" sent out from the Official Weibo Account of the Emperor's Bar. The Official Weibo Account of the Emperor's Bar listed a series of articles about me. Now that was really something. Somehow in the eyes of the "Bar Boss," I must be their enemy now? Last year this group did in fact express support for those who collectively mobilize people to use extreme obscenities for nationalistic purposes. At the time, I publicly criticized them and ended up having my account suspended for that. The Emperor's Bar has a large group of 10 million followers online. I suppose the "Bar Boss" couldn't tolerate this offense. That's because their leader is indeed the greatest under heaven; no one in this world is a worthy opponent for him. I found this quite amusing. But I still want to believe that 99 percent of the members of the Emperor's Bar are reasonable young people. If there are some even-headed people supporting this platform, how could this Bar have continued on for so long? The slogan "when the Emperor's Bar sets out on an expedition, not even a single blade of grass grows" would actually be great as an advertising slogan.

Spring is now here. Spring is a season of awakening; it is also a season of hope. That awakening and hope are embodied in a poem that begins: "The wildfires cannot eliminate the grass, which shall be reborn when the spring winds blow."[24]

MARCH 23, 2020

All those questions, they remain unanswered.

Day 61 of the quarantine. I began to post this diary on Weibo starting on Day One of the Lunar New Year (January 25); that was two days after the lockdown began. Today marks my 59th diary entry.

A bright clear day and the temperature is perfect. This afternoon I was finally able to take the dog to the vet. His skin problem has been acting up again and is now festering all over his body; I can't delay treatment for him any longer. The injury on my finger is also pretty bad; I need to get it checked out. Before long the vet sent me a video of my dog; they said he was so dirty that the tub of water all turned black! They also said they would need to shave him in order to properly treat his skin problem. This dog was born on Christmas Eve of 2003; at the end of the year he will be 17 years old, a bit too old for a dog. All the other dogs I had from back then have all long died. He's the survivor. He still has an appetite and still likes to play, but his vision is going and he doesn't hear so well anymore. Once he got old, his skin condition also started to deteriorate and has become really difficult to treat. During normal times, I make sure to occasionally take him to the vet to get bathed and treated for his skin disease. But this time, because of the quarantine, he was way overdue for a visit. But it's a good thing that everything is improving now; they'll take good care of him at the hospital and I can finally rest easy.

Outside in the streets they are testing the buses before they start running again, and down by the subway station they are cleaning things up and disinfecting everything; everything is getting ready to start operating again. Everyone is passing this information around to each other and we are all excited to see the city coming back to life. And as for the numbers that used to terrify us each day, they are now at zero, as they have been for the past five days in a row.

First thing this morning, my middle brother uploaded a photo to our group chat of someone offering 10-minute "quickcut" haircuts in his neighborhood. They were doing them out on the field right outside my brother's window. The weather is sunny today and residents were lining up, at a distance of about one meter apart, in a long line. My brother said that they had been lining up like that all day long. His neighborhood was once the single most dangerous area in all of Wuhan. My brother has been locked up in his apartment for more than 60 days, but today he seems quite relaxed. For someone like my brother, who has a lot of medical issues, to get through these two months without getting sick is really a gift from God.

According to Mayor Zhou, just before the Lunar New Year approximately five million people left Wuhan. A few days ago there was a notification that most of these people can now reenter the city if they have a health QR code. My housekeeper also sent me a text saying that she should be able to come back sometime in the next day or two. Some of my former classmates who ended up staying on in Hainan island keep sending photos of themselves hanging out on the beach; we originally had planned to have seafood together before the outbreak. We have been trapped at home, they have been trapped outside the city; but now they can all start making their way back to Wuhan.

I'm told that right now it is relatively easy to enter Wuhan, but much more difficult to get out. This reminds me of those people who visited Wuhan just before the lockdown; I wonder what happened to them? Are they still here? I suspect that the two months they were detained here in Wuhan might be the most difficult period of their lives. How many people are there like them in Wuhan? I'm afraid there are probably no precise numbers. I'm just asking out of curiosity, but I discovered it must be a fairly large number; and most of them are still here. For the time being, none of Wuhan's transportation services have resumed service outside the city; that means that no airplanes, trains, buses, or private automobiles are allowed to leave the city limits. I wonder how those people from elsewhere who have been stuck here in Wuhan and their worried family members have gotten through these two months; it must be so hard for all of them.

My neighbor Y told me that two of the volunteers in his Shadow Dream Team are actually out-of-towners who still cannot go home; one of them is from Nanning in Guangxi Province. When he saw the reports about the outbreak in Wuhan, he rushed here to volunteer. When he got here, the quarantine was imposed and now he is stuck here. The other volunteer is from Guangdong and he too has no way to get back home. The volunteer team takes care of their room and board and they also plan on buying them train tickets to get home once this is all over.

One of my doctor friends who has been providing news on the coronavirus throughout this whole period told me today that a few of his friends came to Wuhan on a business trip just before the lockdown; they also got stuck here with no way of going home. All of a sudden it has now been two months; when they came it was still winter and now we are already in spring; they don't even have the appropriate clothes. Another friend owns a company in Beijing; since he got held up in Wuhan, he has been unable to run his company.

During the outbreak, these unfortunate individuals from elsewhere who ended up getting stuck here in Wuhan during the quarantine were completely marginalized. For a long time no one even thought about them. It was only much later in the outbreak that a reporter discovered a few people who had been living in one of the city's underground pedestrian tunnels without anything to drink or eat. Only after that article came out did people realize that there was a group of people like that here in Wuhan who were basically out on the streets. Their situation was really too tragic. After that report was published, the government stepped in and came up with some housing options for those people. But now, after all this time has gone by, it is hard to imagine that they are still here in Wuhan. They are even more anxious for the city to reopen than the other nine million residents of Wuhan. Sometimes I think that if there were more thoughtful people in the world, perhaps they could help the government to come up with some ideas to figure out how to get these people home a little sooner. For instance, we could do a census by scanning everyone's health QR code, determine which province they are from, and then arrange one bus for each province to send them all home to their respective provincial capitals; they could then be quarantined in a hotel designated by the individual; then after 14 days, they could be permitted to return home. That kind of a policy wouldn't be too difficult to implement. If you can dream it, you can do it. That would be an easy option for resolving this problem; and it could save a lot of people from this desperate situation, so what's stopping us from trying?

Ever since yesterday, there has been a lot of news about Beijing refusing to let people from Hubei into the city. It is really hard for me to believe; even now I have trouble believing this is true. I just can't fathom what the difference between a healthy person from Hubei and a healthy person from Beijing could possibly be. If Beijing really refuses Hubei residents entry into the city, it may be the people of Hubei who will be suffering, but it is certainly not anything they should feel shameful about. It is those people who suggested and adopted these policies of exclusion that should feel shame. Of course, it is also our entire civilization that should feel shame. One day we will look back and realize what level our civilization was still stuck at in 2020. For the time being, I'd like to hope this report is not accurate; but it is worth noting here in my diary.

There was also some bad news today: Several days back, a young nurse from Guangxi who had come to Wuhan as a member of one of the relief teams suddenly collapsed at the hospital. It was a good thing that there were several doctors present, so they quickly administered lifesaving treatment. At the time, all the media outlets reported this story; everyone was happy that she was able to escape death. But last night my doctor friend told me that, in the end, she still didn't make it. She lost her life on the front lines of the fight against the coronavirus. Her name is Liang Xiaoxia; this year she would have been 28 years old. Let's forever remember her. I hope she is able to rest in peace.

For the past few days, the calls for people to assume responsibility for what happened have been growing weaker, so much so that even I have started to overlook this issue. There seem to be fewer and fewer in-depth investigative reports, and now there are nearly none.

Last night I read one report entitled "The 41 Missing Coronavirus Reports," which concludes with the following sentence: "By pulling away the deeply hidden thorns and accepting the pain hidden in these dark corners of society, the media uses its limited strength to reveal the truth and expose it to the light. While some reports may have temporarily disappeared, when all is said and done, there will certainly be a place for them in the manuscript of history." Reading that, I was struck with a small revelation: I suspect that perhaps those groups that have suddenly been launching vicious attacks against me might have something to do with those deleted posts?

But when it comes to the topic of assigning responsibility, I still want to believe that people from all levels of society will be on the same page: that this is an essential step we have to take. If we don't investigate who was responsible for such a massive incident, I wonder how the government can ever face its people. I have been following this topic from the beginning. Looking over things carefully, among all those people connected to what happened, some of them should certainly take the initiative and resign; that's what happened after the SARS outbreak. But for some reason, even up until today, not a single official in Hubei has resigned; I guess they know how to play the game. One thing that is interesting: When people passed blame, it was often the politicians who blamed the scientists, who, in turn, blamed the politicians. But now things are getting really interesting; now they are all placing all the responsibility on the United States. A few days ago I saw a series of curious essays by the economist Hua Sheng. In his essay he mentioned a "deepthroat" figure here in Wuhan. If it hadn't been for this "deepthroat," the coronavirus may not have been reported until much later. According to him, this "deepthroat" is the true whistleblower. As I read that essay, images from the Chinese television spy drama *Lurking* kept appearing in my head. A few days ago I told my friend that I was really dying to know who this "deepthroat" was. My friend felt the same. Sounds like the kind of person I could put into one of my novels.

Among the essays that friends keep sending me on WeChat, there was one by Professor Du Junfei from Nanjing University. Professor Du holds a PhD in sociology and his essays often hit on some very important issues. In this essay of his I just read, he points out seven items:

1. After those front-line hospitals first discovered that there was an outbreak, why couldn't they just directly report it online?
2. Once the team of experts arrived in Wuhan, were they really unable to grasp the fact that this was a contagious virus, capable of being transmitted between people?
3. Once news of the outbreak leaked, were those government offices really placing a higher priority on dealing with the leaker than on the actual outbreak?
4. Does the fact that no one is willing to accept responsibility have something to do with the fact that Zhong Nanshan seems to be the only one with the authority to reveal the truth to the public?
5. As the Wuhan outbreak was getting increasingly serious, why couldn't hospital administrators have taken early action to prevent the serious lack of medical supplies?
6. As both the virus and fear began to simultaneously spread, was a full lockdown really the best measure available?
7. After the quarantine was in place, was it really not possible to have some of the confirmed patients transferred to other hospitals with less-strained resources where they would have received better treatment?

Actually, I suspect that Professor Du had even more questions, because after his seventh question, he left a line of ellipses, which seems to indicate that he wasn't finished with his line of questioning. Actually, for those of us here in Wuhan, we have even more questions we could raise. A shame, then, that all those questions, they remain unanswered.

Today is the 59th installment of my diary. I told quite a few people that I would stop at 60; tomorrow will be my last entry. There have been a lot of readers who have been staying up late every night to wait for my next installment to hit the internet; some of them have been so loyal that they complain they have messed up their biological clock. To them I want to say: Just one more day and, after tomorrow, you won't need to wait up anymore. At the same time, I am so thankful that you have all been out there waiting for me.

One more thing I want to say today: This is my individual record written during the coronavirus outbreak; it represents one person's memories. At first I didn't even really look at this as a "diary." That's because I wasn't the one who suggested using that term. It was only later that this record truly turned into a diary, one entry per day. When other people referred to it as a "diary" I didn't object. My initial motivation was just to fulfill a publishing agreement. I thought writing daily essays would be an easy way to do that. I never expected that as I went further down this road, I would completely forget what brought me here to begin with.

MARCH 24, 2020

I have fought the good fight.

Day 62 of the Wuhan quarantine. This is also the 60th installment in my diary; you could also refer to this as my final chapter.

Coincidentally, I saw a notice today announcing that the quarantine is now officially lifted for all districts outside Wuhan; as long as you scan your health QR code, you can now freely move about. For the city of Wuhan, the quarantine will be lifted on April 8th. Wuhan will be coming back to life again quite soon. I initially said that I would continue writing until the city reopens and only stop then. It was only later that I realized that opening the city back up doesn't happen all at once, like when the lockdown was imposed as an emergency action. It is going to be a slow and gradual process, with each district opening one at a time. It is for that reason that I think it is perfectly suitable to bring this diary to a close, now that the virus is slowing down and people are beginning to get back to work. I shared my thoughts on this with some friends and almost all of them supported my decision. And so after completing 54 installments, I decided to extend it up to 60 entries. After going through this entire process, I never imagined that the final chapter would be published just as they announced when they would reopen the city; this is something worth commemorating. That means that this record traces the outbreak from Day 1 of the Lunar New Year all the way up until the announcement lifting the quarantine order; so the record is quite complete. On March 14 my eldest brother did some calculations based on the number of confirmed cases and how those numbers decreased over time; based on his numbers, he thought that Wuhan would be able to reopen by April 8. I never imagined that he would get it right on the nose. He was also quite ecstatic: "My rough model really was able to predict the exact day Wuhan would lift the quarantine."

The sky was really bright this afternoon, but later in the afternoon it turned overcast and even sprinkled a bit. My housekeeper texted me to tell me that she would be probably be here tomorrow. Deep down I heaved sigh of relief. My housekeeper is a pretty good cook; my colleagues used to always come by and end up inviting themselves to stay for dinner. I'm sure once we are allowed to move around freely again they will start coming back again to crash our dinners. My difficult days are now almost behind me.

As for Miss Liang, that nurse from Guangxi, I should say a few additional words of explanation. Last night as I was writing my diary, I received a text from a doctor friend, which his friend had forwarded to him. It was a photo with a caption reading: "That nurse from Guangxi who fainted in our hospital has left us. To her mother, she was still a young girl, just 28 years old. Those people who went against the grain to come to Wuhan to help when everyone else was fleeing have really given their lives for this city." My doctor friend was extremely moved, and I was also quite devastated. Before this, a lot of media outlets had covered the story of this nurse's being saved. In order to confirm that this new development was accurate, I forwarded the picture to a big-shot doctor from Wuhan Union Hospital and asked him if he could verify the story. He responded with a short text: "Brain dead. A real tragedy." I guess my level of medical knowledge is really pathetic; I took that as a confirmation that she had indeed passed away. I didn't want Miss Liang to just quietly disappear without any acknowledgment; I felt I should write something so we would always remember her. And that is how that passage ended up in my diary. Today a lot of people raised suspicions about that news; others went on to refute it as a rumor. This afternoon I decided to get back in touch with those two doctors to see what I could verify. Both of them provided me with very detailed and technical explanations; they both had basically the same stance on the issue, and they suggested that I had better apologize. I agreed. And so, I would here like to offer my sincere apologies to my readers. More important, I would like to apologize to Miss Liang's family. This also shows how much all of us care about Miss Liang. As that text message said, she was one of the people who sacrificed so much for this city. I sincerely hope that one day she will wake up; my doctor friends and I will be closely following her condition. And thanks, everyone, for keeping me in check.

Yesterday a friend of mine sent me an article; he said that someone was calling on me to "participate in a joint signing event with the citizens of Wuhan to prove you are not a running dog for the Americans." When I saw that title I felt it was so disgusting and juvenile that I really didn't know whether to laugh or cry. I won't mention the name of the author here, but I'm told he has a doctorate; I wonder what kind of books he read to get that degree! I was a bit curious if he had also done his undergraduate studies at Peking University, or did he even have an undergraduate degree? Normally speaking, people with even a basic undergraduate education would never stoop so low. Before I even had time to read his essay, someone else told me that someone from the government had already sought the author out to have a talk with him about the essay and asked him to cease this type of behavior. My friend laughed: "Now you're never going to get the chance to make your case." In reality, I still don't fully understand what even happened.

What is really getting interesting is that now politicians from both China and America are going after each other; both sides are really digging into each other with all kinds of nasty speech, while, at the same time, doctors from China and America are joining forces to discuss the best methods for saving patients' lives. The doctors have been discussing which medications are most effective in lowering death rates and which treatment methods have been proven most effective. They are also discussing protective measures, proper quarantine procedures, and other related topics. When the Wuhan outbreak was at its most critical stage, overseas Chinese purchased any and all medical supplies they could get off the shelves and sent them all to China as donations;

now American doctors are facing a shortage of face masks and other personal protective equipment. One overseas Chinese friend told me how sorry she feels about the whole thing. Meanwhile, these doctors are actively discussing how to solve this problem. None of these doctors seem to be politically biased; there is no sense of national identity that comes into play during their discussions; they just share their experiences and share whatever leads they have on the coronavirus. From this you can sense a core goodness and a higher sense of what love is from these doctors; this is a love for humanity, a love for individual human beings. I figure that with every different profession there is indeed a different perspective and a completely different way of looking at things. Personally, I prefer the professional spirit and state of mind of these doctors.

Just because this is my last installment, that doesn't mean that I will stop writing. Weibo will continue to be my platform, and I will continue to express my views on Weibo, just like before. I will also not give up on making sure that those who need to be held accountable take blame for what they have done. A lot of people have left messages on my Weibo account saying that the government will never hold these people accountable; that there is no hope. I have no way of knowing if officials in the government will ever pursue this. But regardless of what actions the government takes, as a Wuhan citizen who has been quarantined here for two months, as someone who has personally experienced and witnessed this tragedy that befell Wuhan, we have a responsibility and a duty to seek justice for those wronged souls. Whoever made mistakes and whoever is responsible, those are the people who should carry this burden. If we abandon the search for justice, if we forget what has happened here during these days, if we one day can no longer even remember Chang Kai's final words, then, my fellow Wuhan people, you will be carrying a much heavier burden than this disaster; you will also be carrying the burden of shame. And the burden of forgetting! If someone wants to one day nonchalantly wipe all this away, I'm afraid that will be an impossibility. Even if I have to etch it out one character at a time, I will carve their names on history's pillar of shame.

I would like to give special thanks to those ultra-leftists who attack me every day. If not for their egging me on, a lazy person like me would have probably stopped writing a long time ago; at the very least I would have lacked the perseverance to write nearly as much as I ended up doing. Without them, how many people would have even read this record I have presented through my entries? What I'm especially happy about is the fact that their attacks have gotten everyone to pay attention. They have summoned together all their teams and every one of them has been writing essays. But what have readers seen through their essays? They have seen those ultra-leftists' mixed-up logic, deformed thoughts, twisted perspectives, crude writing, and low moral character. In short, all that their consistent attacks reveal are their own shortcomings; every day they put their disgusting values on display for all to see. And now everyone has finally woken up to see what these Big V ultra-leftists are really made of.[25]

That's right, that's who they really are; they are all at the level of that supposed "high school student" who wrote a letter to me; actually, that is about as good as they get. Actually, a while back there was already someone who offered a very accurate summary of who these ultra-leftists are; you should still be able to find the essay online. Vile and lowly as they may be, for the past several years now these ultra-leftists have been gradually spreading throughout our society, just like the coronavirus. They are especially active around those government officials, always at their beck and call, which makes many officials particularly susceptible to infection. In the end, they come to shield these ultra-leftists, helping them get stronger and stronger. They expand to the point that their structure resembles a massive underworld operation; they have taken over the internet, which puts up with their howls and storms as they humiliate and insult anyone who goes against them. It is precisely because of this that I need to say it again and again: The presence of these ultra-leftists represents an existential threat to China and her people! They are the greatest hindrance to the Reform Era! If we allow the ultra-leftists to throw their weight around as they wish and spread their disease throughout our society, the reforms will die, and China's future will be doomed.

Finally, this being my final chapter, I need to say a few words of thanks. Thanks to all my readers for their support and encouragement. Their endless posts and essays have deeply moved me and led me to realize: Wow, there are so many people out there who see things the same way as I do. I always thought I was standing alone against an empty backdrop, while in fact there are tall mountains behind me, supporting me. I need to express my appreciation for Er Xiang; she was the one who provided enormous help when my Weibo account was blocked. Without her, I'm afraid I would never have been able to continue this diary. I also would like to thank Caixin and Headlines Today; they always provided platforms for me to publish my essays when I had nowhere else to go. From another perspective, all this help has given me an untold reservoir of psychological comfort. With them beside me throughout these days, I have never felt alone.

> *I have fought the good fight,*
> *I have finished the race,*
> *I have kept the faith.*

THIS PLACE
CALLED WUHAN

This place called Wuhan has always been referred to by people as "River Town." The reason for that naturally has to do with the fact that the city is located on the banks of the Yangtze River. Actually, "River Town" isn't at all a bad name for Wuhan. It is the provincial capital of the Hubei Province, sometimes referred to as the "province of a thousand lakes," because there are at least 100 bodies of water surrounding it. These lakes are like beautiful pearls and jade ornaments adorning the body of Wuhan; when the wind blows, you might even hear the sound of them clinking in the wind. Those old-timers who have lived here long enough can hear it—it is the sound of the billowing river and the ripples on the lakes responding to the wind whipping by.

If you go back to an earlier time, Wuhan was once part of the Kingdom of Chu, which is why Wuhan residents like to refer to this place where they live as "the Land of Chu." People in Wuhan really worship the Chu. That is because the people of Chu were known for their military spirit; they had an unbridled romanticism and a strong will, which are both qualities that Wuhan natives appreciate. Of course, this could also be because people from Wuhan already have Chu genes inside them, which is why they are so proud to be Chu.

Ever since the concept of "big city" came around, Wuhan has always been one of China's best-known cities. I thought about it, and I think Wuhan is just behind the big-six cities of Beijing, Nanjing, Xi'an, Shanghai, Tianjin, and Guangzhou. The first three of those cities all have deep cultural roots because they are former capitals; the latter three have more developed economies, thanks to their locations along the coast. Wuhan never served as the capital of China and it is not on the ocean; it is a city on the water, right in the middle of the Yangtze River. The inland province of Hubei where it is located is different from virtually any other province that is located in the frontier region, which makes it only natural to be ranked below those other six cities.

However, amid this vast nation of China, the fact that Wuhan can maintain its position as the "central land" isn't bad at all. Wuhan's corridors and streets are like rays emanating out and shining down into every corner of this nation. If you were to draw them across the map of China, they would look like the rays of sunlight shooting out in all directions. And Wuhan represents the sun on that map.

Its being located in the heart of China means that transportation in and out of Wuhan is extremely convenient. No matter where you go, it never feels that far; after all, there isn't a huge difference between locations near and far in terms of distance. That has become especially true these past few years as more high-speed rail lines and highways have opened up. No matter where you go, you can reach most major cities in China from Wuhan in around four hours by train. It is even more convenient for Wuhan residents with cars to do short road trips; there are even a lot of places you can go on a daytrip. This is something that a lot of Wuhan people are quite proud of. Owing to its central location, Wuhan is also referred to as the "gateway to nine provinces."

There was a time when people referred to Wuhan (specifically to its

Hankou district) as "the Chicago of the East." That's because the pace of Wuhan's development was quite similar to that of Chicago, although that nickname seems to have gradually disappeared over time. These days there are still some people who would very much like to revisit the dream of their city's being "the Chicago of the East," but after referring to it like that a few times, there wasn't much of a reaction so they all stopped calling it that. I've never been to Chicago, so I can't really say where the similarities and differences actually lie.

If Wuhan is a pearl, then the Yangtze River is the necklace that runs through the pearl, as it goes directly through the heart of the city. The largest tributary of the Yangtze, the Han River, cuts through the downtown district of Wuhan where it meets with the Yangtze near the foot of Tortoise Mountain. Those two rivers divide Wuhan up into three towns: Hankou, Wuchang, and Hanyang. All three of these areas are built on the banks of these rivers, and they are designed to twist and curve alongside the flowing water. That's why most people in Wuhan have such a poor sense of direction. Whenever someone asks for directions elsewhere, most people from Wuhan will respond with phrases like "go up there" or "down there," or they'll say things like "walk down that way" or "take that path up." When they say to "go up," they are referring to the upstream direction of the Yangtze; when they say, "go down," they mean to follow the downstream flow of the river. From that detail alone one can tell that the impact of living on the water is something that is deep in the bones of every resident of Wuhan; even when someone haphazardly points somewhere, you can still sense the presence of the flowing river.

There was a time when Wuhan was clearly trying to build up Hankou into a business district, Wuchang into a cultural district, and Hanyang into an industrial district; this was part of a plan to emphasize the different qualities of each town.

The most bustling areas in the city are all north of the city in Hankou. Places like Jianghan Road, Six Crossings Bridge, and the somewhat famous Hanzheng Road are all located here. I remember back a long time ago that when people living in Wuchang and Hanyang wanted to buy gifts for their family, they would always have to take a bus or a ferry to Hankou. These days the business districts in Wuchang and Hanyang are quite robust, yet people still can't shake the idea that things in Hankou are still better priced and of better quality, so everyone still likes to go north of the river for shopping.

Compared with the bustling Hankou district, Wuchang, located south of the river, is much more subdued. What attracts the most attention about this district is its large number of universities and high-level research facilities. My alma mater, Wuhan University, with its long history and beautiful campus, is located here in Wuchang. Wuhan University has always been highly ranked nationwide for its high level of academic achievements. But following the evolution of the market, several commercial outlets have also popped up in several corners of Wuchang; the district is no longer playing second fiddle to Hankou.

But as for Hanyang, which has always been the industrial district, even today it continues to lag behind Hankou and Wuchang. Sandwiched between the Yangtze and the Han River, it seems to always get less notice than other parts of the city. Its most famous claim to fame was the construction of the Hanyang Arsenal back in the early 20th century. Everyone who ever served in the army is familiar with seeing "Made in Hanyang" stamped on their equipment. Even today, Hanyang continues to be most famous for its manufactured goods. A few years ago Wuhan started developing a brand-new modernized industrial zone and it too is naturally situated in Hanyang.

I'm not sure what year the decision was made to give each district a distinct character; it may have been back when Zhang Zhidong (1837–

1909) was the governor of the region. But over time, modernization has transformed all three towns dramatically; yet somehow what makes each district unique has remained, even if those remnants of the past continue to fade over time.

There are few cities out there that have the kind of scenery that Wuhan has been blessed with; the rich Jianghan Plains frame Wuhan on all sides. The plains surround the city with an openness that is adorned by countless beautiful lakes, leaving the entire region with a feeling of brightness and freshness. Those two great rivers—the Han and the Yangtze—rumble through the center of the city and converge, while countless rolling hills adorn both sides of the river like chess pieces in formation. Wuhan is a city with a strong modern sensibility, yet it remains framed by the mountains and rivers and decorated by the scenery of those hundred lakes. The crimson water and the green hills, gulls from Liudi Lake and high-rise buildings, bridges and cableways, mast-like towers and massive flashing LED screens—all converge and blend together in a moving tapestry. Wuhan has been bestowed with incredible natural gifts from the environment; with a bit of careful planning and some reasonable construction projects, Wuhan could easily become one of the most beautiful cities in the world.

Like a lot of other well-known urban cities, Wuhan is not just a commercial hub; it is also an industrial center and a major site for research and education. It has endured the vicissitudes of history and witnessed its share of blood and tears; it has been through the insult of having foreign concessions established here and it has been home to legendary tales of resistance; it has been through a construction boom and also the ridiculous Cultural Revolution; it has been home to heroes and prostitutes; just as the water never stops flowing, so the traffic never ceases and the neon lights never dim; it boasts of luxury hotels and bustling markets; it has beautiful scenes of green trees against both red walls and environmental pollution; it has its quiet, beautiful side; and it is home to both the nouveau riche and the poor and destitute. All the amenities enjoyed by every modern city, along with all the urban problems that big cities face, are all right here in this place called Wuhan.

I WILL FACE IT ALL
WITH NO MISGIVINGS:
AFTER *WUHAN DIARY*

Fang Fang

It was at this time two years ago that I found myself locked down in Wuhan. At that time, COVID-19 was brutally ravaging the city in which I live. A historically unprecedented citywide quarantine was imposed in Wuhan. Trapped here in the city, every day I heard stories about people who were infected, every day I heard news of people passing away—there were even videos being shared that showed frontline medical workers crying out on the brink of collapse. Almost all of us were in a state of utter terror and panic, gripped by a deep sense of helplessness. None of us knew if we would be next to be infected, or next to die.

At the very start of the lockdown, the Shanghai-based literary journal *Harvest* commissioned me to write a "Record of the Lockdown," which is why I started recording some of the details surrounding the coronavirus on my Sina Weibo account. What I recorded was nothing more than everyday people's lives in the city, some of the incidents that occurred over the course of the battle against the virus, as well as some of my own personal emotions about what was happening. Naturally, there were also criticisms, recommendations, reflections, and calls for accountability. Then, without my realizing it, this record came to be read and shared by countless people. By some estimates, there were tens of millions of readers who stayed up at night waiting for me to post the next installment of my record. (Most of my posts were only uploaded online after midnight.) Some of the more enthusiastic readers even collected all my posts into digital files and renamed them "Fang Fang's Quarantine Diary." That is how people started referring to the collection as a "diary."

In reality, there was a long period of time in which I didn't even realize just how many people were reading my record. I was just driven to "record everything that was happening," writing it all down one day after another. Since I was just recording what was happening, I didn't take time to structure my writing, nor did I go out of my way to revise the prose; I just loosely recorded all the things going on around me on a day-to-day basis. My earlier entries were a bit more carefree; later on, after I learned that there were countless readers following my posts, I started to take things a bit more seriously. Every day I searched online for the latest news concerning COVID-19, received all kinds of videos from my friends, talked to all kinds of people on the phone, and sent questions and carried out interviews with busy doctors and others who were locked down in Wuhan. And so, the time slipped by, one day after another. The process of writing also helped me get through those most difficult days. When I look back and reappraise everything that I wrote during that period, I feel extremely fortunate that I was able to record what happened over a full sixty-day period.

Looking back, no one could have ever anticipated that Wuhan would end up completely locked down from January 23 to April 8, 2020—a total of seventy-six days. But even more difficult to anticipate is the fact that COVID-19 would go on to impact the entire world. Even today, we have yet to see its end.

My own fate also ended up completely transformed by this virus. That is yet another aspect of things that I never could have anticipated.

It was on April 8, 2020, that the Wuhan lockdown order was lifted. Coincidently, it was also on that day that presale notification for the United States and German editions of *Wuhan Diary* appeared online. The fact that this news stirred up a major controversy within China should of course not have come as a surprise because it was the result of people maliciously controlling and manipulating what was happening from behind the scenes. And so, I suddenly found myself accused of all kinds of crimes. What had originally been a record commissioned by the literary journal *Harvest* was now accused of being a work commissioned by the United States; what had been a normal publication process was described as "light-speed publishing." Over the course of recording the lives and emotions of average people living through the COVID-19 crisis in *Wuhan Diary*, I also criticized the government's cover-ups and delays in responding during the early phase of the outbreak, I expressed my sympathy for those people who had died at the hands of COVID-19, and I continually called for accountability. It was one thing for this content to be read by Chinese readers, but once people knew that foreign readers would also be able to see what I wrote, I was immediately labeled as someone who was "handing over a knife" to the West's anti-China forces; in the eyes of some I was a "traitor" who had "sold out her country," I became the leading figure in China representing the anti-China forces, and in the eyes of certain national security organs, I was probably even considered a "spy."

The online violence I was targeted with went on for many months, lasting well over a year. I was targeted with countless acts of slander, name-calling, and abuse. The entire internet lit up with these attacks, which included people trying to incite a group to come to Wuhan and murder me, someone who called upon all martial arts practitioners to beat me, someone who posted denunciation posters in the streets of Wuhan insulting me, and another who openly declared he was going to construct a statue of me that people could publicly spit on and deface to record my shame. There was even a series of countless videos, songs, and cartoons created specifically to insult and attack me. These malicious and defamatory rumors also targeted my family members. But I was unable to respond or fight back. Early on, there were a series of reporters willing to interview me about what had happened, and I answered all their questions about the writing and publication process surrounding *Wuhan Diary*; I provided clear explanations and rebuttals to all the various questions about *Wuhan Diary* raised by various netizens. It was a shame that whenever these interviews were published, they were quickly deleted from the internet. After that happened a few times, no other reporters dared to seek me out for additional interviews. This rendered me completely unable to explain the simple fact that everything written in *Wuhan Diary* is the truth.

The entire situation has been extremely frustrating. The reason I initially tried to explain everything was because I thought that netizens simply didn't understand the truth, which led to a series of misunderstandings. However, once I saw that I was not the only one being silenced and that the rumors about me began to lead the direction of government discourse, I realized this was no misunderstanding—this was all the result of intentional actions taken by certain individuals, who are certainly coming from the ultra-leftist faction in China.

Instead of making a logical assessment of *Wuhan Diary* based on the actual content contained within, the government has instead blindly suppressed the book based on the malicious misinterpretations being spread online by some netizens. That is how the wave of nonphysical abuse against me began. I am unable to print or publish any of my writings within China, I am prohibited from participating in any literary or public events, my name is not allowed to appear in any mainstream publications, professional literary critics have been completely banned from carrying out research on my work, and even when independent or self-published media entities publish my essays, they are either shut down or blocked. I repeatedly receive telephone calls from higher-ups reminding me not to accept any foreign interview requests, that all my communications are being monitored and controlled. Whenever I go out, I receive phone calls "checking up" on me to ask where I am. Not only that, the ultra-leftists attacking me have even used the slogan "besiege the enemy stronghold in order to attack the reinforcements" to describe their campaign of exposing the names of all people (and their family members) who support me online and attacking them. If those individuals or their relatives are found to have ever made any purportedly "inappropriate statements" or had a history of any speech or actions that violated certain regulations, the government takes swift punitive measures against them. These types of underhanded "guilt-by-association" tactics have left me and my friends in an extremely precarious situation. Once these vicious forces coming from outside the government reach a consensus with those in power and join forces, what else can I possibly say? My only option is to say nothing and tell my friends to say nothing. When this kind of power is wielded over you, when you stand before a crowd of people who have lost their reason, whatever you say is pointless.

I asked some of the officials who came to investigate me: You all must have read *Wuhan Diary*—do you really think that it contains rumors? Do you really think it contains anti-government rhetoric? Does it contain any words that attempted to incite people not to cooperate with the battle against the virus? Their almost unanimous response was: no. So I replied, if that's the case and these essays have all been publicly circulated online where everyone can see, then isn't it perfectly normal for these writings to be collected and published in China or abroad? How could this diary be considered an act of "handing over a knife"? How could it be considered a traitorous act or something that will damage national interests? None of them had a response for me.

Quite a few friends have also asked me: Were you trying to do something brave by writing this book? Were you possessed by a certain breed of courage to get you through the writing process? Did you adopt the stance that you were ready to just put it all on the line? Were you swept away by the spirit of justice and righteousness? My response to all those questions is: no. I never looked at what I did as an act that required bravery or courage, and it was certainly not a case of putting it all on the line, nor was there any need for any of this business about justice and righteousness. For a writer trapped in a city being torn apart by a terrible virus, recording what people were going through and the process of fighting COVID-19 is the most natural thing in the world. Over the course of my writing, never did anyone try to stop me nor did anyone signal for me to pay attention to anything in particular. Although many of my essays were deleted by internet censors, in China, that is nothing new; there are countless essays that are censored and deleted all the time. I'm certainly not the only one to be censored, but we all continue writing. So, I never once felt that writing these posts needed any kind of special "courage." My level of political sensitivity has always been quite low; I have never had any interest in officially joining any political party—mostly because of how much I hate attending meetings. In my record of the COVID-19 crisis in Wuhan, there are absolutely no anti-government sentiments; there are no ideas in which I am trying to create tensions with any specific people. As a professional writer finding herself amid a great calamity, recording the unprecedented events unfolding around her is an almost instinctual response; in my profession, writing is how I am accustomed to engaging with the world. As a veteran writer, especially someone like me whose career ran side by side with China's Reform Era, how could I have ever imagined

that a frank and sincere account of what was happening would somehow not be allowed? How could I have imagined that such moderate
words could send shock waves across the country, even tearing groups
of people apart? This is something that I have not only never experienced, but never even witnessed in my lifetime.

For the past two years, I have found myself repeatedly asking these
questions; I've been constantly asking why?

Why did this record of COVID-19 end up having such an unbearable fate, putting me personally in such a terrible position? When you
read the entire diary, you can completely see that I was trying my best
to help the government calm people down, I was trying to console the
people; I was actively putting forth all kinds of suggestions in hopes of
coming to a more effective strategy for fighting the virus. Of course,
there were also criticisms contained in my book. I was encouraging
people and consoling them so they wouldn't be scared. I told them it
would all pass. It is a fact that there were facts hidden and precious
time was lost during the early phase of the outbreak; once the peak
COVID-19 outbreak had passed, reflection and accountability are issues that must be addressed. This is part of the necessary follow-up
work that must be carried out in the aftermath of any major disaster. I
followed the normal thought process of a typical writer over the course
of the sixty days that I composed this book, *Wuhan Diary*. According to
reason, anyone who reads the actual text should see all its main points
very clearly. How could so many people be so easily deceived by the
malicious postings of a few ill-intentioned netizens? How could they
come at me with such force that I have lost so many of my individual
rights? There are many high-ranking Chinese officials who share a very
similar life experience with me, and they too lived through the entire
Reform Era; how could they all be so blind to the truth and make such
a muddleheaded decision in handling this? When I was first inundated

by that initial wave of crazed online attacks, I wasn't afraid, but I was confused. I couldn't figure out why they were doing this, which led me to a place of unusual anger and sadness.

Time passed. I gradually came to realize some things. I realized that I was different from them. Besides our different set of values, the more important thing was that I had a completely different perspective from them when it came to literature.

The kind of writers they recognize are "Chinese writers," but that does not include "independent writers." They believe that "Chinese writers" should be attached to China and should not raise any criticisms about China or they shall be considered traitors to the nation. I believe that "independent writers" should follow their own sensibilities and judgments irrespective of the country in which they live and that they should criticize those things that call for criticism. In their eyes, a "writer" is a label that carries national significance but not literary significance. I suppose this is where we have a difference of opinion. I feel their literary understanding is stuck in a state of misunderstanding; they on the other hand must think that my literary views are completely backward. And so, we have naturally come to stand on opposing sides of this issue.

After thinking about it like this, I have no misgivings. I am neither pessimistic nor depressed; in fact, I'm not even angry. I am calm now and have no misgivings. And that is how I face everything that *Wuhan Diary* has brought me.

My perspective on literature has always clearly told me that authors should be independent writers. Writers don't need to be attached to or in service of anyone; they should certainly never take orders from anyone who wields power, nor should they fear any form of suppression. In fact, writers have always been rebels. Once I stopped flattering them, obeying them, being attached to them; once I decided to be loyal to what my own heart told me to write, I became something else. I became a thorn in their side, my name was added to their blacklist; but I remained unaware of that, at least until after *Wuhan Diary*.

I continue to write from my heart as I always have. I suppose this is the standard that I have always naturally followed ever since I first decided to pursue a career as a writer. Perhaps it is only after experiencing all the turmoil brought on by *Wuhan Diary* that I have finally realized the deeper meaning of the act of writing and what kind of person a true writer should really be.

Time will naturally determine the value of the record contained within *Wuhan Diary*.

Spring 2022

TRANSLATOR'S
AFTERWORD

Reading *Wuhan Diary* in English is a very different experience than how Chinese-speaking readers experienced it when it first appeared online. The diary was initially released in daily installments that were uploaded to various Chinese social media platforms and microblogging sites like Weibo and WeChat. Fang Fang's dispatches were blasted out each night, offering real-time responses to and reflections on events and news reports that had transpired just hours earlier. As the outbreak in Wuhan spread and began to attract more attention both within China and globally, Fang Fang's readership began to grow. More and more Chinese readers from around the world found their way to Fang Fang's postings, which provided a platform to understand what was happening on the ground in Wuhan. Whereas we often think of diaries as an especially private literary form—a place where you record your innermost fears and desires, often alongside a more mundane record of events from everyday life—*Wuhan Diary* was a public platform from the very beginning: a virtual open book.

Part of that openness meant that Fang Fang's diary entries were not read as they are presented here in this volume—that is, compiled into a book-length narrative dominated exclusively by the author's voice and perspective. For Chinese readers, *Wuhan Diary* came delivered in many forms—as daily installments on Weibo and WeChat; as excerpts that were cut, pasted, and forwarded via text message; as memes that were culled from entries and paired with photos; and even as PDF compilations that individuals who wanted to document Fang Fang's entire narrative forwarded to friends via email. Most significantly, on Fang Fang's primary platforms of Weibo and WeChat, the posts would be accompanied by a comments section, which would variously include remarks, criticisms, links to articles, photos, and embedded videos uploaded by an army of actually millions of readers. According to a *Guardian* article from April 10, 2020, "On Weibo, 'Fang Fang Diary' has had 380m views, 94,000 discussions, and 8,210 original posts, peaking last week."[1] At the height of the diary's popularity, many of her posts were getting between 3 and 10 million hits in just the span of two or three days; those message boards emerged as a virtual biosphere of vibrant social debate—a place for readers to converge, share, sometimes argue, and often cry.

While no book, print or electronic, can encapsulate the rich social dimension of *Wuhan Diary*'s sprawling digital footprint, readers will be able to sense the presence of that world because as the diary unfolds, Fang Fang increasingly interacts with her many supporters as well as with the trolls who attack her, both of whom become an increasingly important part of the narrative that she weaves. Indeed, even as *Wuhan Diary* offers manifold insights into the coronavirus outbreak in Wuhan, it offers an equally rich dive into the complex world of the Chinese internet. As the quarantine drags on, Fang Fang finds her life increasingly intertwined into a virtual world of texts, online news clips, and social media posts. But what makes *Wuhan Diary* such a remarkable document is the way in which Fang Fang merges the firsthand perspective of someone going through the uncertainty, fear, and isolation of life under the shadow of a strange new virus, with online reports, news coverage, texts, and messages received from relatives, friends, colleagues, former classmates from her youth, and neighbors. The result is a hybrid form that alternates between the quotidian and the epic, the mundane boredom of life under lockdown and the ever-expansive network of the World Wide Web. Fang Fang's diary at times serves as a clearinghouse for suggestions and recommendations on everything from online shopping tips to how to actually save the lives of people with chronic health conditions unable to get care amid the outbreak.

Another remarkable facet of *Wuhan Diary* consists of Fang Fang's repeated calls for action and appeals for accountability. This is another area where how we in the West read the book is different than how Chinese readers read it. In the United States and many other Western countries, media thrives on pundits, politicians, and activists criticizing one another, often along party and political lines. Many American and European readers of *Wuhan Diary* therefore may not fully appreciate the extraordinary courage that Fang Fang displays in her repeated, unflinching calls for local and national officials and specialists who "dropped the ball" to stand up and take responsibility for their missteps. In a society where "keeping your head low and staying out of trouble" serves as the guiding principle for many writers and intellectuals, Fang Fang dared to speak out—and when her critics came after her, she spoke even more loudly.

This also marks a major shift in the tone of the diary itself; for as the COVID-19 outbreak gradually comes under control in Wuhan, Fang Fang goes from chronicling the coronavirus to calling out officials and specialists for their negligence, mistakes, and lack of action. Eventually, Fang Fang homes in on the topic of accountability. Of course, a price must be paid for her outspokenness; as *Wuhan Diary* progresses and Fang Fang's calls for justice grow stronger, so too do the attacks of the invisible army of "internet trolls" who have been hounding her. These two forces are, of course, connected. And, for the final third of the diary, much of her focus is spent deflecting the myriad online attacks that she confronts each and every day.

The ultra-leftist groups attacking Fang Fang in China first came after her in 2017 after the publication of her award-winning novel *A Soft Burial*. The novel offered a penetrating exploration of amnesia as an allegory for suppressing lost pages in modern Chinese history—in this case, the era of the country's land reform campaign of the late 1940s and early 1950s. Because of that novel's refusal to read that history along black-and-white binary lines, it became the target of a fierce smear campaign by ultra-leftist groups in China. The novel was eventually pulled from shelves and Fang Fang herself became the target of countless online attacks. Fast-forward to 2020, and those same ultra-leftist groups have now found a new target—*Wuhan Diary*. The depth and vitriol of these attacks were such that, even as this HarperVia edition of the book was being prepared, leftist attackers waged a media war in China, claiming the book was to be "weaponized" as a tool for the United States to criticize China!

As I was translating *Wuhan Diary*, "weaponizing" the book, or using it as a tool to criticize China, was surely the last thing on my mind. In contemporary Chinese literature, Fang Fang has been the single most powerful voice to emerge from Wuhan in decades. When the coronavirus outbreak occurred, many people looked to her for solace, information, and a path forward. She became, more than anyone else, a voice that people could look to for an honest appraisal of what was happening every day in Wuhan during the age of COVID-19. Even as the world slumbered, Fang Fang's voice was crying out daily. Her cries needed to be heard around the world, both as a personal testament to the horrors the people of Wuhan were enduring and as a warning of what might come to the world if precautions were not taken. So, instead of weaponizing *Wuhan Diary*, I instead felt the pressing need for the United States, and the world for that matter, to learn from Fang Fang. Part of that lesson comes from Fang Fang's compassion and bravery, but another side comes from her audacity—the audacity to bear witness, the audacity to refuse to be silenced even when thousands of vicious attacks are raining down on her head, and the audacity to speak truth to power.

In a country with 1.4 billion people, crowded with hundreds of satellite television stations, newspapers, websites, and state media, somehow this lone figure cut through all the noise and emerged as *the* voice of Wuhan. Her words became the city's heartbeat and its conscience. Her diary became a lightning rod for activism and criticism, compassion and malice, love and hate— all playing out every day in the seemingly endless comments thread that trailed behind her every post.

I first encountered Fang Fang's fiction back in the mid-1990s when I read several of her stories and novellas, including *Black Hole*. I followed her career for more than two decades before a mutual friend put us in touch regarding the translation of her controversial novel *A Soft Burial*. I fell in love with the novel and had actually been translating that work for her when news of the novel coronavirus began gaining attention all over the world. Knowing that Fang Fang is a longtime resident of Wuhan, I texted her several times to check in on her and make sure she and her family were okay, but she never mentioned anything about her diary. It wasn't until mid-February—roughly two weeks into the diary—that a close friend recommended that I take a look. By then, the diary had already "gone viral," so to speak, in unfortunate synchronicity with the virus, and was all over the Chinese internet. I read a few entries and was immediately drawn in.

I had been closely following news of the coronavirus outbreak since January; I even co-organized one of the first public forums on COVID-19 in the United States with members of the Fielding School of Public Health at the University of California, Los Angeles. But, frankly speaking, as someone with no medical training, I felt quite helpless in the face of the coronavirus. What can *I* do, what can *any* individual do, in the face of a global threat like COVID-19? But as soon as I read a few entries from Fang Fang's *Wuhan Diary*, I immediately knew what I could do. *This* was something I could contribute.

I immediately wrote to Fang Fang, suggesting that I temporarily table my translation work on *A Soft Burial* and, instead, translate *Wuhan Diary* first. Fang Fang initially hesitated; after all, her diary wasn't even finished, and the coronavirus events were still playing out in unpredictable ways. Eventually, however, we both agreed that this was a story that needed to be told and that the world needed to hear Fang Fang's testimony. The writing was on the wall, so to speak; the virus was spreading; and I felt an urgent need to get Fang Fang's words out as quickly as possible. I put other projects aside and started to furiously translate, often producing more than 5,000 words a day. At the time, I had no way of knowing that this would evolve into one of the more simultaneously rewarding and excruciating projects I had ever undertaken. It was also, in many ways, the strangest.

Let's start with the strange. Over the course of my translation, it was as if I were living simultaneously in three different temporalities. When you delve deeply into a translation, part of your psyche becomes embroiled in the author's world. You swim in her language, breathing it, internalizing it, before rendering it into English. This is especially the case for a time-sensitive project like this one, on which I was translating for more than 10 hours a day, 7 days a week, always a month behind Fang Fang, although racing desperately to catch up. Yet beyond the language was Fang Fang's inner world; translation allows you to enter that world in a much deeper way than simple reading. But Fang Fang's world was of the past—I started translating *Wuhan Diary* on February 25, exactly one month after she began writing. So, everything I was translating was already a month behind, yet as coronavirus cases began to rise in the city of Los Angeles where I live, Fang Fang's words increasingly felt like they were dispatches from the future. She was showing us where we were going, anticipating how society was likely to respond, and warning us where the many pitfalls lie.

So for 46 days, from February 25 through April 10, 2020, I translated roughly 5,000 words a day (minus a week's break to recover from illness), living amid an unfolding pandemic, translating a diary written one month in the past, which somehow, simultaneously, offered glimpses into our future. Along the way, I experienced many moments when these different temporalities seemed to clash, in eerie and jarring ways. Take, for instance, Fang Fang's outrage about the 40,000-family Lunar New Year event held in Baibuting, which resulted in widespread infections throughout Wuhan. Fang Fang published that entry on January 28; the day I was translating it, which was over a month later, on March 7, one of the headlines in the United States was "Trump Says Campaign Rallies Won't Stop Over Coronavirus Fears." How I wish that the people attending those rallies could read Fang Fang's diary. Even at the time of this writing on April 11, mass church gatherings are still being held in many American states. On January 27, Fang Fang wrote an entire entry about the scarcity of face masks (there was no debate about the need to wear them, as that was already an obvious fact); however, the United States didn't officially recommend that face masks be worn in public until April 3. And then an eerie incident occurred that still haunts me: On March 4, I had a doctor's appointment and happened to just mention *Wuhan Diary* to my physician. At the time, I had recently translated the February 15 diary entry about Liu Fan; I told my doctor about how the coronavirus had wiped out this entire family of four in a matter of days. My doctor looked at me with skepticism and asked, "Isn't it just like the flu? I've never heard of anything like that." Almost exactly two weeks later, news of the coronavirus ravaging the Fusco family of Freehold, New Jersey, made headlines—four family members were lost in less than a week. I had grown up in Freehold and even went to high school with Peter Fusco; he lost two brothers, a sister, and his mother to the novel coronavirus, while three additional members of his family were also infected. Shocked, and still feeling helpless, I quickened the pace of my work.

Yet the strangest aspect of this project was the way my life gradually began to mimic Fang Fang's. When I began work on *Wuhan Diary*, the outbreak in Wuhan felt like a world away for most people. As I translated those first entries, life initially continued as usual in Los Angeles. As a professor of Chinese studies, I frequently discussed with my students what was happening in Wuhan. Eventually, some international students started to wear face masks on campus, but most people in Los Angeles continued on with their normal lives and their usual routines: work, school, concerts, sporting events, parties. Meanwhile, I began to get anxious. Living in Fang Fang's world had made me hypersensitive to what was surely coming, so I started considering canceling campus events that I was scheduled to host and I even discussed with my wife whether we should pull our kids out of school.

We eventually did decide to keep them home, and a week later, on March 13, the huge Los Angeles Unified School District announced its temporary shutdown; roughly halfway through my translation work, Los Angeles also fell under quarantine, which California's governor called his "Stay at Home Order." So there was Fang Fang, quarantined in Wuhan writing her daily diary, while I sat halfway around the world, quarantined in Los Angeles, translating her diary. I began almost every day with a flurry of texts back and forth between Fang Fang, our agent, and our publisher; that would usually last from around 6:00 a.m. until close to 9:00 a.m.; and then it would be time to translate. Over the course of the project, I developed an extremely close relationship with Fang Fang, and often my heart would break when she would recount stories of all the vicious and vile attacks that had been waged against her online by various ultra-leftist groups. I always tried to be empathetic and understanding of what she was going through: It was hard for me to imagine being quarantined in one's beloved city that had become the epicenter of a major outbreak, being trapped in one's home where one of the few lifelines you have to the outside world is your computer, and knowing that every time you turn it on you receive literally thousands of threats and attacks. But then, Fang Fang and I had one more thing in common: On April 8, they came after me.

After receiving a series of texts from friends warning me about what was happening, I checked my Weibo account to find more than 600 messages and comments filled with hateful comments and threats against my family and me. These were all in response to news that an English edition of Fang Fang's *Wuhan Diary* was to be published and that I was the translator. *Wuhan Diary* was going global—and Fang Fang's detractors did not like that one bit. Aligned with the internet trolls' attacks to my own Weibo site were dozens of perfectly timed articles alleging everything from the book's being part of a CIA plot to attack China to various conspiracy theories regarding the pace of the translation (which to some seemed "impossibly quick"), to allegations that Fang Fang was "selling out" to the Americans. The headline of one of these disturbing articles rhetorically asked, "So, Fang Fang, How Does It Taste to Feed Off a Steamed Bun Dipped in the Blood of the Wuhan People?" The author of that article seemed oblivious to the fact that all her profits from this publication will go to relief charities in Wuhan. Coincidentally enough, April 8 also marked the day on which the quarantine in Wuhan was finally lifted.

And that brings us up to the present and to what each of us can take away from *Wuhan Diary*. For me, Fang Fang's courage to stand up, speak truth to power, and demand accountability has been a revelation. I got a small taste of the price she pays when the "trolls" turned on me, but I also know that it is but a tiny fraction of the thousands of attacks she faces day after day. If, as the trolls allege, Fang Fang's *Wuhan Diary* is indeed to be "weaponized," I hope it will be a weapon to show the power an individual possesses to cut through the noise and perhaps to effect real change. *Wuhan Diary* was the lightning rod and Fang Fang was the voice for Wuhan during its darkest hour; but in the West where is *our* lightning rod? Whose voice can *we* look to that will cut through the noise and demand truth and accountability? Against all odds, Fang Fang rose to the occasion . . . and so can we.

I would like to acknowledge my profound admiration and thanks to Fang Fang; working with her on this project was an experience that I will always treasure. J. L., our agent, provided unflinching support for this project from day one, and even when we hit bumps in the road, she was always there to defend us and fight for this project. I feel fortunate to have had her with us along this journey. Thanks to Juan Milà at HarperVia for championing this important project and for all his editorial feedback. Judith Curr was a staunch supporter from day one and I appreciate her efforts in helping Fang Fang's voice to reach a wider readership. I also wish to acknowledge the efforts of the editorial, design, and promotion teams at HarperCollins, who also worked on this book from their homes, especially Terri Leonard, Lisa Zuniga, and Kim Nir. Thanks to my colleagues and friends Michael Emmerich, Satoko Shimazaki, Esther Jou, King-kok Cheung, Hongling Zhang, Yongli Li,

Jeffrey Wasserstrom, Li Cheng, John Nathan, King Yu, and all my students at UCLA. Thanks to my parents and my brother, John Berry, who provided support and advice along the way. Special thanks to Professor David Der-wei Wang, whom I am fortunate to have always had in my corner. Finally, thanks to the support of my children, who put up with hearing "Daddy needs to work on the book!" many more times than they would have liked while quarantined at home. And enormous thanks to my wife, Suk-Young Kim. Despite her own teaching duties and deadlines, she took on extra childcare responsibilities so that I could complete this project as quickly as possible; the world needs to know. I dedicate my translation to the memory of all the victims of COVID-19.

Michael Berry
Los Angeles, April 11, 2020,
under quarantine

BETWEEN HISTORY AND THE FUTURE: *WUHAN DIARY* TWO YEARS ON

Michael Berry

From January 25 through March 25, 2020, veteran Wuhan-based writer Fang Fang posted a series of online diary entries that would divide a nation and incite one of the most controversial cultural incidents in decades. Originally published on the Chinese social media platforms of Weibo and WeChat, *Wuhan Diary: Dispatches from a Quarantined City* chronicled the first citywide lockdown due to COVID-19. The diary provided a space where more than 50 million readers converged to understand what was transpiring in Wuhan during the height of the outbreak. It was there in the pages of *Wuhan Diary* that readers found someone who gave voice to their sorrow and rage, providing a bastion of solace and consolation. For those millions of Chinese readers during the early months of 2020, *Wuhan Diary* became the most important account of the unfolding tragedy. Fang Fang provided real-time reports on the nature of this strange new virus, sharing information she received from doctor friends on the condition at hospitals across the city, offering gentle suggestions to her readers, and crying with them during the death of Li Wenliang. Countless followers stayed up each night until the wee hours of the morning anxiously waiting for Fang Fang to upload her next installment online. She became the voice of Wuhan. As award-winning novelist Yan Lianke mused, "Imagine this: the author Fang Fang did not exist in today's Wuhan. . . . What would we have heard? What would we have seen?"[1] For countless Chinese readers, Fang Fang became the eyes through which they navigated the darkest days of the coronavirus outbreak in Wuhan. When Fang Fang began to write her diary, the virus still did not have an official name, residents still did not know how the virus was transmitted, and no one knew just how long the lockdown, which was the first of its kind, would last. The diary was very much a "first look," a raw and unfiltered attempt to document, process, and make sense of the unprecedented events unfolding around her, which at that time must have felt almost cataclysmic. The role this first look played was multifold: Fang Fang's diary functioned as an online clearinghouse of basic and breaking medical information about the virus, information that was of great interest to Chinese-speaking readers all over the world but carried an especially vital place for those fellow residents of Hubei province. As Zhu Jianguo observed, during the early stage of the COVID-19 outbreak, the diary actually played a direct and crucial role in raising widespread awareness about the virus and aiding China in its ability to take precautionary measures. This reveals the power of a "first look" to also wield potential for action, activism, and engagement.

But in early April as news broke that *Wuhan Diary* was to be published in English and German, public discourse around the book underwent a radical shift. A sophisticated disinformation campaign was unleashed against the book, which included a series of conspiracy theory-like accusations, anti–Fang Fang diss songs, political cartoons mocking the diary, hastily prepared academic articles attacking the book, thousands of online troll attacks, and even death threats. As the English translator of *Wuhan Diary*, I too was targeted with hate mail and death threats, which continued on an almost daily basis for more than 18 months.

Wuhan Diary, which was once embraced by millions, has now been largely washed from Chinese social media, plans for a print version of the book in China were scrapped, and an army of dozens of "politically correct" diaries have risen up to take its place and tell the "official story." By the time the English translation of *Wuhan Diary* was first published in e-book format in mid-May, which was remarkably quick by normal publication standards, I already felt like we were too late—the United States was already in the clutches of COVID-19. I silently wondered if there was an invisible "expiration date" tied to a first look; like daily headline news, was there a time in which Fang Fang's account would no longer be relevant?

Two years later, detractors of the book in China claim *Wuhan Diary* missed its mark: for them, the failure of the West in controlling COVID-19 has accentuated China's success, rendering early mistakes (which Fang Fang highlighted in her diary) laughable as compared to the catastrophic losses suffered by countries like the United States. Others view *Wuhan Diary* as a historical document—an explosive of-the-moment record of how a global crisis first unfolded, an eyewitness account that offered the world its first glimpse of the damage this invisible virus is capable of unleashing and what a global lockdown might look like. It is this aspect of the "first look" that is particularly important: while the entire world would eventually adjust to life under lockdown, there is no way to recapture the fear, trepidation, anger, and feelings of confusion, isolation, loss, and sadness that residents in Wuhan experienced during January and February 2020. In this context, Fang Fang's account provided a crucial archive of raw emotion, a record of responses, a museum of memories; it is this initial emotional response to COVID-19 that can never be reconstructed. In this sense, Fang Fang's account is a crucial touchstone for future readers to understand the affective dimensions of the early lockdown.

But for me, the most remarkable aspect of *Wuhan Diary* two years later is just how prophetic the book would prove to be. The year 2020 was not just the year of COVID-19, it was also a year of discrimination and racial tension, disinformation campaigns, fake news, conspiracy theories, political division, and online violence, and all of those key-words played a central role in Fang Fang's diary. It is in this context that *Wuhan Diary* offered the world not only a "first look" at the novel coro-navirus, but also a "future look." Of course, there is an experiential sym-metry in the ways that Fang Fang described experiences that seemed novel in January 2020—like wearing face masks, trying to reserve a delivery spot for online grocery deliveries, and the mundane aspects of life under quarantine, which she boiled down to "eating, sleeping, and binge watching." However, on a much more profound level, Fang Fang was able to pinpoint the deeper fault lines extending out from behind the dark shadow of this virus.

The COVID-19 outbreak in the United States has been racialized on a number of different levels, from a sharp increase in instances of prejudice and hate crimes against Asian Americans to the ways in which Black and Hispanic communities have been disproportionately afflicted with this virus. But even before the United States had a single documented case of the coronavirus, Fang Fang had already discussed the overt discrimination against Wuhan natives throughout China. Early on in the outbreak in China, one of the first responses to what was then broadly referred to in Chinese media as "Wuhan pneumonia" was widespread discrimination against Wuhan residents living, work-ing, and traveling in other parts of China. It was a cogent warning of how rapidly disease unleashes paranoia, fear, discrimination, and an urge to isolate and "quarantine" racial, ethnic, and regional groups that are labeled as "infected." She also made it clear that the virus itself does not differentiate when it comes to race or class; as early as January 28,

2020, Fang Fang wrote, "the virus doesn't discriminate between ordinary people and high-ranking leaders," advice that those who attended the White House Rose Garden super-spreader event on September 26, 2020, would have done well to heed.

Fang Fang also wrote at length about the politicization of the virus in China, but she certainly could have never predicted the obscene level of political polarity that would coalesce around simple commonsense preventive measures like the wearing of face masks or getting vaccinated in the United States. According to Fang Fang's account, she first wore a face mask on January 18, 2020, when she visited a friend in the hospital. At the time, there were still no official announcements about an outbreak, yet in response to rumors of a new SARS-like illness spreading in Wuhan, Fang Fang began to don a mask. Compare that to countries like the United States where "mask wars" have continued to rage despite basic scientific evidence about the important role they play in stopping the spread of COVID-19.

Fang Fang's diary also traced the disturbing intersection of COVID-19 with disinformation campaigns, fake news, and conspiracy theories. As online attacks against the book mounted, *Wuhan Diary* became pulled into an increasingly complex vortex of conspiracy theories involving everything from the US-China Trade War to the origins of the COVID-19 virus. Along the way, the wild accusations ranged from allegations that Fang Fang and I were CIA agents to the diary being part of a sophisticated anti-China plot to damage the nation's global image. Over the ensuing two years, those theories not only failed to die down, but they became even more unbridled, with Chinese social media posts in early 2021 blaming Fang Fang for the United States's failure to control COVID-19! (They claimed that Fang Fang's calls for Chinese government accountability lulled the US into a state of complacency, thinking that the outbreak was a result of human failure.) The protracted nature of the attacks against *Wuhan Diary* also speaks to the continued relevance and power that a "first look" can wield, which in this case went on to shape so much of the subsequent discourse about the Wuhan outbreak. The conspiracy theories that arose fueled waves of online hate and the aforementioned death threats, all of which were further exacerbated by the fact that millions of people were out of work, locked down at home, angry, and frustrated. Imagine my surprise when, a few months later, I began to see a nearly identical pattern of online hate, disinformation, and conspiracy theories sweeping the United States— from QAnon to "Stop the Steal"—with many of the most egregious lies echoing through, if not emanating from, the highest office in the land.

Two years later, the meaning of *Wuhan Diary* lies not only in its account of COVID-19, but also in the fierce public and online debates that surrounded the book. These debates circulating around *Wuhan Diary* became a public referendum on the very nature of civil society in China. It was not about Fang Fang, but about what kind of country Chinese citizens wanted for themselves: A nation where someone can publish a diary without fear or threats of reprisal? Or a nation where only one "politically correct" version of truth is permissible? It was a war between those who advocated for a more open and pluralistic society and a "you're with us or against us" faction that viewed the world in simplistic black-and-white terms. The debates over this issue in China were fierce and unprecedented; I received numerous letters from Chinese netizens who told me they had stopped talking to friends or relatives due to disagreements over *Wuhan Diary*. The book became a lightning rod issue that was literally tearing families apart. A few months later, the United States would also be torn apart as it too navigated similar questions about civil society, which would go from online forums and presidential Twitter feeds to the very halls of the Capital Building during the January 6 insurrection.

Finally, 2020 was also a year that stood out for the stunning lack of accountability for those who mishandled the virus. One of the most remarkable aspects of Fang Fang's *Wuhan Diary* are her repeated appeals for specialists and officials who mishandled the outbreak to stand up, take responsibility for their mistakes, apologize, and resign. In *Wuhan Diary*, Fang Fang raged against those officials who suppressed information about the virus early on, public security personnel who muzzled the whistleblower Li Wenliang, and the public health officials who claimed person-to-person transmission of the coronavirus was not possible. As Fang Fang writes: "who were the leaders that in order to save face decided to twist the truth when reporting to their superiors and hide the truth from the public, who was it that put political correctness above the lives of our people, how many people contributed to this disaster? Whoever had a hand in this should take responsibility: the people need someone to assume accountability. At the same time, the government should urge officials from various departments whose actions misguided the public, leading to massive numbers of deaths, to resign." Make no mistake, China did mishandle some details of the novel coronavirus outbreak early on in Wuhan; this is now part of the public record. The police officers that wrongly accused Li Wenliang of "spreading rumors" publicly apologized. And once the central government took control of the "battle against the virus," they quickly adopted a clear and strong policy that effectively flattened the curve and ultimately squashed the outbreak in China. Their actions may have fallen short by Fang Fang's standards, but there was some degree of accountability in China. Numerous officials *were* dismissed from office or demoted as a direct consequence for their mishandling of the COVID-19 response in Wuhan. When the United States looks back upon its own failed response to the COVID-19 crisis, especially during that first crucial year in 2020, and takes stock of the string of missteps, from a dismantled pandemic response team, broken CDC test kits, chronic shortages of PPE and ventilators, delays in testing even when it was declared "anyone who wants a test can get a test," a stunning lack of federal policy concerning COVID-19, early flaws to the vaccination roll-out, a cesspool of lies, distraction, and disinformation, and a mounting death toll, we must ask who will hold *our* leaders accountable? If Fang Fang, writing under an authoritarian regime, under constant attack by thousands of internet trolls, was able to demand that her government live up to a higher standard of truth, transparency, and accountability, what is our excuse?

Two years on in China, Fang Fang's initial calls for accountability have been all but forgotten, buried under a smoke screen of attacks and threats against the author. Thanks to one of the most sophisticated and protracted personal attack campaigns waged against an individual, Fang Fang is now alternately referred to as "the witch of lies," a "traitor to China," a "secret CIA agent," and an entitled, out-of-touch *gongzhi* (a derogatory reference to "public intellectuals") who exploited the Chinese people to gain fame and profit. Then in January 2022, the Chinese city of Xi'an faced a strict lockdown reminiscent of what the people of Wuhan had experienced two years earlier . . . a few months later Shanghai would fall under an even stricter lockdown.. Suddenly Fang Fang's name became to reappear on Chinese social media. Residents of Xi'an began to cry out: "Who will be our Fang Fang?" "We need Fang Fang!" "A shame that Xi'an doesn't have its own Fang Fang." Clearly, the final word on the story of *Wuhan Diary* has not yet been written. The book began as a raw and explosive "first look" at the first citywide lockdown during the pandemic; it provided a "future look," anticipating the complex intersection between the virus and discrimination, cyberhate, and political extremism; it went on to become an important historical record documenting the first page of our COVID-19 era; and, though widely maligned by online trolls and disinformation campaigns, has still been able to break through the darkness, as we saw in Xi'an and Shanghai, and serve as a beacon for truth, transparency, courage, and accountability.[2]

February 24, 2021
Revised February 24, 2022

NOTES

All notes are the translator's.

JANUARY

1. Yuan is sometimes referenced as RMB, which is short for renminbi, or as Chinese Yuan Renminbi (CNY). During the period that Fang Fang kept her diary, from January 25 to March 24, 2020, the approximate exchange rate was 1 USD=7 RMB.

2. Chinese Premier Li Keqiang visited Wuhan on January 27, 2020, to inspect the situation on the ground. During his visit, the Wuhan mayor, Zhou Xianwang, nimbly removed his cap and smoothly handed it off to one of his assistants just moments before the premier spoke in public. Videos of what was described as Mayor Zhou's "disappearing hat performance" went viral on the Chinese internet.

3. This is a reference to a comic coronavirus song that became an online hit in China during the early outbreak. The full lyrics read: "On those sunny days when we till the crops, It's hard to get a good night's rest! We sleep all morning; We sleep all afternoon; We sleep today, we sleep tomorrow; and the day after tomorrow too; We sleep for our country and our family; carrying on with the cause no matter how difficult it may be; I'd rather sit home and gain weight, than go anywhere outside; Putting on some pounds is a luxury, going out leads to disaster; I beg you to follow the rules, and take care of yourself; Staying in bed every day is our pride, and it helps the nation save on face masks."

4. Huoshenshan Hospital, literally "Fire God Mountain Hospital," is an emergency hospital facility constructed in Wuhan between January 23 and February 2, 2020. The speedy construction was carried out to accommodate the rapidly rising cases of novel coronavirus in Wuhan. The construction of the hospital was live-streamed nationwide and served as a symbol of China's aggressive response to fight the coronavirus outbreak. The hospital is run under the management of the People's Liberation Army and staffed by 1,400 PLA medical personnel. The hospital was modeled after the Xiaotangshan Hospital, which was constructed in Beijing to deal with the SARS outbreak in 2003.

5. Jiang Zidan (b. 1954) is a Chinese writer who published her first essay in 1978. She has gone on to publish dozens of books, including short story collections, essays, and novels, including *A Date with Time* (*Suiyue zhi yue*) and *When I Am Alone* (*Yige ren de shihou*). She has also served as the editor for several leading literary journals, including *Tianya*.

6. The 7th CISM Military World Games was held in Wuhan, China, from October 18 to 27, 2019. It was a competitive sporting event in which military athletes from member countries of the International Military Sports Council competed.

FEBRUARY

1. Huanan Seafood Market is a live animal and seafood market located in the Jianghan District of Wuhan. During the initial outbreak of the novel coronavirus, some two-thirds of the first group of 41 patients were identified as having visited the market. Several specialists have pointed to evidence that the source of the virus may be tied to bats or pangolins (scaly anteaters) sold at the market. The market was closed on January 1, 2020, after the outbreak began.

2. Wang Guangfa (b. 1964) is a respiratory specialist at Peking University First Hospital. He is also a professor at Peking University and serves on numerous national health committees.

3. Zhong Nanshan (b. 1936) is a Chinese epidemiologist who came under the national spotlight in 2003 for his role in heading China's response to the SARS epidemic. In 2020 he was appointed as a leading advisor for managing the novel coronavirus outbreak.

4. Chen Cun (b. 1954) is a Shanghai-based writer who serves as vice chair of the Shanghai Writers Association. He began publishing in 1973 and has written numerous short stories, essays, and novels, including *The Blue Flag* (*Lan qi*) and *Chinese Youth* (*Zhongguo qingnian*).

5. *The City of Wuchang* (*Wuchang cheng*) was originally published in 2011 by People's Literature Publishing House. The novel portrays historical events that occurred in the city before and after 1927 through the story of Chen Mingwu and Ma Weifu, who are coming of age amid a backdrop of war and violence.

6. This is an inverted line from the poem "Encountering Sorrow" ("Li sao") from *Songs of the South* (*Chu ci*). Attributed to the poet Qu Yuan, "Encountering Sorrow" dates from the Warring States period and recounts the poet's spiritual voyage to fantasy realms while lamenting his betrayal by various court factions.

7. In February 2020, after the novel coronavirus outbreak in Wuhan, the China National Health Commission, in conjunction with local authorities, began building the Huoshenshan Hospital, the Leishenshan Hospital, and 11 other temporary hospitals across the area. These large, mobile hospital facilities were established to quickly expand the ability to care for the large influx of patients infected with COVID-19.

8. Yan Zhi (b. 1972) is the CEO of Zall Smart Commerce Group. He is also a member of the People's Congress and a graduate of Wuhan University. Yan Zhi is listed on the

Forbes List of the wealthiest people in the world and has also been recognized for his philanthropic activities. Besides his contributions to business and government, Yan Zhi is also a member of the China Writers Association and editor of *Chinese Poetry* (*Zhongguo shige*).

9. Li Wenliang (1986–2020) was an ophthalmologist at Wuhan Central Hospital. On December 30, 2019, he sent out a message on the social media platform WeChat, warning colleagues about a new virus similar to SARS. His messages were later shared online and on January 3, 2020, Dr. Li was accused by police of spreading false information over the internet and forced to sign a self-confession. After returning to work at Wuhan Central Hospital, Dr. Li contracted the disease and died on February 7, 2020. His death sparked a widespread response across Chinese social media, with the former "whistleblower" hailed by many as a national hero.

10. *A Thousand Arrows Piercing the Heart* (*Wanjian chuanxin*) is a popular novella by Fang Fang. The work was also adapted in 2012 into a feature-length film *Feng Shui* (*Wanjian chuanxin*) by Wang Jing, which won numerous awards in China.

11. Many of the doctors, nurses, and medical volunteers who traveled to Wuhan during the height of the COVID-19 outbreak shaved their heads as a means of reducing the risk of cross-contamination. Another safety method employed was the use of adult diapers so that medical workers would not need to risk infection when using the restroom.

12. These lines are taken from Wang Changling's poem "Seeing Off Imperial Censor Chai" ("Song Chai shiyu"), which dates from the Tang Dynasty.

13. *One Person, One City* (*Yigeren he yizuo chengshi*) was a 2002 CCTV documentary series directed by Wei Dajun and written by Li Hui and Feng Jicai. The series contained 17 episodes to approach various cities in China through the personal lens of famous writers; including Liu Xinwu (Beijing), Sun Ganlu (Shanghai), and Zhang Xianliang (Yinchuan). The episode on Wuhan featured Fang Fang.

14. Tang Xiaohe (b. 1941) was born in Wuchang and is regarded as one of China's leading oil painters active during the Mao period. Many of his revolutionary-themed paintings were widely reprinted and circulated as posters and murals; many of his works have been included in the collection of the China Art Gallery.

15. Lei Feng (1940–1962) was a "model soldier" serving in the People's Liberation Army who was espoused by Mao Zedong and elevated to the role of national hero for his willingness to sacrifice for others, display modesty, and work hard without any hope for credit or reward. Decades after his tragic death, schoolchildren throughout China are still taught to "learn from the spirit of Lei Feng."

16. Zhang Manling (b. 1948) is a film director, producer, and writer. She was the first Chinese woman to be featured on the cover of *TIME* magazine during the Reform Era. She is the award-winning author of numerous books and screenplays.

17. *Sacrificed Youth* (*Qingchun ji*) was a 1985 film adapted from Zhang Manling's novella *A Beautiful Place* (*Yige meili de difang*). The film was directed by Zhang Nuanxin (1940–1995) and explored themes of sexual awakening and minority cultures through the lens of an "educated youth" sent to Yunnan during the Cultural Revolution.

18. According to traditional Chinese custom, the "Seventh Day" (*tou qi*) is a rite that occurs seven days after a death. It is believed that on the Seventh Day the soul of the deceased will return home. On that day, the deceased person's family is expected to prepare a meal for the dead and then retreat to the bedroom or somewhere out of sight, so that the wandering soul won't run into their family members and get nostalgic, which could threaten the deceased person's ability to be reborn.

19. Liu Shouxiang (1958–2020) was a Chinese watercolor painter who also served as professor at the Hubei Institute of Film Arts. He was the founding director the Art Education Department at his Institute and he held individual exhibitions in Germany, Hong Kong, and Taipei, along with his work being exhibited in major collections all over the world. Professor Liu died of COVID-19 on February 13, 2020, at the Jinyintan Hospital in Wuhan.

20. Xiang Ligang (b. 1963) is a political commentator specializing in the field of communications. He is active on Chinese social media, with over 1 million followers on Weibo.

21. Liu Fan (1961–2020) was the first nurse to die due to COVID-19 in China. She worked at Wuchang Hospital in Wuhan where she served as deputy chief nurse. Her death was widely covered by the media in China and gained a massive amount of attention due to the fact that her parents and brother also died due to novel coronavirus. Early on, her death was subject to a variety of online rumors and speculations.

22. Duan Zhengcheng (1934–2020) was a professor at Huazhong University of Science and Technology. He was a leading specialist in his field and an academician of the Chinese Academy of Engineering. He also worked as an industrial engineer and inventor, specializing in automation. His contributions were varied and spanned many industries ranging from automotive to laser surgery. He died on February 15, 2020, from the novel coronavirus.

23. Haizi (1964–1989) was an iconic poet who started writing poetry in 1982. He took his life by laying down on a set of railroad tracks on March 26, 1989, at the age of 25. He was one of the most influential poets of the 1980s and his work has continued to be reprinted since his death. In this passage, Fang Fang playfully cites a line from his famous poem, "Tonight in Delingha" ("Jinye zai Delingha"), the final line of which reads, "Sister, tonight I care not about mankind, I care only about you."

24. Chang Kai (1965–2020) was a filmmaker working with the Hubei Film Studio, where his work involved preserving and dissemination of traditional Chinese opera films. His sister Liu Fan and his parents also died from the novel coronavirus.

25. Pan Xiangli (b. 1966) holds a PhD in literature and is a writer and editor based in Shanghai. Pan is also the vice chair of the Shanghai Writers Association. She is the author of numerous books, including *That Age When You Still Believe in Love* (*Xiangxin ai de nianji*) and *The Lotus That Penetrates the Heart* (*Chuan xin lian*).

26. *A Soft Burial* (*Ruan mai*) is a novel by Fang Fang published in 2017. It explores the decades-long trauma and pain of the Land Reform Movement on a family, using amnesia as a metaphor for the loss of historical memory. The novel was subject to vicious attacks by ultra-leftist groups in China and was subsequently banned.

27. In China the term "ultra-leftists" refers to political groups with strong nationalist views and ties to the leftist movement of the Cultural Revolution (1966–1976). They represent the more conservative faction of the Chinese Communist Party and are often critical of capitalism and the West.

28. Liu Zhiming (1968–2020) was a 1991 graduate of the Medical College of Wuhan University. He was a neurosurgeon and director of the Department of Neurosurgery at Third Municipal Hospital of Wuhan before being appointed president of Wuchang Hospital in 2015. Dr. Liu died on February 18, 2020, due to lung failure after being afflicted with the novel coronavirus.

29. Xiang Xinran (b. 1940) is regarded as one of China's leading architects. His best-known projects include the reconstruction of the Yellow Crane Tower and the new addition to the Hubei Provincial Museum. He has also served as a member of the People's Congress.

30. Liu Daoyu (b. 1933) is a well-known educator, chemist, and social activist. He has served as the chancellor of Wuhan University and various high-level roles within the Chinese Ministry of Education. Besides his research accomplishments in the field of chemistry, he has also authored numerous books on education and career planning.

31. While still preliminary, more recent studies have suggested that one reason so many healthcare practitioners have not only been infected but also suffered severe symptoms from COVID-19 may have to do with them being exposed to a higher "viral load." In "Viral Dynamics in Mild and Severe Cases of COVID-19," published on March, 19, 2020, a study of coronavirus patients in Nanchang, China, indicated a preliminary correlation between the severity of symptoms and the amount of virus present in the nose.

32. "If Wuhan has a true media, would there have been an outbreak?" ("Ruguo Wuhan de meiti shi zhenzheng de meiti, Wuhan haihui baofa yiqing ma?") published on the website "Daily Focus" ("Jiaodian ribao") on February 26, 2020. http://www.jdxwrb .com/pingshuo/1596.html?from=singlemessage&isappinstalled=0#10006-weixin-1 -52626-6b3bffd01fdde4900130bc5a2751b6d1.

33. On January 24, 2020, *Hubei Daily* reporter Zhang Ouya went to his Weibo social media account to call for the political leaders of Wuhan to be replaced with stronger leaders, like those who led the fight against SARS in Beijing during 2003. Zhang's employer, *Hubei Daily*, issued a swift apology to various government bodies for the post.

34. Zhang Guangnian (1913–2002), also known as Guang Weiran, was a Chinese poet and military leader. He joined the Chinese Communist Party in 1929. He wrote the poem that would become the basis for the lyrics of the *Yellow River Cantata* (*Huanghe dahechang*) in 1939. He also served as editor of *People's Literature* (*Renmin wenxue*).

35. Dai Jianye (b. 1956) is a professor of Traditional Chinese Literature at Huazhong Normal University. He is the author and editor of numerous books, including *Laozi's Philosophy of Life* (*Laozi de rensheng zhexue*), and a popular columnist. On February 26, 2020, he published an essay supporting Fang Fang entitled "Shouldn't Old Men Like Us Feel at Least a Little Bit Ashamed When Facing Fang Fang?" ("Miandui Fang Fang, women zhexie yemen nandao jiu meiyou yidian kuiyi?"); the essay was later removed from the internet.